Prostate Cancer

Translational Medicine Series

1. Prostate Cancer: Translational and Emerging Therapies, *edited by Nancy A. Dawson and W. Kevin Kelly*
2. Breast Cancer: Translational Therapeutic Strategies, *edited by Gary Lyman and Harold Burstein*

Prostate Cancer

Translational and Emerging Therapies

Edited by

Nancy A. Dawson
University of Maryland
Baltimore, Maryland, U.S.A.

W. Kevin Kelly
Yale University
New Haven, Connecticut, U.S.A.

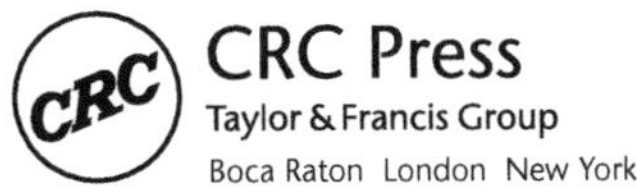

CRC Press
Taylor & Francis Group
Boca Raton London New York

CRC Press is an imprint of the
Taylor & Francis Group, an **informa** business

CRC Press
Taylor & Francis Group
6000 Broken Sound Parkway NW, Suite 300
Boca Raton, FL 33487-2742

First issued in paperback 2019

ISBN-13: 978-0-8493-7185-1 (hbk)
ISBN-13: 978-0-367-39018-1 (pbk)

A CIP record for this book is available from the British Library.

Library of Congress Cataloging-in-Publication Data available on application

Visit the Taylor & Francis Web site at
http://www.taylorandfrancis.com

and the CRC Press Web site at
http://www.crcpress.com

Preface

Prostate cancer is the most common malignancy in men and its incidence will dramatically increase over the next several decades due to the "baby boomers" reaching maturity. While the majority of patients can be cured with local radiotherapy or surgical modalities, many will progress with metastatic disease for which there is, currently, a limited number of treatment options. However, research in prostate cancer has made significant progress over the last decade, providing us with a better understanding of the critical events that lead to the development and progression of this disease and novel targets for therapies. This book will provide state-of-the-art information on evolving translational therapies in prostate cancer, which will translate into better outcomes for our patients.

It is appropriate that Drs. Nelson and De Marzo set the stage and describe the initial events of the development and progression of prostate cancer and identify the key elements that could be potential targets for preventing prostate cancer. However, identifying the target does not always lead to an effective therapy, as Dr. Sausville illustrates, and clinical investigations with these new targeted therapies require the integration of unique tumor markers, imaging modalities, and trial designs to show the clinical or biologic effect of the drug. Many therapies have overcome these hurdles and are now showing clinical benefit in patients.

Some agents that have shown promise include the endothelial receptor antagonists, vitamin D analogs, monoclonal antibodies to the prostate-specific membrane antigen, angiogenesis inhibitors, and many other small molecules such as the tyrosine kinase inhibitors. Drs. Qian and Pili and his colleagues describe a new class of agents called posttranscription modifiers, which include the histone deacetylase inhibitors and demethylation agents, while others have been investigating antisense oligonuclitides to inhibit specific proteins and kinases such as Bcl-2, clusterin, and other vital proteins that are critical in the growth of prostate cancer. Therapies that inhibit telomerase, proteasomes, and heat shock proteins have been promising avenues for the treatment of prostate cancer and these therapies are described by Drs. Burger, Dreicer, and Solit.

Immunologic and gene therapy approaches continue to be pursued and the data showing that these therapies may one day be a standard treatment is strengthening. Dr. Small and his researchers update us on the exciting data of several novel vaccine approaches and other new modalities that modify the immune response.

Investigators are also developing a better understanding of the pathophysiology of osteoblastic metastasis and androgen receptor. Dr. Hamdy and associates have reviewed the advancements in bone-targeted therapies and new agents that will be entering into the clinics while Dr. Mellinghoff highlights novel therapies that will inhibit the androgen receptor.

For decades, hormone-refractory prostate cancer was thought to be resistant to chemotherapy; however recent data has shown that prostate cancer is sensitive to chemotherapy and improves survival, which has renewed the interest in identifying novel cytotoxic drugs for this disease. Dr. Hussain reviews this ongoing research and highlights the new agents that are in clinical trials—many of which are in Phase III testing.

Compared to a decade ago, we have made great advancements in the understanding of prostate cancer and the targets that may treat this disease, but this was only possible from the strong support of dedicated researchers and patients.

Nancy A. Dawson
W. Kevin Kelly

Contents

Contributors

Tania Alachalabi Medical Oncology Branch, Center for Cancer Research, National Cancer Institute, National Institutes of Health, Bethesda, Maryland, U.S.A.

Tomasz M. Beer Division of Hematology & Medical Oncology and the OHSU Cancer Insitute, Oregon Health & Science University, Portland, Oregon, U.S.A.

Angelika M. Burger Department of Pharmacology and Experimental Therapeutics, Marlene and Stewart Greenebaum Cancer Center, University of Maryland School of Medicine, Baltimore, Maryland, U.S.A.

Michael Carducci The Sidney Kimmel Comprehensive Cancer Center, The Johns Hopkins University School of Medicine, Baltimore, Maryland, U.S.A.

Kim N. Chi BC Cancer Agency, Vancouver, British Columbia, Canada

Michael C. Cox Medical Oncology Branch, Center for Cancer Research, National Cancer Institute, National Institutes of Health, Bethesda, Maryland, U.S.A.

William L. Dahut Medical Oncology Branch, Center for Cancer Research, National Cancer Institute, National Institutes of Health, Bethesda, Maryland, U.S.A.

Angelo M. De Marzo Department of Pathology, The Sidney Kimmel Comprehensive Cancer Center and Brady Urological Institute, The Johns Hopkins University School of Medicine, Baltimore, Maryland, U.S.A.

Chaitanya Divgi Nuclear Medicine Service, Department of Radiology, Memorial Sloan-Kettering Cancer Center, New York, New York, U.S.A.

Robert Dreicer Department of Solid Tumor Oncology, The Glickman Urologic Institute and The Taussig Cancer Center, Cleveland Clinic Foundation, Cleveland, Ohio, U.S.A.

Colby L. Eaton Academic Urology, University of Sheffield, Royal Hallamshire Hospital, Sheffield, U.K.

William D. Figg Medical Oncology Branch, Center for Cancer Research, National Cancer Institute, National Institutes of Health, Bethesda, Maryland, U.S.A.

Lawrence Fong University of California, San Francisco, California, U.S.A.

Martin E. Gleave Vancouver Hospital D-9, Vancouver, British Columbia, Canada

Freddie C. Hamdy Academic Urology, University of Sheffield, Royal Hallamshire Hospital, Sheffield, U.K.

Arif Hussain University of Maryland Greenebaum Cancer Center, Baltimore, Maryland, U.S.A.

Antonio Jimeno The Sidney Kimmel Comprehensive Cancer Center, The Johns Hopkins University School of Medicine, Baltimore, Maryland, U.S.A.

Lloyd R. Kelland Antisoma Research Laboratories, St. Georges Hospital Medical School, Cranmer Terrace, London, U.K.

Steven Larson Nuclear Medicine Service, Department of Radiology, Memorial Sloan-Kettering Cancer Center, New York, New York, U.S.A.

Kate D. Linton Academic Urology, University of Sheffield, Royal Hallamshire Hospital, Sheffield, U.K.

Ingo K. Mellinghoff Department of Pharmacology, University of California, Los Angeles, California, U.S.A.

Malcolm J. Moore Department of Medicine and Pharmacology, Princess Margaret Hospital, University of Toronto, Toronto, Ontario, Canada

Michael J. Morris Genitourinary Oncology Service, Department of Medicine, Memorial Sloan-Kettering Cancer Center, New York, New York, U.S.A.

Anne Myrthue Division of Hematology & Medical Oncology and the OHSU Cancer Insitute, Oregon Health & Science University, Portland, Oregon, U.S.A.

William G. Nelson The Sidney Kimmel Comprehensive Cancer Center and Brady Urological Institute, The Johns Hopkins University School of Medicine, Baltimore, Maryland, U.S.A.

Neeta Pandit-Taksar Nuclear Medicine Service, Department of Radiology, Memorial Sloan-Kettering Cancer Center, New York, New York, U.S.A.

Roberto Pili The Sidney Kimmel Comprehensive Care Center, The Johns Hopkins University School of Medicine, Baltimore, Maryland, U.S.A.

David Z. Qian The Sidney Kimmel Comprehensive Care Center, The Johns Hopkins University School of Medicine, Baltimore, Maryland, U.S.A.

Neal Rosen Department of Medicine, Pharmacology and Chemistry, Memorial Sloan-Kettering Cancer Center, New York, New York, U.S.A.

Edward A. Sausville University of Maryland, Marlene and Stewart Greenebaum Cancer Center, Baltimore, Maryland, U.S.A.

Howard I. Scher Genitourinary Oncology Service, Department of Medicine, Memorial Sloan-Kettering Cancer Center, New York, New York, U.S.A.

Richard Schraeder University of Maryland Greenebaum Cancer Center, Baltimore, Maryland, U.S.A.

Jonathan W. Simons Department of Hematology and Oncology, Winship Cancer Institute, Emory University School of Medicine, Atlanta, Georgia, U.S.A.

Susan F. Slovin Genitourinary Oncology Service, Department of Medicine, Memorial Sloan-Kettering Cancer Center, New York, New York, U.S.A.

Eric J. Small University of California, San Francisco, California, U.S.A.

David B. Solit Department of Medicine and the Human Oncology and Pathogenesis Program, Memorial Sloan-Kettering Cancer Center, New York, New York, U.S.A.

Srikala S. Sridhar Department of Medicine, Juravinski Cancer Center, McMaster University, Hamilton, Ontario, Canada

James V. Tricoli Diagnostic Biomarkers and Technology Branch, Division of Cancer Treatment and Diagnosis, Cancer Diagnosis Program, National Cancer Institute, Rockville, Maryland, U.S.A.

Henry T. Tsai Department of Hematology and Oncology, Winship Cancer Institute, Emory University School of Medicine, Atlanta, Georgia, U.S.A.

1 The Molecular Pathogenesis and Pathophysiology of Prostate Cancer

William G. Nelson
The Sidney Kimmel Comprehensive Cancer Center and Brady Urological Institute, The Johns Hopkins University School of Medicine, Baltimore, Maryland, U.S.A.

Angelo M. De Marzo
Department of Pathology, The Sidney Kimmel Comprehensive Cancer Center and Brady Urological Institute, The Johns Hopkins University School of Medicine, Baltimore, Maryland, U.S.A.

INTRODUCTION

At the dawn of the new millennium, prostate cancer has become a major scourge for men as they age in the developed world. In the United States, autopsy series have revealed small prostate cancers in as many as 29% of men between age 30 and 40, and 64% of men between age 60 and 70 (1). With the current widespread use of serum prostate-specific antigen (PSA) testing and digital rectal examination in the United States for prostate cancer screening, the lifetime risk of a prostate cancer diagnosis has risen to about one in six, whereas the lifetime risk of death from prostate cancer is on the order of 1 in 30 (2). Fortunately, since about 1994 or so, with increased diagnosis and treatment of prostate cancer, age-adjusted prostate cancer death rates have fallen steadily (2). Whether this trend reflects a benefit of prostate cancer screening and/or early prostate cancer treatment on prostate cancer mortality has not been fully resolved (3,4). Nonetheless, while some men with prostate cancer do not appear to be at high risk for symptomatic or life-threatening prostate cancer progression, others continue to face the threat of death from the disease.

Over the past decade, new insights into the molecular mechanisms underlying the pathogenesis of prostate cancer have generated remarkable new opportunities for the discovery and development of new approaches to prostate cancer detection, diagnosis, prevention, and treatment. In this chapter, we review the molecular pathogenesis and pathophysiology of prostate cancer, providing a conceptual basis for the coming innovations in prostate cancer care.

ANATOMY AND FUNCTION OF THE HUMAN PROSTATE

All male mammals have sex accessory glands called prostates; in *Homo sapiens*, the prostate surrounds the urethra and produces secretions that form about a third of the volume ejaculated during sexual intercourse. Adjacent to the bladder and rectum, the prostate is enveloped by a thin "capsule" consisting of collagen, elastin, adipose tissue, and smooth muscle (5). The gland contains three distinct zones that are visible by transrectal ultrasonography or magnetic resonance imaging, and can be recognized by microscopic examination: the central zone, ~25% of the prostate, which contains the ejaculatory ducts; the transition zone, ~10% of the prostate, which sits near the urethra; and the peripheral zone, ~65% of the prostate, which occupies the posterolateral region of the prostate (6,7). The peripheral zone of the prostate is the region of the gland most susceptible to neoplastic transformation and cancer development; the transition zone is the region that develops benign prostatic hyperplasia in the vast majority of cases.

Prostate tissues contain an epithelium, the source of secretions for the ejaculate, and a stroma, occupied by fibroblasts, smooth muscle cells, nerves, and blood vessels. The prostate epithelium is composed of basal cells, columnar secretory cells, and rare neuroendocrine cells. Basal cells, some of which are believed to serve as the multipotent epithelial stem cells, typically express cytokeratin K5, p63, Notch1, and little or no androgen receptors (8,9). Cytokeratin K14 is variably expressed in basal cells. Cytokeratins K8 and K18 can be detected in basal cells, but at much lower levels than in luminal cells. Columnar cells, terminally differentiated to produce ejaculate secretions, express high levels of androgen receptors, NKX3.1, PSA, cytokeratins K8, and K18, prostate-specific membrane antigen (PSMA), and prostate-specific acid phosphatase (PAP). Neuroendocrine cells produce chromogranin A, neuron-specific enolase, and synaptophysin, and are found scattered throughout the prostate epithelium in both the basal and luminal compartments (9–11).

The study of prostate epithelial stem cells has become an area of very active investigation. Although definitive proof is lacking, the best evidence to date is that epithelial stem cells are likely located in the basal epithelial compartment, and that at least some of the basal cells, perhaps the stem cells, can give rise to luminal epithelial cells (8,9,12–15). Furthermore, a rare population of prostate epithelial cells expressing CD133 and stereotypical basal cell markers, but not expressing androgen receptors, can be isolated experimentally and shown to be able to generate daughter cells with some characteristics of luminal secretory epithelial cells (16,17). Thus far, however, fully differentiated luminal secretory cells and neuroendocrine cells have not been produced in in vitro cell culture systems from any less differentiated prostate epithelial cell. Hence, the isolation of the pluripotent prostate epithelial stem cell capable of producing progeny that can differentiate in vitro in a manner recapitulating terminal differentiation in vivo has remained elusive. Finally, bone marrow stem cells have been found to contribute to the prostate epithelium, either by producing progeny that differentiate into epithelial cells or by fusing with existing epithelial cells, after inflammatory damage to the gland in a mouse model (18). In addition to the intrinsic regulation of epithelial cell growth and differentiation, epithelial interactions with the stroma play key roles in the development, growth, and maintenance of the prostate (13). For example, stromal cells, which express the androgen receptor and elaborate keratinocyte growth factor, help to regulate epithelial homeostasis via paracrine signaling (19,20).

The normal growth and development of the prostate requires both androgenic steroids and a functioning androgen receptor. The major circulating androgenic hormone, testosterone, is produced by Leydig cells in the testes in response to stimulation by leutinizing hormone. Testosterone is converted by 5α-reductase (nicotinamide-adenine dinucleotidephosphate-dependent Δ^4-3-ketosteroid 5α-oxidoreductase) to 5α-dihydrotestosterone (DHT), a more potent androgen, which can bind androgen receptors and promote dissociation of the receptors from chaperone proteins, leading to receptor dimerization and post-translational modification, transport into the cell nucleus, and activation of target gene transcription (21–23). In prostatic epithelial cells, androgen receptor target genes, such as *PSA*, have androgen response element DNA sequences, capable of binding the activated androgen receptor, within the promoter and enhancer regions (24,25). In addition to this "genomic" androgen receptor-dependent signaling pathway culminating in specific gene transactivation, increased research attention has recently been afforded "nongenomic" signaling pathways activated by androgens, which appear to trigger responses rapidly (within minutes to hours), and may or may not always involve androgen receptors (26). One such "nongenomic" androgen receptor signaling pathway, described in association with prostate cancer cell growth, features a cell surface complex containing the androgen receptor, the estrogen receptor, and the C-SRC (Rous sarcoma virus oncoprotein homolog) kinase (27).

THE CELLULAR ORIGIN OF PROSTATE CANCER

Prostatic epithelial cells, typically in the peripheral zone of the prostate, are the favored targets for neoplastic transformation, leading to the appearance of prostatic intraepithelial neoplasia (PIN) lesions and prostate cancers. The transformed prostate epithelial cells tend to maintain phenotypic features characteristic of differentiated columnar secretory cells (i.e., exhibit the morphology of an adenocarcinoma), including the expression of androgen receptor, NKX3.1, PSA, PSMA, and PAP, while prostate cancers with attributes of basal cells are exceedingly rare. Many prostate adenocarcinomas contain some neuroendocrine cells sprinkled throughout the tumor tissue, yet pure neuroendocrine carcinomas and/or small cell carcinomas are also uncommon (28). Nevertheless, unlike normal columnar secretory cells, transformed prostate epithelial cells respond to androgenic stimulation by proliferation rather than by terminal differentiation (21). This paradox may be partially explained by the proposal that the target cell for neoplastic transformation in the prostate may be an "intermediate" cell, in transit from a basal stem cell to a differentiated columnar secretory cell, with properties of both basal cells and differentiated luminal cells, permitting some proliferation despite attempts at differentiation (9,29). A new potential explanation for the tendency for androgens to promote terminal differentiation in the normal prostate epithelium but proliferation in prostate adenocarcinomas has been generated by the discovery of fusion transcripts from translocated genes in many prostate cancer cases (30). These translocations place nonandrogen-regulated androgenic stimulatory gene sequences, such as those encoding ETS transcription factors, immediately 3′ of androgen-regulated differentiation genes, such as *TMPRSS2*, permitting the expression of the products of growth regulatory genes in response to androgenic stimulation from translation of the fusion transcripts (30).

PIN, a lesion in which neoplastic prostate epithelial cells appear to proliferate within the confines of otherwise normal glandular structures, is found in at least 5% of men who undergo prostate biopsies (31). PIN, a likely precursor to prostate cancer, is commonly detected in prostates that also contain prostate cancer, tends to rise in the peripheral zone of the prostate, where cancers tend to develop, and is often adjacent to prostate cancer. Furthermore, both PIN and prostate cancer cells have similar molecular phenotypes and share some somatic genome abnormalities (32,33). The notion that high-grade PIN lesions might be prostate cancer precursors has stimulated interest in possibly treating men with high-grade PIN to prevent prostate cancer. However, the natural history of PIN, including what frequency of PIN lesions progress to prostate cancer and how quickly prostate cancers emerge from PIN lesions, is not well understood, Also, although like cancer cells, PIN cells typically exhibit phenotypic features of columnar secretory epithelial cells while undergoing exuberant proliferation, unlike cancer cells, in PIN, the chromosomal translocations involving ETS transcription factors genes and androgen-regulated differentiation genes like *TMPRSS2* appear rare (30).

These emerging insights into the cellular origin of prostate cancer, and into the functions of androgen signaling in normal and neoplastic prostate cells, have profound implications for the contribution(s) of androgenic hormones to the pathogenesis of prostate cancer. For the normal prostate, where androgen signaling promotes terminal differentiation, androgenic hormones may act to suppress prostatic carcinogenesis, providing an explanation for the progressive appearance of prostatic carcinomas accompanying the progressive decline in androgenic hormone levels with age. The generation of PIN lesions may then proceed via an androgen-independent process. However, if the progression of PIN to prostate cancer involves chromosomal translocations creating somatic androgen-regulation growth-stimulatory fusion gene, prostate cancers will be androgen-dependent, or at least androgen-sensitive.

GENETIC SUSCEPTIBILITY TO PROSTATE CANCER

Twin studies, comparing the propensity for concordant prostate cancer development between monozygotic twins, sharing all of their genes, and dizygotic twins, sharing half of their genes, have consistently suggested a significant role for heredity in prostatic carcinogenesis (34–37). In the well-known study of 44,788 pairs of twins in Sweden, Denmark, and Finland, 42% of the prostate cancer cases (with a 95% CI of 29–50%) were attributed to inheritance (34). In another twin study from America, heredity was thought to contribute to as many as 57% of prostate cancer cases, with environmental influences accounting for as much as 43% of cases (35). Familial clusters of prostate cancer also occur frequently, in which men with prostate cancer report having family members affected by the disease (38–45). Of course, clustering of prostate cancer cases in families could be a result of shared susceptibility genes, shared exposures to carcinogens or to infectious agents, or some sort of detection bias (e.g., male relatives of a man with prostate cancer tend are more likely to undergo screening for the disease). Complex segregation analyses, attempting to distinguish between these explanations, have supported a significant role for heredity in prostate cancer family clusters, with rare autosomal dominant genes predicted to be responsible for as many as 43% of prostate cancer cases diagnosed before age 55 and some 9% of all prostate cancer cases, and additional X-linked genes predicted to account for the disease in some families (46,47). Several genome-wide screens of polymorphic DNA markers undertaken with hereditary prostate cancer families have identified genomic regions of linkage, with likely complex gene–gene interactions, further highlighting the contributions of heredity to prostate cancer for many men who develop the disease (48–51).

The search for prostate cancer susceptibility genes has been hampered by the clinical features of the disease itself. Because prostate cancer typically strikes older men (ages 50–70 years), there are few multigenerational families suitable for genetic analyses. Also, many men who appear unaffected by prostate cancer at a younger age (and thus not be designated a "case" in genetic studies) might later be diagnosed with prostate cancer at an older age. Furthermore, the likelihood of being diagnosed with prostate cancer often reflects the use of prostate cancer screening via serum PSA testing. Finally, the lifetime risk of prostate cancer in the developed world is so high that many men in prostate cancer families with the disease may represent phenocopies, i.e., suffer with sporadic, rather than genetic, prostate cancer.

So far, *RNASEL* and *MSR1* have been identified as candidate prostate cancer susceptibility genes, though mutations in these genes do not likely account for the majority of familial prostate cancer cases (52,53). *RNASEL* encodes a latent endoribonuclease that functions as part of an interferon-inducible 2′,5′-oligoadenylate-dependent RNA decay pathway to degrade viral and cellular RNA upon viral infection (54–58). In one hereditary prostate cancer family, four brothers were found to carry *RNASEL* mutations resulting in protein truncation at amino acid position 265 ($aa256^{glu \rightarrow X}$), while in another family, four of six brothers with prostate cancer carried *RNASEL* mutations affecting the initiator methionine codon ($aa1^{met \rightarrow ile}$) (52). In addition, in one case–control study, a common polymorphic variant *RNASEL* allele encoding a less active enzyme (with an amino acid change $aa462^{arg \rightarrow glu}$) was correlated with increasing prostate cancer risk ($p = 0.011$) (59). In this study, the polymorphic *RNASEL* allele accounted for as many as 13% of all prostate cancer cases. Other studies have not detected such associations (60–62).

MSR1 encodes subunits of a trimeric class A macrophage scavenger receptor capable of binding bacterial lipopolysaccharide and lipoteichoic acid, and oxidized high- and low-density serum lipoproteins (oxidized HDL and LDL) (63,64). The receptor itself is expressed by macrophages, regulated by inflammatory cytokines, and functions in innate immunity against microbial infections (64–66). For *MSR1*, not only mutations have been linked to prostate cancer susceptibility in some prostate cancer families, but one mutant allele, encoding a receptor subunit polypeptide with an $aa293^{arg \rightarrow X}$ expected to have "dominant negative" function, has been detected in ~3% of nonHPC prostate cancer cases but only 0.4% of unaffected men ($p < 0.05$) (53,67,68). Other studies have not detected strong linkage of prostate cancer risk to *MSR1* (69–71). Nonetheless, the identification of *RNASEL* and *MSR1* as candidate prostate cancer susceptibility genes has intensified interest in the possibility that infection and/or inflammation might contribute to the pathogenesis of human prostate cancer. In mice, targeted disruption of *RNASEL* leads to diminished interferon-a activity and increased susceptibility to viral infection, while targeted disruption of *MSR-A* leads to increased vulnerability to infection with *Listeria monocytogenes, Staphylococcus aureus, Escherichia coli,* and *Herpes simplex* virus type 1 (63,65,72–74).

If infection and/or inflammation plays a role in prostatic carcinogenesis, then polymorphic variants of other genes encoding participants in inflammatory responses to infections, or encoding participants in cell and tissue defenses against promutagenic damage inflicted by inflammatory cells, might be expected to show associations with prostate cancer risk. Thus far, increased or decreased prostate cancer risk has been reported for variants of *IL-8, IL-10, VEGF, MIC-1, IL-1RN,* and *TLR4,* providing further support for the notion that the regulation of inflammation may influence prostate cancer development (75–81). Macrophages and polymorphonuclear leukocytes control and eradicate pathogenic infections by elaborating microbicidal reactive oxygen and nitrogen species. Of course, these reactive species threaten "collateral" cell and genome damage at the site(s) of infection. For defense against the somatic mutations threatened by such damage, mammalian cells possess pathways both for detoxification of damaging species and for repair of genome damage. Of interest in this regard, polymorphic variants of *MnSOD*, encoding a detoxification enzyme, and *OGG1*, encoding an oxidative genome damage repair enzyme, have been reported to be affect the risk of prostate cancer development (82–85). Also, an inactivating mutation at *BRCA2*, encoding a genome damage response participant, has been correlated with prostate cancer appearing at an early age, and various mutations at *CHEK2*, encoding a contributor to the *p53* genome damage signaling pathway, have been associated with both sporadic and hereditary prostate cancer (86,87).

Even though androgenic hormones promote normal prostate growth and development, and fuel the growth and survival of prostate cancers, consistent associations of variants of genes encoding participants in androgen signaling pathways have been difficult to demonstrate. For *AR*, encoding the androgen receptor, the focus has been on polymorphic polyglutamine repeats, varying in lengths from 11 to 31 amino acids, and polymorphic polyglycine repeats, varying in lengths from 10 to 22 amino acids. Androgen receptors with shorter polyglutamine repeats, more commonly expressed by African-Americans, a group with high prostate cancer risks, may possess increased transcriptional transactivation activity (88–91). Genetic epidemiology studies of prostate cancer risk associated with shorter androgen receptor polyglutamine repeats have tended to support more of a contribution of such receptors to prostate cancer progression (manifest as prostate cancer stage at presentation) than to the development of prostate cancer itself (92–95). *SRD5A2*, encoding the type 2 5α-reductase, the enzyme that generates DHT from testosterone in the prostate, has several polymorphic variants that may affect prostate cancer risk (96–98). Some of the variants encode enzymes that respond differently to clinically used drugs, like finasteride and dustasteride, which are being tested as prostate cancer prevention drugs (22).

EPIDEMIOLOGY OF PROSTATE CANCER

Although there is a well-established contribution of heredity to prostate cancer development, the environment remains a major source of exposures driving prostatic carcinogenesis. Prostate cancer incidence and mortality vary widely throughout the world, with high rates of prostate cancer incidence and mortality in the United States and in Western Europe, and low prostate cancer in Asia (99). The geographic differences in prostate cancer incidence and mortality are likely attributable to aspects of lifestyle like the diet, as ethnic Asians in America exhibit higher prostate cancer risks than ethnic Asians who remain in Asia (45,100,101). Animal fat intake, particularly the consumption of red meats, has been associated with increased prostate cancer risk in a number of population-based prospective cohort studies (102–104). Such meats may be a source of exposure to prostate carcinogens: the grilling or charbroiling of red meats promotes the formation of both heterocyclic aromatic amines and polycyclic aromatic hydrocarbons (105–108). 2-Amino-1-methyl-6-phenylimidazopyridine (PhIP), one of the heterocyclic aromatic amine carcinogens that can form by cooking meats at high temperatures, causes prostate cancer in rats (109,110).

Vegetables and anti-oxidant micronutrients appear to reduce prostate cancer risks. Intake of tomato products, containing the anti-oxidant carotenoid lycopene, has been associated with decreased prostate cancer risks in population studies, and with reduced oxidative genome damage in the prostate in a clinical study (111–114). Intake of cruciferous vegetables, containing sulforaphane and other isothiocyanates, may also reduce prostate cancer risk (115–117). As for anti-oxidant micronutrients, in randomized clinical trials in which prostate cancer incidence constituted secondary end points, treatment with vitamin E and selenium have tended to reduce prostate cancer risks (118–120). To validate this protective effect against prostate cancer development in a clinical study for which prostate cancer incidence is the primary trial end point, a clinical trial of supplementation with vitamin E and selenium to prevent prostate cancer (the Select Trial), involving 32,400 men, has been launched as is now fully accrued (121). The tendency for anti-oxidants to reduce prostate cancer risk, and for polymorphic variants of oxidative damage protection enzymes to also affect the risk of prostate cancer development, strongly suggests that reactive oxygen and/or nitrogen species, perhaps elaborated by inflammatory cells, might play causative roles in prostatic carcinogenesis.

INFLAMMATION AND PROSTATE CANCER

Chronic or recurrent inflammation contributes to the pathogenesis of a large fraction human cancers arising in epithelial cells of different organs, the barriers limiting exposure to the microbial world. Inflammation, most often asymptomatic, is well recognized to be quite common in prostates from high-risk prostate cancer regions of the world, and prostatic inflammation has long been postulated to have an association with prostate cancer (122). Symptomatic prostatitis, a syndrome affecting ~9% of men at some point in their lives, has been correlated with increased prostate cancer risk, but this risk association has been challenged by the contention that men with prostatitis are more likely to be screened and evaluated for prostate cancer than men with no urinary symptoms (123,124). Exudative sexually transmitted infections, some of which lead to prostate inflammation and an elevation of serum PSA values, appear to increase prostate cancer risks (125–127). Despite the association of prostate cancer and sexually transmitted infections, a consistent etiologic pathogen has not been identified, raising the possibility that the inflammatory response itself, rather than the infecting microorganism, might promote neoplastic transformation of prostate epithelial cells. Supporting this notion, decreased prostate cancer risks have been reported in association with nonsteroidal anti-inflammatory drug use (128–131). Also, frequent ejaculations, which would tend to clear prostate ducts of both pathogens and inflammatory cells, have been correlated with diminished prostate cancer risk (132).

Inflammatory processes tend to cause collateral damage to tissue and organ architecture. In the prostate, such damage appears to result in a specific lesion termed proliferative inflammatory atrophy (PIA) which may be a direct precursor to PIN and to prostate cancer (133). PIA lesions are characterized by luminal epithelial cells which are reduced in size and not fully differentiated into columnar secretory cells. Focal atrophy lesions have long been described by prostate pathologists (122,134); the term PIA refers to focal atrophy lesions with exuberantly proliferating epithelial cells that are associated with acute and/or chronic inflammation and that are often adjacent to or contiguous with prostate cancers (133,135–137). For those atrophic lesions not associated with obvious inflammatory infiltrates, the term proliferative atrophy (PA) has been applied. The epithelial cells in PIA/PA lesions, many of which have a phenotype reminiscent of intermediate cells, with phenotypic properties of both basal and columnar secretory luminal cells, typically also express high levels of stress response markers such as GSTP1, GSTA1, cyclooxygenase 2 (COX-2), and p16 (138–140). Loss of GSTP1 expression in rare PIA/PA lesions, attributable to de novo *GSTP1* CpG island hypermethylation, may be what leads to the development of PIN and prostate cancer (32,141,142). Focal atrophy lesions, including PIA/PA, exhibit many morphological patterns; a new classification scheme has recently been established and validated (143).

The hypothesis that inflammation in some way causes or promotes prostate cancer development presents considerable new opportunities and new challenges to prostate cancer researchers. The cause(s) of prostate inflammation are not well understood. Of course, infectious agents may trigger innate and adaptive immune responses leading to cell and tissue damage. Identifying such pathogens will likely be difficult, as infections may first occur in men as early as in puberty (1). Also, in addition to infections, estrogen exposure has been associated with prostate inflammation in rats (144–147). Could estrogens drive a nonbacterial autoimmune prostatitis in *Homo sapiens*? Prostatic inflammation appears common in regions of the world with high prostate cancer risks. However, whether less prostate inflammation is characteristic of regions of the world with lower prostate cancer risks has not been tested.

Inflammatory processes in the prostate are difficult to detect and monitor without direct tissue sampling. To gain insight into the natural history of prostate infections, inflammatory responses, PIA lesions, PIN lesions, etc., new prostate imaging strategies, permitting serial evaluation, will likely be needed. Some atrophic and inflammatory lesions may be visible by magnetic resonance imaging (148). Otherwise, new biomarkers of prostate inflammation that can be assayed in blood, urine, or prostate fluid, may provide useful tools for population studies of the association between prostate inflammation and prostate cancer. Already, the systematic analysis of single nucleotide polymorphisms in genes encoding regulators of immune/inflammatory responses, and participants in oxidative genome damage defense and repair, are ongoing at a rapid pace. This may provide hints as to critical pathways for the development of prostate cancer in the setting of prostate inflammation. Ultimately, the key question will be whether treatment of prostate infection or inflammation serves to prevent prostate cancer. Unfortunately, the development of such prevention strategies has been hindered somewhat recently by concerns about the long-term safety of chronic exposure to anti-inflammatory drugs (149).

SOMATIC GENOME CHANGES IN PROSTATE CANCER CELLS

Prostate cancer cells typically contain many somatic genome alterations, including gene mutations, gene deletions, gene amplifications, chromosomal rearrangements/gene fusions, and changes in DNA methylation. The mechanisms by which such gene lesions accumulate have not been established, but several aspects of prostatic carcinogenesis hint at prolonged exposures to genome damaging stresses as the culprit, including: (i) the early age of appearance of prostate cancers (30% of men by age 40 years) despite a much older age of diagnosis (age 60–70 years), providing a prolonged (30 years or more) window for genome damaging exposures, (ii) the known genetic and environmental influences on prostatic carcinogenesis, implicating chronic prostatic inflammation in disease pathogenesis, (iii) the possibility that dietary carcinogens, such as those from overcooked meats, might act as mutagens for the prostatic epithelium, and (iv) the consistent protective effects of anti-oxidants against prostate cancer development. With these influences, the marked heterogeneity of somatic genome lesions, prostate cancer case to prostate cancer case, and prostate cancer lesion to prostate cancer lesion within one prostate cancer case is not surprising (150). The diversity of somatic genome abnormalities has provided impetus and opportunity to the discovery and development of molecular biomarkers useful not only for prostate cancer detection and diagnosis, but also for prostate cancer prognosis and therapy-response prediction (150).

Epigenetic genome alterations may be the first to appear during prostate cancer development (150). Several genes have now been reported to carry somatic hypermethylation of CpG island sequences in prostate cancers, likely causing epigenetic gene silencing, preventing gene transcription in response to appropriate signals (151–153). The most intensively studied, and universally appearing (>90–95% of cases), epigenetic alteration in prostate cancer has been somatic hypermethylation of the CpG island at *GSTP1*, encoding the π-class glutathione S-transferase (GST), a member of a large family of enzymes responsible for detoxification of reactive chemical species via conjugation with glutathione (141,154). GSTP1 likely poses a significant barrier to procarcinogenic genome damage: disruption of the π-class GST genes in mice leads to increased skin tumors after treatment with the carcinogen 7,12-dimethylbenzanthracene, and human prostate cancer cells with silenced *GSTP1* genes appear vulnerable to genome damage by PhIP-related carcinogens, such as those that appear in charbroiled meats (155,156). In the normal human prostate, GSTP1 is expressed by basal epithelial cells, but not by most columnar secretory cells; prostate epithelial cells subjected to genome damaging stresses, such as the cells comprising PIA lesions, elevate GSTP1 expression, along with the expression of GSTA1, to very high levels (133,139). As a consequence of CpG island hypermethylation, with the accompanying assembly of a repressive chromatin structure, *GSTP1* expression is lost in prostate cancer cells in almost all prostate cancer cases (141,157). Absence of GSTP1 expression and *GSTP1* CpG island hypermethylation may appear as early as in PIA and PIN lesions, before most other somatic genome lesions arise (142). Thus far, the molecular mechanisms by which epigenetic alterations appear during the development of prostate cancers remain elusive. For *GSTP1*, epigenetic silencing may be subject to selection during prostatic carcinogenesis by increasing the probability of other genetic lesions in response to carcinogenic exposures.

Progressive shortening of telomeres, repeat DNA sequences at the termini of chromosomes, also appears to be an early, and nearly universal, somatic genome change arising during the pathogenesis of prostate cancer. Telomeres are thought to protect against loss of chromosome sequences during DNA replication, a phenomenon termed the "end-replication" problem (158,159). Telomerase, an enzyme that acts to extend telomere sequences, maintains chromosomal length despite DNA replication and mitosis (160). During the development of most cancers, either as a consequence of inadequate telomerase action or some sort of telomere sequence damage, chromosome telomeres are often critically shortened to the point where genetic instability, with illegitimate DNA recombination, ensues (161,162). In some studies, mice carrying disrupted genes needed for a functioning telomerase show increased numbers of cancers, such as when crossed to mice with defective *p53* genes, while in other studies, telomerase deficient mice with shortened telomeres are somewhat resistant to carcinogenesis, because telomerase function may be needed to support the emergence and proliferation of transformed cells (163–165). In the human prostate, short telomere repeat sequences are characteristic of cells both in PIN lesions and prostate cancer, and telomerase expression is common in prostate cancer cells (33,166,167).

NKX3.1, which encodes a prostate-specific homeobox gene required for normal gland development, frequently undergoes somatic allelic deletion during prostatic carcinogenesis (168–171). The gene product, which appears to have preserved, but reduced, expression in prostate cancer cells, may function via DNA binding and transcriptional *trans*-regulation (172,173). Mice carrying one or two disrupted *Nkx3.1* alleles manifest increases oxidative genome damage, and prostatic epithelial hyperplasia and dysplasia (170,174,175). In one study of human prostate cancers, deletions at 8p21, the location of *NKX3.1*, occurred early and commonly during carcinogenesis, in some 63% of PIN lesions and >90% of prostate cancers (169). In another study, diminished NKX3.1 expression was evident in 90% of cancers, with *NKX3.1* deletions detected in 63% of cases and *NKX3.1* DNA methylation changes detected in 83% of cases (176). In contrast, somatic *NKX3.1* mutations appear quite rare in prostate cancers (177). In addition to somatic alterations targeting *NKX3.1*, a germline *NKX3.1* variant has been reported to segregate with prostate cancer in hereditary prostate cancer families (178).

PTEN, phosphatase and tensin homolog a tumor suppressor gene encoding a lipid phosphatase that functions as an inhibitor of the phosphatidylinositol 3′-kinase/protein kinase B (PI3K/Akt) signaling pathway needed for cell cycle progression and cell survival, may be a common somatic target for alteration in prostate cancers and in many other cancers (179–192). PTEN is expressed by normal prostate epithelial cells, but is decreased in many prostate cancers, with regions of prostate cancer cells often displaying little or no PTEN expression at all (189). Mice carrying one intact and one disrupted *Pten* allele exhibit prostatic hyperplasia and dysplasia, and crosses of *Pten*$^{+/-}$ mice with *Nkx3.1*$^{+/-}$ mice have revealed that *Pten*$^{+/-}$ *Nkx3.1*$^{+/-}$ mice and *Pten*$^{+/-}$ *Nkx3.1*$^{-/-}$ mice develop invasive carcinoma (193,194). *Pten* defects also cooperate with *SV40 T-antigen* in *TRAMP* (transgenic adenocarcinoma of the prostrate) mice prone to prostatic tumorigenesis, as well as with *p53* defects, to cause more virulent prostate cancers (195,196). The phenotypic effects of *Pten* insufficiency in the mouse models is the likely the result of deregulated Akt activation, because forced prostate expression of Akt in transgenic mice also causes intraepithelial neoplasia (197). The Akt signaling pathway has been aggressively targeted by new inhibitors now in or soon to be introduced into clinical trials for prostate cancer treatment, including the mTOR inhibitors rapamycin and its analogs CCI-779 (temsirolimus) and RAD001 (everolimus). In the transgenic mice expressing Akt in prostate cells, mTOR inhibitor treatment completely reversed the neoplastic epithelial cell phenotype (198).

Decreased levels of p27, a cyclin-dependent kinase inhibitor encoded by *CDKN1B*, are characteristic of prostate cancers (199–204). Nonetheless, the mechanism(s) by which p27 levels are diminished in PIN and prostate cancer cells have not been established. Somatic deletion of *CDKN1B* have been described for only 23% of localized prostate cancers, 30% of prostate cancer lymph node metastases, and 47% of distant prostate cancer metastases (205,206). *CDKN1B* may also be the target of repression by the Akt signaling pathway, exhibiting decreased p27 polypeptide levels in response to inappropriate Akt activation accompanying PTEN deficiency (207–209). In mouse models, disruption of *Cdkn1b* alleles results in prostatic hyperplasia, and *Pten*$^{+/-}$*Cdkn1b*$^{-/-}$ mice develop prostate cancer by 3 mo of age (210).

Androgenic hormones promote the growth and survival of prostate cancer cells. As such, the mainstay systemic treatments for prostate cancer have long involved androgen deprivation, the use of anti-androgens, or a combination of androgen deprivation and anti-androgens (211–214). One explanation for the benefits of treatments targeting the androgen signaling axis may be provided by the finding of recurrent chromosomal deletions and translocations in prostate cancers resulting in the production of fusion transcripts of the 5′ untranslated region of *TMPRSS2*, an androgen-regulated gene, and *ERG* or to *ETV1*, likely growth-stimulating ETS family members (30). Such chromosomal rearrangements have been detected in 79% of prostate cancer cases, but seem to be rarely present in prostate cancer precursor lesions (30). If chromosomal rearrangements have resulted in the capture of growth regulatory genes by transcriptional regulatory DNA sequences permitting androgen receptor transcriptional transactivation in prostate cancer cells, then treatments that interfere with androgen receptor function can be expected to also interfere with prostate cancer growth and survival.

However, for advanced and/or metastatic prostate cancers, androgen-independent prostate cancer cells typically emerge despite treatment to ultimately threaten life. Remarkably, androgen-independent prostate cancers most often maintain androgen receptor expression and androgen receptor signaling even in the presence of anti-androgens or in a milieu with reduced androgen levels (215–217). Somatic alterations of *AR*, encoding the androgen receptor, have been reported for many prostate cancers, especially for androgen-independent prostate cancers (218–231). In human prostate cancer xenograft models, progression to androgen-independence has been associated with increased expression of androgen receptors, leading to an increased sensitivity of the receptors to low levels of androgenic hormones (232). Whether increased androgen receptor expression is a consequence of *AR* amplification or some other process, or is common in prostate cancer cases that progress despite androgen deprivation therapy, has not been fully resolved. Some *AR* mutations lead to the production of androgen receptors with altered ligand specificity, which can result in agonist behavior for anti-androgens. Such mutations may well be the basis for the well-described "anti-androgen withdrawal" syndrome, in which men with prostate cancer appear to benefit from discontinuation of anti-androgen therapy (225,233–236). An examination of 44 mutant androgen receptors from prostate cancers revealed that 16% of the receptors were unable to activate target gene transcription, 45% displayed altered transcriptional regulation, 32% retained partial transcriptional regulatory activity, and the remaining 7% exhibited normal behavior (237). For many prostate cancer cases, progression to androgen independence may not involve *AR* gene alterations, but rather be a result of androgen receptor activation, despite low or absent levels of androgens, by other signaling pathways capable of modifying the androgen receptor and/or its associated transcriptional co-regulators (21,238–242).

GENE EXPRESSION CHANGES IN PROSTATE CANCER

New technology platforms have permitted global analyses of gene expression changes in prostate cancers, providing opportunities for biomarker and therapeutic target discovery (243–254). Among the first and most consistently overexpressed genes detected in prostate cancers was *AMACR*, encoding α-methylacyl-CoA racemase, an enzyme essential for conversion of *R*- to *S*-stereoisomers during the β-oxidation of certain lipids (255). Germline *AMACR* mutations are associated with a syndrome of adult-onset neuropathy (256). In the prostate, anti-AMACR immunostaining studies have revealed that AMACR is rarely expressed by normal prostate cells, but tends to be expressed at high levels in PIN lesions and in prostate cancer cells, supporting the use of anti-AMACR immunohistochemistry as an adjunctive tool for prostate cancer diagnosis by histopathology (257–259). *Hepsin*, encoding a transmembrane serine protease, is also overexpressed in prostate cancers (243,244,249). In a mouse model, forced overexpression of Hepsin in the prostate resulted in basement membrane abnormalities and progressive defects in epithelial-substrate adherence in the prostate (260). When these mice were crossed to mice prone to develop prostate tumors, more aggressive prostate cancers resulted (260).

PROSTATE CANCER PROGRESSION TO METASTASIS

Although many prostate cancers diagnosed in the current era of serum PSA screening may pose little threat to life or to health, metastatic prostate cancer remains a significant cause of death in the developed world. As discussed above, prostatic carcinogenesis appears to be characterized by prolonged exposure to genome damaging species, such as dietary carcinogens and inflammatory oxidants, which trigger genetic and epigenetic alterations leading to neoplastic transformation and malignant progression. What is the molecular basis for the "lethal phenotype" of prostate cancer? In one recent autopsy series of men dying of prostate cancer, cancer deposits were found in the prostate (though small), in skeletal structures (including the skull and dura), in the liver, in the lung, in lymph nodes, in the adrenals, and in pelvic soft tissues, though not in the brain (261).

To reach various metastatic sites, prostate cancer cells clearly have to travel via lymphatics and via the circulation, and have to be able to survive and grow in varied microenvironments. Unfortunately, the molecular bases for these phenotypic attributes are not well understood. One area of controversy concerns whether (1) different rare cells emerge in primary prostate cancers with different genotypes, phenotypes, and predestined fates as metastases or whether (2) a single cancer cell with a defined genotype capable of supporting different phenotypes dominates the metastatic process. Molecular studies of metastatic lesions tend to support the latter model: different metastatic cancer deposits at different sites in individual prostate cancer cases seem to contain similar somatic genomic/epigenomic abnormalities, but exhibit a marked heterogeneity in phenotype, assessed via morphologic appearance, immunohistochemical staining for androgen receptor and PSA, and transcriptome profiling (152,262–264). These findings appear most consistent with a mechanism by which prostate cancer cells capable of metastasis form early in the prostate during disease pathogenesis, but adapt to environments at metastatic sites. The efficiency of adaptation may be responsible for the patterns of metastases characteristic of prostate cancer. If such a model was correct, then primary prostate cancers prone to recurrence and metastasis despite local therapy should be able to be distinguished by genotypic or phenotypic properties (e.g., the use of molecular biomarkers). Furthermore, local therapy would be expected to interrupt the continuous shedding of prostate cancer cells capable of metastasis into lymphatics or the circulation and attenuate life-threatening prostate cancer progression. Of interest in this regard, in a randomized clinical trial comparing prostate surgery to watchful waiting for men with prostate cancer, removal of the prostate was associated with a substantial reduction in the risk of prostate cancer metastasis as well as of prostate cancer mortality (265,266).

A stereotypical feature of prostate cancer progression is the propensity of prostate cancer to cause bony metastases. Prostate cancer cells likely arrive at bony sites via the circulation; prostate cancer cells are well known to be present in bone marrow in many prostate cancer cases, including in men thought to have localized disease (267–269). The means by which prostate cancer cells in the bone marrow survive to produce progeny, and then undermine the coordinated behavior of osteoblasts and osteoclasts to produce destructive bony lesions, have not been discerned (270). However, PTHrP, RANKL, osteoprotegerin, TGFβ, bone morphogenetic proteins, matrix metalloproteinases, and endothelin-1 have all been indicted in animal model studies as candidate participants in the development of prostate cancer bone metastases (271–273). The emerging understanding of this process has led to several new treatments targeting bone metastases, including the bisphosphonate zoledronic acid, and the endothelin receptor antagonist atrasentan (274,275).

CONCLUSIONS

Accumulating insights into the cellular and molecular mechanisms underlying the development of prostate cancer, and the progression of prostate cancer to threaten life, offer many exciting new opportunities for reducing prostate cancer morbidity and mortality. The possibility that inflammation contributes to early prostatic carcinogenesis has provided both a rationale for the use of anti-inflammatory agents and anti-oxidants for prostate cancer prevention, and an impetus to hunt for prostate pathogens that may initiate the pathogenesis of the disease. New revelations regarding chromosomal rearrangements producing fusion transcripts between androgen-regulated genes and growth control genes have the potential of explaining not only the initial sensitivity of prostate cancer to androgen deprivation therapy, but also the tendency for maintenance of ligand-independent androgen receptor activation even in androgen-independent prostate cancer. The implication of genes encoding participants in Akt signaling pathways in prostate cancer growth and survival will support testing of inhibitors targeting this pathway as new systemic prostate cancer treatments. Finally, a growing understanding of the deregulation of bone biology at prostate cancer bony metastases has already led to new and improved therapeutic approaches to reduce the morbidity of prostate cancer progression.

REFERENCES

1. Sakr WA, Grignon DJ, Crissman JD, et al. High grade prostatic intraepithelial neoplasia (HGPIN) and prostatic adenocarcinoma between the ages of 20–69: an autopsy study of 249 cases. In Vivo 1994; 8:439–443.
2. Jemal A, Murray T, Ward E, et al. Cancer statistics, 2005. CA Cancer J Clin 2005; 55: 10–30.
3. Bartsch G, Horninger W, Klocker H, et al. Prostate cancer mortality after introduction of prostate-specific antigen mass screening in the Federal State of Tyrol, Austria. Urology 2001; 58:417–424.
4. Hankey BF, Feuer EJ, Clegg LX, et al. Cancer surveillance series: interpreting trends in prostate cancer. Part I. Evidence of the effects of screening in recent prostate cancer incidence, mortality, and survival rates. J Natl Cancer Inst 1999; 91:1017–1024.

5. Brooks JD. Anatomy of the lower urinary tract and male genitalia. In: Walsh PC, ed. Campbel's Urology. Vol. 1. Philadelphia, PA: Saunders, 2002:41–80.
6. McNeal JE. The zonal anatomy of the prostate. Prostate 1981; 2:35–49.
7. McNeal JE. Normal histology of the prostate. Am J Surg Pathol 1988; 12:619–633.
8. Wang XD, Shou J, Wong P, French DM, Gao WQ. Notch1-expressing cells are indispensable for prostatic branching morphogenesis during development and re-growth following castration and androgen replacement. J Biol Chem 2004; 279:24733–24744.
9. De Marzo AM, Nelson WG, Meeker AK, Coffey DS. Stem cell features of benign and malignant prostate epithelial cells. J Urol 1998; 160:2381–2392.
10. Parsons JK, Gage WR, Nelson WG, De Marzo AM. p63 protein expression is rare in prostate adenocarcinoma: implications for cancer diagnosis and carcinogenesis. Urology 2001; 58:619–624.
11. van Leenders G, Dijkman H, Hulsbergen-van de Kaa C, Ruiter D, Schalken J. Demonstration of intermediate cells during human prostate epithelial differentiation in situ and in vitro using triple-staining confocal scanning microscopy. Lab Invest 2000; 80:1251–1258.
12. Bonkhoff H, Remberger K. Differentiation pathways and histogenetic aspects of normal and abnormal prostatic growth: a stem cell model. Prostate 1996; 28:98–106.
13. van Leenders GJ, Schalken JA. Epithelial cell differentiation in the human prostate epithelium: implications for the pathogenesis and therapy of prostate cancer. Crit Rev Oncol Hematol 2003; 46:S3–S10.
14. Rizzo S, Attard G, Hudson DL. Prostate epithelial stem cells. Cell Prolif 2005; 38: 363–374.
15. Hudson DL. Epithelial stem cells in human prostate growth and disease. Prostate Cancer Prostatic Dis 2004; 7:188–194.
16. Richardson GD, Robson CN, Lang SH, Neal DE, Maitland NJ, Collins AT. CD133, a novel marker for human prostatic epithelial stem cells. J Cell Sci 2004; 117:3539–3545.
17. Collins AT, Berry PA, Hyde C, Stower MJ, Maitland NJ. Prospective identification of tumorigenic prostate cancer stem cells. Cancer Res 2005; 65:10946–10951.
18. Palapattu GS, Meeker AK, Harris T, et al. Epithelial architectural destruction is necessary for bone marrow derived cell contribution to regenerating prostate epithelium. Urology. J Urol 2006; 176:813–818.
19. Planz B, Wang Q, Kirley SD, Lin CW, McDougal WS. Androgen responsiveness of stromal cells of the human prostate: regulation of cell proliferation and keratinocyte growth factor by androgen. J Urol 1998; 160:1850–1855.
20. Peehl DM, Rubin JS. Keratinocyte growth factor: an androgen-regulated mediator of stromal–epithelial interactions in the prostate. World J Urol 1995; 13:312–317.
21. Feldman BJ, Feldman D. The development of androgen-independent prostate cancer. Nat Rev Cancer 2001; 1:34–45.
22. Makridakis NM, di Salle E, Reichardt JK. Biochemical and pharmacogenetic dissection of human steroid 5 alpha-reductase type II. Pharmacogenetics 2000; 10:407–413.
23. Brinkmann AO, Blok LJ, de Ruiter PE, et al. Mechanisms of androgen receptor activation and function. J Steroid Biochem Mol Biol 1999; 69:307–313.
24. Roche PJ, Hoare SA, Parker MG. A consensus DNA-binding site for the androgen receptor. Mol Endocrinol 1992; 6:2229–2235.
25. Schuur ER, Henderson GA, Kmetec LA, Miller JD, Lamparski HG, Henderson DR. Prostate-specific antigen expression is regulated by an upstream enhancer. J Biol Chem 1996; 271:7043–7051.
26. Gatson JW, Kaur P, Singh M. Dihydrotestosterone differentially modulates the MAPK and the PI-3 kinase/akt pathways through the nuclear and novel membrane androgen receptor in C6 cells. Endocrinology 2006; 147:2028.
27. Migliaccio A, Di Domenico M, Castoria G, et al. Steroid receptor regulation of epidermal growth factor signaling through Src in breast and prostate cancer cells: steroid antagonist action. Cancer Res 2005; 65:10585–10593.
28. Oesterling JE, Hauzeur CG, Farrow GM. Small cell anaplastic carcinoma of the prostate: a clinical, pathological and immunohistological study of 27 patients. J Urol 1992; 147:804–807.

29. van Leenders GJ, Gage WR, Hicks JL, et al. Intermediate cells in human prostate epithelium are enriched in proliferative inflammatory atrophy. Am J Pathol 2003; 162:1529–1537.
30. Tomlins SA, Rhodes DR, Perner S, et al. Recurrent fusion of TMPRSS2 and ETS transcription factor genes in prostate cancer. Science 2005; 310:644–648.
31. McNeal JE, Bostwick DG. Intraductal dysplasia: a premalignant lesion of the prostate. Hum Pathol 1986; 17:64–71.
32. Brooks JD, Weinstein M, Lin X, et al. CG island methylation changes near the GSTP1 gene in prostatic intraepithelial neoplasia. Cancer Epidemiol Biomarkers Prev 1998; 7:531–536.
33. Meeker AK, Hicks JL, Platz EA, et al. Telomere shortening is an early somatic DNA alteration in human prostate tumorigenesis. Cancer Res 2002; 62:6405–6409.
34. Lichtenstein P, Holm NV, Verkasalo PK, et al. Environmental and heritable factors in the causation of cancer—analyses of cohorts of twins from Sweden, Denmark, and Finland. N Engl J Med 2000; 343:78–85.
35. Page WF, Braun MM, Partin AW, Caporaso N, Walsh P. Heredity and prostate cancer: a study of World War II veteran twins. Prostate 1997; 33:240–245.
36. Ahlbom A, Lichtenstein P, Malmstrom H, Feychting M, Hemminki K, Pedersen NL. Cancer in twins: genetic and nongenetic familial risk factors. J Natl Cancer Inst 1997; 89:287–293.
37. Gronberg H, Damber L, Damber JE. Studies of genetic factors in prostate cancer in a twin population. J Urol 1994; 152:1484–1487; discussion 1487–1489.
38. Morganti G, Gianferrari L, Cresseri A, Arrigoni G, Lovati G. Recherches clinicostastisiques et genetiques sur les neoplasies de la prostate. Acta Genet 1956; 6:304–305.
39. Steinberg GD, Carter BS, Beaty TH, Childs B, Walsh PC. Family history and the risk of prostate cancer. Prostate 1990; 17:337–347.
40. Lesko SM, Rosenberg L, Shapiro S. Family history and prostate cancer risk. Am J Epidemiol 1996; 144:1041–1047.
41. Ghadirian P, Howe GR, Hislop TG, Maisonneuve P. Family history of prostate cancer: a multi-center case-control study in Canada. Int J Cancer 1997; 70:679–681.
42. Glover FE Jr, Coffey DS, Douglas LL, et al. Familial study of prostate cancer in Jamaica. Urology 1998; 52:441–443.
43. Rodriguez C, Calle EE, Miracle-McMahill HL. Family history and risk of fatal prostate cancer. Epidemiology 1997; 8:653–657.
44. Spitz MR, Currier RD, Fueger JJ, Babaian RJ, Newell GR. Familial patterns of prostate cancer: a case–control analysis. J Urol 1991; 146:1305–1307.
45. Whittemore AS, Kolonel LN, Wu AH, et al. Prostate cancer in relation to diet, physical activity, and body size in blacks, whites, and Asians in the United States and Canada. J Natl Cancer Inst 1995; 87:652–661.
46. Carter BS, Beaty TH, Steinberg GD, Childs B, Walsh PC. Mendelian inheritance of familial prostate cancer. Proc Natl Acad Sci USA 1992; 89:3367–3371.
47. Monroe KR, Yu MC, Kolonel LN. Evidence of an X-linked or recessive genetic component to prostate cancer risk. Nat Med 1995; 1:827–829.
48. Smith JR, Freije D, Carpten JD, et al. Major susceptibility locus for prostate cancer on chromosome 1 suggested by a genome-wide search. Science 1996; 274:1371–1374.
49. Stanford JL, McDonnell SK, Friedrichsen DM, et al. Prostate cancer and genetic susceptibility: a genome scan incorporating disease aggressiveness. Prostate 2006; 66:317–325.
50. Slager SL, Zarfas KE, Brown WM. Genome-wide linkage scan for prostate cancer aggressiveness loci using families from the University of Michigan Prostate Cancer Genetics Project. Prostate 2006; 66:173–179.
51. Chang BL, Lange EM, Dimitrov L, et al. Two-locus genome-wide linkage scan for prostate cancer susceptibility genes with an interaction effect. Hum Genet 2006; 118:716–724.
52. Carpten J, Nupponen N, Isaacs S, et al. Germline mutations in the ribonuclease L gene in families showing linkage with HPC1. Nat Genet 2002; 30:181–184.
53. Xu J, Zheng SL, Komiya A, et al. Germline mutations and sequence variants of the macrophage scavenger receptor 1 gene are associated with prostate cancer risk. Nat Genet 2002; 32:321–325.

54. Silverman RH, Jung DD, Nolan-Sorden NL, Dieffenbach CW, Kedar VP, SenGupta DN. Purification and analysis of murine 2-5A-dependent RNase. J Biol Chem 1988; 263:7336–7341.
55. Jacobsen H, Czarniecki CW, Krause D, Friedman RM, Silverman RH. Interferon-induced synthesis of 2-5A-dependent RNase in mouse JLS-V9R cells. Virology 1983; 125:496–501.
56. Floyd-Smith G, Slattery E, Lengyel P. Interferon action: RNA cleavage pattern of a (2′–5′)oligoadenylate—dependent endonuclease. Science 1981; 212:1030–1032.
57. Clemens MJ, Williams BR. Inhibition of cell-free protein synthesis by pppA2′p5′A2′p5′A: a novel oligonucleotide synthesized by interferon-treated L cell extracts. Cell 1978; 13:565–572.
58. Zhou A, Hassel BA, Silverman RH. Expression cloning of 2-5A-dependent RNAase: a uniquely regulated mediator of interferon action. Cell 1993; 72:753–765.
59. Casey G, Neville PJ, Plummer SJ, et al. RNASEL Arg462Gln variant is implicated in up to 13% of prostate cancer cases. Nat Genet 2002; 32:581–583.
60. Wang L, McDonnell SK, Elkins DA, et al. Analysis of the RNASEL gene in familial and sporadic prostate cancer. Am J Hum Genet 2002; 71:116–123.
61. Kotar K, Hamel N, Thiffault I, Foulkes WD. The RNASEL 471delAAAG allele and prostate cancer in Ashkenazi Jewish men. J Med Genet 2003; 40:e22.
62. Wiklund F, Jonsson BA, Brookes AJ, et al. Genetic analysis of the RNASEL gene in hereditary, familial, and sporadic prostate cancer. Clin Cancer Res 2004; 10:7150–7156.
63. Platt N, Gordon S. Is the class A macrophage scavenger receptor (SR-A) multifunctional?—The mouse's tale. J Clin Invest 2001; 108:649–654.
64. Shirai H, Murakami T, Yamada Y, Doi T, Hamakubo T, Kodama T. Structure and function of type I and II macrophage scavenger receptors. Mech Ageing Dev 1999; 111:107–121.
65. Thomas CA, Li Y, Kodama T, Suzuki H, Silverstein SC, El Khoury J. Protection from lethal gram-positive infection by macrophage scavenger receptor-dependent phagocytosis. J Exp Med 2000; 191:147–156.
66. Ishiguro T, Naito M, Yamamoto T, et al. Role of macrophage scavenger receptors in response to *Listeria monocytogenes* infection in mice. Am J Pathol 2001; 158:179–188.
67. Dejager S, Mietus-Snyder M, Friera A, Pitas RE. Dominant negative mutations of the scavenger receptor: native receptor inactivation by expression of truncated variants. J Clin Invest 1993; 92:894–902.
68. Xu J, Zheng SL, Komiya A, et al. Common sequence variants of the macrophage scavenger receptor 1 gene are associated with prostate cancer risk. Am J Hum Genet 2003; 72:208–212.
69. Miller DC, Zheng SL, Dunn RL, et al. Germ-line mutations of the macrophage scavenger receptor 1 gene: association with prostate cancer risk in African-American men. Cancer Res 2003; 63:3486–3489.
70. Seppala EH, Ikonen T, Autio V, et al. Germ-line alterations in MSR1 gene and prostate cancer risk. Clin Cancer Res 2003; 9:5252–5256.
71. Wang L, McDonnell SK, Cunningham JM, et al. No association of germline alteration of MSR1 with prostate cancer risk. Nat Genet 2003; 35:128–129.
72. Zhou A, Paranjape J, Brown TL, et al. Interferon action and apoptosis are defective in mice devoid of 2′,5′-oligoadenylate-dependent RNase L. EMBO J 1997; 16:6355–6363.
73. Suzuki H, Kurihara Y, Takeya M, et al. A role for macrophage scavenger receptors in atherosclerosis and susceptibility to infection. Nature 1997; 386:292–296.
74. Peiser L, Gough PJ, Kodama T, Gordon S. Macrophage class A scavenger receptor-mediated phagocytosis of *Escherichia coli*: role of cell heterogeneity, microbial strain, and culture conditions in vitro. Infect Immunol 2000; 68:1953–1963.
75. McCarron SL, Edwards S, Evans PR, et al. Influence of cytokine gene polymorphisms on the development of prostate cancer. Cancer Res 2002; 62:3369–3372.
76. Lindmark F, Zheng SL, Wiklund F, et al. H6D polymorphism in macrophage-inhibitory cytokine-1 gene associated with prostate cancer. J Natl Cancer Inst 2004; 96:1248–1254.
77. Xu J, Lowey J, Wiklund F, et al. The interaction of four genes in the inflammation pathway significantly predicts prostate cancer risk. Cancer Epidemiol Biomarkers Prev 2005; 14:2563–2568.

78. Chen YC, Giovannucci E, Lazarus R, Kraft P, Ketkar S, Hunter DJ. Sequence variants of Toll-like receptor 4 and susceptibility to prostate cancer. Cancer Res 2005; 65:11771–11778.
79. Lindmark F, Zheng SL, Wiklund F, et al. Interleukin-1 receptor antagonist haplotype associated with prostate cancer risk. Br J Cancer 2005; 93:493–497.
80. Sun J, Wiklund F, Zheng SL, et al. Sequence variants in Toll-like receptor gene cluster (TLR6-TLR1-TLR10) and prostate cancer risk. J Natl Cancer Inst 2005; 97:525–532.
81. Zheng SL, Augustsson-Balter K, Chang B, et al. Sequence variants of toll-like receptor 4 are associated with prostate cancer risk: results from the cancer Prostate in Sweden Study. Cancer Res 2004; 64:2918–2922.
82. Woodson K, Tangrea JA, Lehman TA, et al. Manganese superoxide dismutase (*MnSOD*) polymorphism, alpha-tocopherol supplementation and prostate cancer risk in the alpha-tocopherol, beta-carotene cancer prevention study (Finland). Cancer Causes Control 2003; 14:513–518.
83. Li H, Kantoff PW, Giovannucci E, et al. Manganese superoxide dismutase polymorphism, prediagnostic antioxidant status, and risk of clinical significant prostate cancer. Cancer Res 2005; 65:2498–2504.
84. Chen L, Elahi A, Pow-Sang J, Lazarus P, Park J. Association between polymorphism of human oxoguanine glycosylase 1 and risk of prostate cancer. J Urol 2003; 170:2471–2474.
85. Xu J, Zheng SL, Turner A, et al. Associations between hOGG1 sequence variants and prostate cancer susceptibility. Cancer Res 2002; 62:2253–2257.
86. Edwards SM, Kote-Jarai Z, Meitz J, et al. Two percent of men with early-onset prostate cancer harbor germline mutations in the BRCA2 gene. Am J Hum Genet 2003; 72:1–12.
87. Dong X, Wang L, Taniguchi K, et al. Mutations in CHEK2 associated with prostate cancer risk. Am J Hum Genet 2003; 72:270–280.
88. Chamberlain NL, Driver ED, Miesfeld RL. The length and location of CAG trinucleotide repeats in the androgen receptor N-terminal domain affect transactivation function. Nucl Acids Res 1994; 22:3181–3186.
89. Kazemi-Esfarjani P, Trifiro MA, Pinsky L. Evidence for a repressive function of the long polyglutamine tract in the human androgen receptor: possible pathogenetic relevance for the (CAG)n-expanded neuronopathies. Hum Mol Genet 1995; 4:523–527.
90. Irvine RA, Ma H, Yu MC, Ross RK, Stallcup MR, Coetzee GA. Inhibition of p160-mediated coactivation with increasing androgen receptor polyglutamine length. Hum Mol Genet 2000; 9:267–274.
91. Beilin J, Ball EM, Favaloro JM, Zajac JD. Effect of the androgen receptor CAG repeat polymorphism on transcriptional activity: specificity in prostate and non-prostate cell lines. J Mol Endocrinol 2000; 25:85–96.
92. Hsing AW, Gao YT, Wu G, et al. Polymorphic CAG and GGN repeat lengths in the androgen receptor gene and prostate cancer risk: a population-based case–control study in China. Cancer Res 2000; 60:5111–5116.
93. Hakimi JM, Schoenberg MP, Rondinelli RH, Piantadosi S, Barrack ER. Androgen receptor variants with short glutamine or glycine repeats may identify unique subpopulations of men with prostate cancer. Clin Cancer Res 1997; 3:1599–1608.
94. Giovannucci E, Stampfer MJ, Krithivas K, et al. The CAG repeat within the androgen receptor gene and its relationship to prostate cancer. Proc Natl Acad Sci USA 1997; 94:3320–3323.
95. Stanford JL, Just JJ, Gibbs M, et al. Polymorphic repeats in the androgen receptor gene: molecular markers of prostate cancer risk. Cancer Res 1997; 57:1194–1198.
96. Makridakis N, Ross RK, Pike MC, et al. A prevalent missense substitution that modulates activity of prostatic steroid 5alpha-reductase. Cancer Res 1997; 57:1020–1022.
97. Makridakis NM, Ross RK, Pike MC, et al. Association of mis-sense substitution in SRD5A2 gene with prostate cancer in African-American and Hispanic men in Los Angeles, USA. Lancet 1999; 354:975–978.
98. Nam RK, Toi A, Vesprini D, et al. V89L polymorphism of type-2, 5-alpha reductase enzyme gene predicts prostate cancer presence and progression. Urology 2001; 57:199–204.
99. Hsing AW, Tsao L, Devesa SS. International trends and patterns of prostate cancer incidence and mortality. Int J Cancer 2000; 85:60–67.

100. Haenszel W, Kurihara M. Studies of Japanese migrants. I. Mortality from cancer and other diseases among Japanese in the United States. J Natl Cancer Inst 1968; 40:43–68.
101. Shimizu H, Ross RK, Bernstein L, Yatani R, Henderson BE, Mack TM. Cancers of the prostate and breast among Japanese and white immigrants in Los Angeles Country. Br J Cancer 1991; 63:963–966.
102. Le Marchand L, Kolonel LN, Wilkens LR, Myers BC, Hirohata T. Animal fat consumption and prostate cancer: a prospective study in Hawaii. Epidemiology 1994; 5:276–282.
103. Giovannucci E, Rimm EB, Colditz GA, et al. A prospective study of dietary fat and risk of prostate cancer [see comments]. J Natl Cancer Inst 1993; 85:1571–1579.
104. Gann PH, Hennekens CH, Sacks FM, Grodstein F, Giovannucci EL, Stampfer MJ. Prospective study of plasma fatty acids and risk of prostate cancer. J Natl Cancer Inst 1994; 86:281–286.
105. Gross GA, Turesky RJ, Fay LB, Stillwell WG, Skipper PL, Tannenbaum SR. Heterocyclic aromatic amine formation in grilled bacon, beef and fish and in grill scrapings. Carcinogenesis 1993; 14:2313–2318.
106. Morgenthaler PM, Holzhauser D. Analysis of mutations induced by 2-amino-1-methyl-6-phenylimidazo[4,5-b]pyridine (PhIP) in human lymphoblastoid cells. Carcinogenesis 1995; 16:713–718.
107. Knize MG, Salmon CP, Mehta SS, Felton JS. Analysis of cooked muscle meats for heterocyclic aromatic amine carcinogens. Mutat Res 1997; 376:129–134.
108. Lijinsky W, Shubik P. Benzo(a)pyrene and other polynuclear hydrocarbons in charcoal-broiled meat. Science 1964; 145:53–55.
109. Stuart GR, Holcroft J, de Boer JG, Glickman BW. Prostate mutations in rats induced by the suspected human carcinogen 2-amino-1-methyl-6-phenylimidazo[4,5-b]pyridine. Cancer Res 2000; 60:266–268.
110. Shirai T, Sano M, Tamano S, et al. The prostate: a target for carcinogenicity of 2-amino-1-methyl-6-phenylimidazo[4,5-b]pyridine (PhIP) derived from cooked foods. Cancer Res 1997; 57:195–198.
111. Giovannucci E, Ascherio A, Rimm EB, Stampfer MJ, Colditz GA, Willett WC. Intake of carotenoids and retinol in relation to risk of prostate cancer. J Natl Cancer Inst 1995; 87:1767–1776.
112. Gann PH, Ma J, Giovannucci E, et al. Lower prostate cancer risk in men with elevated plasma lycopene levels: results of a prospective analysis. Cancer Res 1999; 59: 1225–1230.
113. Giovannucci E, Rimm EB, Liu Y, Stampfer MJ, Willett WC. A prospective study of tomato products, lycopene, and prostate cancer risk. J Natl Cancer Inst 2002; 94:391–398.
114. Chen L, Stacewicz-Sapuntzakis M, Duncan C, et al. Oxidative DNA damage in prostate cancer patients consuming tomato sauce-based entrees as a whole-food intervention. J Natl Cancer Inst 2001; 93:1872–1879.
115. Cohen JH, Kristal AR, Stanford JL. Fruit and vegetable intakes and prostate cancer risk. J Natl Cancer Inst 2000; 92:61–68.
116. Zhang Y, Kensler TW, Cho CG, Posner GH, Talalay P. Anticarcinogenic activities of sulforaphane and structurally related synthetic norbornyl isothiocyanates. Proc Natl Acad Sci USA 1994; 91:3147–3150.
117. Zhang Y, Talalay P, Cho CG, Posner GH. A major inducer of anticarcinogenic protective enzymes from broccoli: isolation and elucidation of structure. Proc Natl Acad Sci USA 1992; 89:2399–2403.
118. Clark LC, Combs GF Jr, Turnbull BW, et al. Effects of selenium supplementation for cancer prevention in patients with carcinoma of the skin: a randomized controlled trial. Nutritional Prevention of Cancer Study Group [see comments] [published erratum appears in JAMA 1997; 277(19):1520]. JAMA 1996; 276:1957–1963.
119. Clark LC, Dalkin B, Krongrad A, et al. Decreased incidence of prostate cancer with selenium supplementation: results of a double-blind cancer prevention trial. Br J Urol 1998; 81:730–734.
120. Heinonen OP, Albanes D, Virtamo J, et al. Prostate cancer and supplementation with alpha-tocopherol and beta-carotene: incidence and mortality in a controlled trial [see comments]. J Natl Cancer Inst 1998; 90:440–446.

121. Hoque A, Albanes D, Lippman SM, et al. Molecular epidemiologic studies within the selenium and vitamin E cancer prevention trial (SELECT). Cancer Causes Control 12:627–633.
122. Gardner WA, Bennett BD. The prostate overview: recent insights and speculations. In: Weinstein RS, Garnder WA, eds. Pathology and Pathobiology of the Urinary Bladder and Prostate. Baltimore: Williams and Wilkens, 1992:129–148.
123. Giovannucci E. Medical history and etiology of prostate cancer. Epidemiol Rev 2001; 23:159–162.
124. Dennis LK, Lynch CF, Torner JC. Epidemiologic association between prostatitis and prostate cancer. Urology 2002; 60:78–83.
125. Hayes RB, Pottern LM, Strickler H, et al. Sexual behaviour, STDs and risks for prostate cancer. Br J Cancer 2000; 82:718–725.
126. Dennis LK, Dawson DV. Meta-analysis of measures of sexual activity and prostate cancer. Epidemiology 2002; 13:72–79.
127. Sutcliffe S, Zenilman JM, Ghanem KG, et al. Sexually transmitted infections and prostatic inflammation/cell damage as measured by serum prostate specific antigen concentration. J Urol. 2006; 15:939–948.
128. Roberts RO, Jacobson DJ, Girman CJ, Rhodes T, Lieber MM, Jacobsen SJ. A population-based study of daily nonsteroidal anti-inflammatory drug use and prostate cancer. Mayo Clin Proc 2002; 77:219–225.
129. Norrish AE, Jackson RT, McRae CU. Non-steroidal anti-inflammatory drugs and prostate cancer progression. Int J Cancer 1998; 77:511–515.
130. Nelson JE, Harris RE. Inverse association of prostate cancer and non-steroidal anti-inflammatory drugs (NSAIDs): results of a case-control study. Oncol Rep 2000; 7:169–170.
131. Platz EA, Rohrmann S, Pearson JD, et al. Nonsteroidal anti-inflammatory drugs and risk of prostate cancer in the Baltimore Longitudinal Study of Aging. Cancer Epidemiol Biomarkers Prev 2005; 14:390–396.
132. Leitzmann MF, Platz EA, Stampfer MJ, Willett WC, Giovannucci E. Ejaculation frequency and subsequent risk of prostate cancer. JAMA 2004; 291:1578–1586.
133. De Marzo AM, Marchi VL, Epstein JI, Nelson WG. Proliferative inflammatory atrophy of the prostate: implications for prostatic carcinogenesis. Am J Pathol 1999; 155: 1985–1992.
134. Franks LM. Atrophy and hyperplasia in the prostate proper. J Pathol Bacteriol 1954; 68:617–621.
135. Putzi MJ, De Marzo AM. Morphologic transitions between proliferative inflammatory atrophy and high-grade prostatic intraepithelial neoplasia. Urology 2000; 56:828–832.
136. Shah R, Mucci NR, Amin A, Macoska JA, Rubin MA. Postatrophic hyperplasia of the prostate gland: neoplastic precursor or innocent bystander? Am J Pathol 2001; 158:1767–1773.
137. Ruska KM, Sauvageot J, Epstein JI. Histology and cellular kinetics of prostatic atrophy. Am J Surg Pathol 1998; 22:1073–1077.
138. De Marzo AM, Marchi VL, Yang ES, Veeraswamy R, Lin X, Nelson WG. Abnormal regulation of DNA methyltransferase expression during colorectal carcinogenesis. Cancer Res 1999; 59:3855–3860.
139. Parsons JK, Nelson CP, Gage WR, Nelson WG, Kensler TW, De Marzo AM. GSTA1 expression in normal, preneoplastic, and neoplastic human prostate tissue. Prostate 2001; 49:30–37.
140. Zha S, Gage WR, Sauvageot J, et al. Cyclooxygenase-2 is up-regulated in proliferative inflammatory atrophy of the prostate, but not in prostate carcinoma. Cancer Res 2001; 61:8617–8623.
141. Lin X, Tascilar M, Lee WH, et al. GSTP1 CpG island hypermethylation is responsible for the absence of GSTP1 expression in human prostate cancer cells. Am J Pathol 2001; 159:1815–1826.
142. Nakayama M, Bennett CJ, Hicks JL, et al. Hypermethylation of the human glutathione S-transferase-pi gene (GSTP1) CpG island is present in a subset of proliferative inflam-

matory atrophy lesions but not in normal or hyperplastic epithelium of the prostate: a detailed study using laser-capture microdissection. Am J Pathol 2003; 163:923–933.
143. De Marzo AM, et al. A working group classification of focal prostate atrophy lesions. Am J Surg Pathol 2006; In press.
144. Naslund MJ, Coffey DS. The differential effects of neonatal androgen, estrogen and progesterone on adult rat prostate growth. J Urol 1986; 136:1136–1140.
145. Gilleran JP, Putz O, DeJong M, et al. The role of prolactin in the prostatic inflammatory response to neonatal estrogen. Endocrinology 2003; 144:2046–2054.
146. Tangbanluekal L, Robinette CL. Prolactin mediates estradiol-induced inflammation in the lateral prostate of Wistar rats. Endocrinology 1993; 132:2407–2416.
147. Robinette CL. Sex-hormone-induced inflammation and fibromuscular proliferation in the rat lateral prostate. Prostate 1988; 12:271–286.
148. Lovett K, Rifkin MD, McCue PA, Choi H. MR imaging characteristics of noncancerous lesions of the prostate. J Magn Reson Imaging 1992; 2:35–39.
149. Bresalier RS, Sandler RS, Quan H, et al. Cardiovascular events associated with rofecoxib in a colorectal adenoma chemoprevention trial. N Engl J Med 2005; 352:1092–1102.
150. Gonzalgo ML, Isaacs WB. Molecular pathways to prostate cancer. J Urol 2003; 170:2444–2452.
151. Herman JG, Baylin SB. Gene silencing in cancer in association with promoter hypermethylation. N Engl J Med 2003; 349:2042–2054.
152. Yegnasubramanian S, Kowalski J, Gonzalgo ML, et al. Hypermethylation of CpG islands in primary and metastatic human prostate cancer. Cancer Res 2004; 64: 1975–1986.
153. Bastian PJ, Yegnasubramanian S, Palapattu GS, et al. Molecular biomarker in prostate cancer: the role of CpG island hypermethylation. Eur Urol 2004; 46:698–708.
154. Lee WH, Morton RA, Epstein JI, et al. Cytidine methylation of regulatory sequences near the pi-class glutathione S-transferase gene accompanies human prostatic carcinogenesis. Proc Natl Acad Sci USA 1994; 91:11733–11737.
155. Henderson CJ, Smith AG, Ure J, Brown K, Bacon EJ, Wolf CR. Increased skin tumorigenesis in mice lacking pi class glutathione S-transferases. Proc Natl Acad Sci USA 1998; 95:5275–5280.
156. Nelson CP, Kidd LC, Sauvageot J, et al. Protection against 2-hydroxyamino-1-methyl-6-phenylimidazo[4,5-b]pyridine cytotoxicity and DNA adduct formation in human prostate by glutathione S-transferase P1. Cancer Res 2001; 61:103–109.
157. Lin X, Nelson WG. Methyl-CpG-binding domain protein-2 mediates transcriptional repression associated with hypermethylated GSTP1 CpG islands in MCF-7 breast cancer cells. Cancer Res 2003; 63:498–504.
158. McEachern MJ, Krauskopf A, Blackburn EH. Telomeres and their control. Annu Rev Genet 2000; 34:331–358.
159. Maser RS, DePinho RA. Connecting chromosomes, crisis, and cancer. Science 2002; 297:565–569.
160. Greider CW, Blackburn EH. Identification of a specific telomere terminal transferase activity in Tetrahymena extracts. Cell 1985; 43:405–413.
161. O'Hagan RC, Chang S, Maser RS, et al. Telomere dysfunction provokes regional amplification and deletion in cancer genomes. Cancer Cell 2002; 2:149–155.
162. Hackett JA, Feldser DM, Greider CW. Telomere dysfunction increases mutation rate and genomic instability. Cell 2001; 106:275–286.
163. Chin L, Artandi SE, Shen Q, et al. p53 deficiency rescues the adverse effects of telomere loss and cooperates with telomere dysfunction to accelerate carcinogenesis. Cell 1999; 97:527–538.
164. Wiemann SU, Satyanarayana A, Buer J, Kamino K, Manns MP, Rudolph KL. Contrasting effects of telomere shortening on organ homeostasis, tumor suppression, and survival during chronic liver damage. Oncogene 2005; 24:1501–1509.
165. Blasco MA, Rizen M, Greider CW, Hanahan D. Differential regulation of telomerase activity and telomerase RNA during multi-stage tumorigenesis. Nat Genet 1996; 12:200–204.

166. Meeker AK, Gage WR, Hicks JL, et al. Telomere length assessment in human archival tissues: combined telomere fluorescence in situ hybridization and immunostaining. Am J Pathol 2002; 160:1259–1268.
167. Sommerfeld HJ, Meeker AK, Piatyszek MA, Bova GS, Shay JW, Coffey DS. Telomerase activity: a prevalent marker of malignant human prostate tissue. Cancer Res 1996; 56:218–222.
168. He WW, Sciavolino PJ, Wing J, et al. A novel human prostate-specific, androgen-regulated homeobox gene (NKX3.1) that maps to 8p21, a region frequently deleted in prostate cancer. Genomics 1997; 43:69–77.
169. Emmert-Buck MR, Vocke CD, Pozzatti RO, et al. Allelic loss on chromosome 8p12–21 in microdissected prostatic intraepithelial neoplasia. Cancer Res 1995; 55:2959–2962.
170. Bhatia-Gaur R, Donjacour AA, Sciavolino PJ, et al. Roles for Nkx3.1 in prostate development and cancer. Genes Dev 1999; 13:966–977.
171. Bieberich CJ, Fujita K, He WW, Jay G. Prostate-specific and androgen-dependent expression of a novel homeobox gene. J Biol Chem 1996; 271:31779–31782.
172. Chen H, Nandi AK, Li X, Bieberich CJ. NKX-3.1 interacts with prostate-derived ETS factor and regulates the activity of the PSA promoter. Cancer Res 2002; 62:338–340.
173. Steadman DJ, Giuffrida D, Gelmann EP. DNA-binding sequence of the human prostate-specific homeodomain protein NKX3.1. Nucl Acids Res 2000; 28:2389–2395.
174. Abdulkadir SA, Magee JA, Peters TJ, et al. Conditional loss of Nkx3.1 in adult mice induces prostatic intraepithelial neoplasia. Mol Cell Biol 2002; 22:1495–1503.
175. Ouyang X, DeWeese TL, Nelson WG, Abate-Shen C. Loss-of-function of Nkx3.1 promotes increased oxidative damage in prostate carcinogenesis. Cancer Res 2005; 65:6773–6779.
176. Asatiani E, Huang WX, Wang A, et al. Deletion, methylation, and expression of the NKX3.1 suppressor gene in primary human prostate cancer. Cancer Res 2005; 65:1164–1173.
177. Voeller HJ, Augustus M, Madike V, Bova GS, Carter KC, Gelmann EP. Coding region of NKX3.1, a prostate-specific homeobox gene on 8p21, is not mutated in human prostate cancers. Cancer Res 1997; 57:4455–4459.
178. Zheng SL, Ju JH, Chang BL, et al. Germ-line mutation of NKX3.1 cosegregates with hereditary prostate cancer and alters the homeodomain structure and function. Cancer Res 2006; 66:69–77.
179. Wu X, Senechal K, Neshat MS, Whang YE, Sawyers CL. The PTEN/MMAC1 tumor suppressor phosphatase functions as a negative regulator of the phosphoinositide 3-kinase/Akt pathway. Proc Natl Acad Sci USA 1998; 95:15587–15591.
180. Steck PA, Pershouse MA, Jasser SA, et al. Identification of a candidate tumour suppressor gene, MMAC1, at chromosome 10q23.3 that is mutated in multiple advanced cancers. Nat Genet 1997; 15:356–362.
181. Li DM, Sun H. PTEN/MMAC1/TEP1 suppresses the tumorigenicity and induces G1 cell cycle arrest in human glioblastoma cells. Proc Natl Acad Sci USA 1998; 95: 15406–15411.
182. Teng DH, Hu R, Lin H, et al. MMAC1/PTEN mutations in primary tumor specimens and tumor cell lines. Cancer Res 1997; 57:5221–5225.
183. Myers MP, Pass I, Batty IH, et al. The lipid phosphatase activity of PTEN is critical for its tumor supressor function. Proc Natl Acad Sci USA 1998; 95:13513–13518.
184. Myers MP, Stolarov JP, Eng C, et al. P-TEN, the tumor suppressor from human chromosome 10q23, is a dual-specificity phosphatase. Proc Natl Acad Sci USA 1997; 94:9052–9057.
185. Maehama T, Dixon JE. The tumor suppressor, PTEN/MMAC1, dephosphorylates the lipid second messenger, phosphatidylinositol 3,4,5-trisphosphate. J Biol Chem 1998; 273:13375–13378.
186. Suzuki H, Freije D, Nusskern DR, et al. Interfocal heterogeneity of PTEN/MMAC1 gene alterations in multiple metastatic prostate cancer tissues. Cancer Res 1998; 58:204–209.
187. Cairns P, Okami K, Halachmi S, et al. Frequent inactivation of PTEN/MMAC1 in primary prostate cancer. Cancer Res 1997; 57:4997–5000.

188. Sun H, Lesche R, Li DM, et al. PTEN modulates cell cycle progression and cell survival by regulating phosphatidylinositol 3,4,5,-trisphosphate and Akt/protein kinase B signaling pathway. Proc Natl Acad Sci USA 1999; 96:6199–6204.
189. McMenamin ME, Soung P, Perera S, Kaplan I, Loda M, Sellers WR. Loss of PTEN expression in paraffin-embedded primary prostate cancer correlates with high Gleason score and advanced stage. Cancer Res 1999; 59:4291–4296.
190. Gray IC, Stewart LM, Phillips SM, et al. Mutation and expression analysis of the putative prostate tumour-suppressor gene PTEN. Br J Cancer 1998; 78:1296–1300.
191. Wang SI, Parsons R, Ittmann M. Homozygous deletion of the PTEN tumor suppressor gene in a subset of prostate adenocarcinomas. Clin Cancer Res 1998; 4:811–815.
192. Whang YE, Wu X, Suzuki H, et al. Inactivation of the tumor suppressor PTEN/MMAC1 in advanced human prostate cancer through loss of expression. Proc Natl Acad Sci USA 1998; 95:5246–5250.
193. Di Cristofano A, Pesce B, Cordon-Cardo C, Pandolfi PP. Pten is essential for embryonic development and tumour suppression. Nat Genet 1998; 19:348–355.
194. Kim MJ, Cardiff RD, Desai N, et al. Cooperativity of Nkx3.1 and Pten loss of function in a mouse model of prostate carcinogenesis. Proc Natl Acad Sci USA 2002; 99:2884–2889.
195. Kwabi-Addo B, Giri D, Schmidt K, et al. Haploinsufficiency of the Pten tumor suppressor gene promotes prostate cancer progression. Proc Natl Acad Sci USA 2001; 98:11563–11568.
196. Abate-Shen C, Banach-Petrosky WA, Sun X, et al. Nkx3.1; Pten mutant mice develop invasive prostate adenocarcinoma and lymph node metastases. Cancer Res 2003; 63:3886–3890.
197. Majumder PK, Yeh JJ, George DJ, et al. Prostate intraepithelial neoplasia induced by prostate restricted Akt activation: the MPAKT model. Proc Natl Acad Sci USA 2003; 100:7841–7846.
198. Majumder PK, Febbo PG, Bikoff R, et al. mTOR inhibition reverses Akt-dependent prostate intraepithelial neoplasia through regulation of apoptotic and HIF-1-dependent pathways. Nat Med 2004; 10:594–601.
199. Yang RM, Naitoh J, Murphy M, et al. Low p27 expression predicts poor disease-free survival in patients with prostate cancer. J Urol 1998; 159:941–945.
200. Cheville JC, Lloyd RV, Sebo TJ, et al. Expression of p27kip1 in prostatic adenocarcinoma. Mod Pathol 1998; 11:324–328.
201. Cordon-Cardo C, Koff A, Drobnjak M, et al. Distinct altered patterns of p27KIP1 gene expression in benign prostatic hyperplasia and prostatic carcinoma. J Natl Cancer Inst 1998; 90:1284–1291.
202. Cote RJ, Shi Y, Groshen S, et al. Association of p27Kip1 levels with recurrence and survival in patients with stage C prostate carcinoma. J Natl Cancer Inst 1998; 90:916–920.
203. De Marzo AM, Meeker AK, Epstein JI, Coffey DS. Prostate stem cell compartments: expression of the cell cycle inhibitor p27Kip1 in normal, hyperplastic, and neoplastic cells. Am J Pathol 1998; 153:911–919.
204. Guo Y, Sklar GN, Borkowski A, Kyprianou N. Loss of the cyclin-dependent kinase inhibitor p27(Kip1) protein in human prostate cancer correlates with tumor grade. Clin Cancer Res 1997; 3:2269–2274.
205. Kibel AS, Christopher M, Faith DA, Bova GS, Goodfellow PJ, Isaacs WB. Methylation and mutational analysis of p27(kip1) in prostate carcinoma. Prostate 2001; 48:248–253.
206. Kibel AS, Faith DA, Bova GS, Isaacs WB. Loss of heterozygosity at 12P12–13 in primary and metastatic prostate adenocarcinoma. J Urol 2000; 164:192–196.
207. Gottschalk AR, Basila D, Wong M, et al. p27Kip1 is required for PTEN-induced G1 growth arrest. Cancer Res 2001; 61:2105–2111.
208. Graff JR, Konicek BW, McNulty AM, et al. Increased AKT activity contributes to prostate cancer progression by dramatically accelerating prostate tumor growth and diminishing p27Kip1 expression. J Biol Chem 2000; 275:24500–24505.
209. Nakamura N, Ramaswamy S, Vazquez F, Signoretti S, Loda M, Sellers WR. Forkhead transcription factors are critical effectors of cell death and cell cycle arrest downstream of PTEN. Mol Cell Biol 2000; 20:8969–8982.

210. Di Cristofano A, De Acetis M, Koff A, Cordon-Cardo C, Pandolfi PP. Pten and p27KIP1 cooperate in prostate cancer tumor suppression in the mouse. Nat Genet 2001; 27:222–224.
211. Huggins C, Stevens RE, Hodges CV. Studies on prostate cancer: II the effects of castration on advanced carcinoma of the prostate gland. Arch Surg 1941; 43:209–222.
212. Iversen P, Tyrrell CJ, Kaisary AV, et al. Bicalutamide monotherapy compared with castration in patients with nonmetastatic locally advanced prostate cancer: 6.3 years of followup. J Urol 2000; 164:1579–1582.
213. Crawford ED, Eisenberger MA, McLeod DG, et al. A controlled trial of leuprolide with and without flutamide in prostatic carcinoma. N Engl J Med 1989; 321:419–424.
214. Laufer M, Denmeade SR, Sinibaldi VJ, Carducci MA, Eisenberger MA. Complete androgen blockade for prostate cancer: what went wrong? J Urol 2000; 164:3–9.
215. Amler LC, Agus DB, LeDuc C, et al. Deregulated expression of androgen-responsive and nonresponsive genes in the androgen-independent prostate cancer xenograft model CWR22-R1. Cancer Res 2000; 60:6134–6141.
216. Mousses S, Wagner U, Chen Y, et al. Failure of hormone therapy in prostate cancer involves systematic restoration of androgen responsive genes and activation of rapamycin sensitive signaling. Oncogene 2001; 20:6718–6723.
217. van der Kwast TH, Schalken J, Ruizeveld de Winter JA, et al. Androgen receptors in endocrine-therapy-resistant human prostate cancer. Int J Cancer 1991; 48:189–193.
218. Visakorpi T, Hyytinen E, Koivisto P, et al. In vivo amplification of the androgen receptor gene and progression of human prostate cancer. Nat Genet 1995; 9:401–406.
219. Koivisto P, Kononen J, Palmberg C, et al. Androgen receptor gene amplification: a possible molecular mechanism for androgen deprivation therapy failure in prostate cancer. Cancer Res 1997; 57:314–319.
220. Haapala K, Hyytinen ER, Roiha M, et al. Androgen receptor alterations in prostate cancer relapsed during a combined androgen blockade by orchiectomy and bicalutamide. Lab Invest 2001; 81:1647–1651.
221. Marcelli M, Ittmann M, Mariani S, et al. Androgen receptor mutations in prostate cancer. Cancer Res 2000; 60:944–949.
222. Taplin ME, Bubley GJ, Ko YJ, et al. Selection for androgen receptor mutations in prostate cancers treated with androgen antagonist. Cancer Res 1999; 59:2511–2515.
223. Taplin ME, Bubley GJ, Shuster TD, et al. Mutation of the androgen-receptor gene in metastatic androgen-independent prostate cancer. N Engl J Med 1995; 332:1393–1398.
224. Tilley WD, Buchanan G, Hickey TE, Bentel JM. Mutations in the androgen receptor gene are associated with progression of human prostate cancer to androgen independence. Clin Cancer Res 1996; 2:277–285.
225. Veldscholte J, Ris-Stalpers C, Kuiper GG, et al. A mutation in the ligand binding domain of the androgen receptor of human LNCaP cells affects steroid binding characteristics and response to anti-androgens. Biochem Biophys Res Commun 1990; 173:534–540.
226. Suzuki H, Sato N, Watabe Y, Masai M, Seino S, Shimazaki J. Androgen receptor gene mutations in human prostate cancer. J Steroid Biochem Mol Biol 1993; 46:759–765.
227. Suzuki H, Akakura K, Komiya A, Aida S, Akimoto S, Shimazaki J. Codon 877 mutation in the androgen receptor gene in advanced prostate cancer: relation to antiandrogen withdrawal syndrome. Prostate 1996; 29:153–158.
228. Schoenberg MP, Hakimi JM, Wang S, et al. Microsatellite mutation (CAG24→18) in the androgen receptor gene in human prostate cancer. Biochem Biophys Res Commun 1994; 198:74–80.
229. Newmark JR, Hardy DO, Tonb DC, et al. Androgen receptor gene mutations in human prostate cancer. Proc Natl Acad Sci USA 1992; 89:6319–6323.
230. Gaddipati JP, McLeod DG, Heidenberg HB, et al. Frequent detection of codon 877 mutation in the androgen receptor gene in advanced prostate cancers. Cancer Res 1994; 54:2861–2864.
231. Evans BA, Harper ME, Daniells CE, et al. Low incidence of androgen receptor gene mutations in human prostatic tumors using single strand conformation polymorphism analysis. Prostate 1996; 28:162–171.

232. Chen CD, Welsbie DS, Tran C, et al. Molecular determinants of resistance to antiandrogen therapy. Nat Med 2004; 10:33–39.
233. Kelly WK, Scher HI. Prostate specific antigen decline after antiandrogen withdrawal: the flutamide withdrawal syndrome. J Urol 1993; 149:607–609.
234. Tan J, Sharief Y, Hamil KG, et al. Dehydroepiandrosterone activates mutant androgen receptors expressed in the androgen-dependent human prostate cancer xenograft CWR22 and LNCaP cells. Mol Endocrinol 1997; 11:450–459.
235. Veldscholte J, Voorhorst-Ogink MM, Bolt-de Vries J, van Rooij HC, Trapman J, Mulder E. Unusual specificity of the androgen receptor in the human prostate tumor cell line LNCaP: high affinity for progestagenic and estrogenic steroids. Biochim Biophys Acta 1990; 1052:187–194.
236. Culig Z, Hobisch A, Cronauer MV, et al. Mutant androgen receptor detected in an advanced-stage prostatic carcinoma is activated by adrenal androgens and progesterone. Mol Endocrinol 1993; 7:1541–1550.
237. Shi XB, Ma AH, Xia L, Kung HJ, de Vere White RW. Functional analysis of 44 mutant androgen receptors from human prostate cancer. Cancer Res 2002; 62:1496–1502.
238. Sadar MD, Gleave ME. Ligand-independent activation of the androgen receptor by the differentiation agent butyrate in human prostate cancer cells. Cancer Res 2000; 60:5825–5831.
239. Nazareth LV, Weigel NL. Activation of the human androgen receptor through a protein kinase A signaling pathway. J Biol Chem 1996; 271:19900–19907.
240. Hobisch A, Eder IE, Putz T, et al. Interleukin-6 regulates prostate-specific protein expression in prostate carcinoma cells by activation of the androgen receptor. Cancer Res 1998; 58:4640–4645.
241. Craft N, Shostak Y, Carey M, Sawyers CL. A mechanism for hormone-independent prostate cancer through modulation of androgen receptor signaling by the HER-2/neu tyrosine kinase. Nat Med 1999; 5:280–285.
242. Scher HI, Sawyers CL. Biology of progressive, castration-resistant prostate cancer: directed therapies targeting the androgen-receptor signaling axis. J Clin Oncol 2005; 23:8253–8261.
243. Dhanasekaran SM, Barrette TR, Ghosh D, et al. Delineation of prognostic biomarkers in prostate cancer. Nature 2001; 412:822–826.
244. Luo J, Duggan DJ, Chen Y, et al. Human prostate cancer and benign prostatic hyperplasia: molecular dissection by gene expression profiling. Cancer Res 2001; 61:4683–4688.
245. Luo JH, Yu YP, Cieply K, et al. Gene expression analysis of prostate cancers. Mol Carcinog 2002; 33:25–35.
246. Stamey TA, Warrington JA, Caldwell MC, et al. Molecular genetic profiling of Gleason grade 4/5 prostate cancers compared to benign prostatic hyperplasia. J Urol 2001; 166:2171–2177.
247. Welsh JB, Sapinoso LM, Su AI, et al. Analysis of gene expression identifies candidate markers and pharmacological targets in prostate cancer. Cancer Res 2001; 61:5974–5978.
248. Waghray A, Schober M, Feroze F, Yao F, Virgin J, Chen YQ. Identification of differentially expressed genes by serial analysis of gene expression in human prostate cancer. Cancer Res 2001; 61:4283–4286.
249. Magee JA, Araki T, Patil S, et al. Expression profiling reveals hepsin overexpression in prostate cancer. Cancer Res 2001; 61:5692–5696.
250. Nelson PS, Han D, Rochon Y, et al. Comprehensive analyses of prostate gene expression: convergence of expressed sequence tag databases, transcript profiling and proteomics. Electrophoresis 2000; 21:1823–1831 [pii].
251. Xu J, Stolk JA, Zhang X, et al. Identification of differentially expressed genes in human prostate cancer using subtraction and microarray. Cancer Res 2000; 60:1677–1682.
252. Walker MG, Volkmuth W, Sprinzak E, Hodgson D, Klingler T. Prediction of gene function by genome-scale expression analysis: prostate cancer-associated genes. Genome Res 1999; 9:1198–1203.
253. Rhodes DR, Barrette TR, Rubin MA, Ghosh D, Chinnaiyan AM. Meta-analysis of microarrays: interstudy validation of gene expression profiles reveals pathway dysregulation in prostate cancer. Cancer Res 2002; 62:4427–4433.

254. Huang GM, Ng WL, Farkas J, et al. Prostate cancer expression profiling by cDNA sequencing analysis. Genomics 1999; 59:178–186.
255. Schmitz W, Albers C, Fingerhut R, Conzelmann E. Purification and characterization of an alpha-methylacyl-CoA racemase from human liver. Eur J Biochem 1995; 231:815–822.
256. Ferdinandusse S, Denis S, Clayton PT, et al. Mutations in the gene encoding peroxisomal alpha-methylacyl-CoA racemase cause adult-onset sensory motor neuropathy. Nat Genet 2000; 24:188–191.
257. Rubin MA, Zhou M, Dhanasekaran SM, et al. Alpha-methylacyl coenzyme A racemase as a tissue biomarker for prostate cancer. JAMA 2002; 287:1662–1670.
258. Luo J, Zha S, Gage WR, et al. Alpha-methylacyl-CoA racemase: a new molecular marker for prostate cancer. Cancer Res 2002; 62:2220–2226.
259. DeMarzo AM, Nelson WG, Isaacs WB, Epstein JI. Pathological and molecular aspects of prostate cancer. Lancet 2003; 361:955–964.
260. Klezovitch O, Chevillet J, Mirosevich J, Roberts RL, Matusik RJ, Vasioukhin V. Hepsin promotes prostate cancer progression and metastasis. Cancer Cell 2004; 6:185–195.
261. Rubin MA, Putzi M, Mucci N, et al. Rapid ("warm") autopsy study for procurement of metastatic prostate cancer. Clin Cancer Res 2000; 6:1038–1045.
262. Roudier MP, True LD, Higano CS, et al. Phenotypic heterogeneity of end-stage prostate carcinoma metastatic to bone. Hum Pathol 2003; 34:646–653.
263. Shah RB, Mehra R, Chinnaiyan AM, et al. Androgen-independent prostate cancer is a heterogeneous group of diseases: lessons from a rapid autopsy program. Cancer Res 2004; 64:9209–9216.
264. Suzuki H, Freije D, Nusskern DR, et al. Interfocal heterogeneity of PTEN/MMAC1 gene alterations in multiple metastatic prostate cancer tissues. Cancer Res 1998; 58:204–209.
265. Holmberg L, Bill-Axelson A, Helgesen F, et al. A randomized trial comparing radical prostatectomy with watchful waiting in early prostate cancer. N Engl J Med 2002; 347:781–789.
266. Bill-Axelson A, Holmberg L, Ruutu M, et al. Radical prostatectomy versus watchful waiting in early prostate cancer. N Engl J Med 2005; 352:1977–1984.
267. Ellis WJ, Pfitzenmaier J, Colli J, Arfman E, Lange PH, Vessella RL. Detection and isolation of prostate cancer cells from peripheral blood and bone marrow. Urology 2003; 61:277–281.
268. Melchior SW, Corey E, Ellis WJ, et al. Early tumor cell dissemination in patients with clinically localized carcinoma of the prostate. Clin Cancer Res 1997; 3:249–256.
269. Gao CL, Dean RC, Pinto A, et al. Detection of circulating prostate specific antigen expressing prostatic cells in the bone marrow of radical prostatectomy patients by sensitive reverse transcriptase polymerase chain reaction. J Urol 1999; 161:1070–1076.
270. Keller ET, Brown J. Prostate cancer bone metastases promote both osteolytic and osteoblastic activity. J Cell Biochem 2004; 91:718–729.
271. Lynch CC, Hikosaka A, Acuff HB, et al. MMP-7 promotes prostate cancer-induced osteolysis via the solubilization of RANKL. Cancer Cell 2005; 7: 485–496.
272. Yin JJ, Mohammad KS, Kakonen SM, et al. A causal role for endothelin-1 in the pathogenesis of osteoblastic bone metastases. Proc Natl Acad Sci USA 2003; 100:10954–10959.
273. Guise TA, Yin JJ, Mohammad KS. Role of endothelin-1 in osteoblastic bone metastases. Cancer 2003; 97:779–784.
274. Saad F, Gleason DM, Murray R, et al. Long-term efficacy of zoledronic acid for the prevention of skeletal complications in patients with metastatic hormone-refractory prostate cancer. J Natl Cancer Inst 2004; 96:879–882.
275. Carducci MA, Padley RJ, et al. Effect of endothelin-A receptor blockade with atrasentan on tumor progression in men with hormone-refractory prostate cancer: a randomized, phase II, placebo-controlled trial. J Clin Oncol 2003; 21:679–689.

2 Targeted Therapies for Cancer: Definitions and Attributes

Edward A. Sausville

University of Maryland, Marlene and Stewart Greenebaum Cancer Center, Baltimore, Maryland, U.S.A.

This chapter will endeavor to place the recent interest in developing "targeted" treatments for cancer in a context that starts from our evolving understanding of the biology of cancer, and yet is mindful of the practicalities encountered in actually developing a drug for cancer treatment. In addition, examples of different target types will be illustrated. This chapter will therefore introduce concepts that will be illustrated in subsequent chapters of this book, directed at specific opportunities to define and exploit molecular targets in prostate cancer.

EMPIRICAL VS. TARGETED AGENTS FOR CANCER

Candidate anti-cancer drugs have been historically selected on the basis of empirically defined anti-proliferative activity in cancer cells. These frequently grow in artificial tissue culture, or as tumors propagated or occurring naturally in animals. The vast majority of agents selected in this fashion have had either some aspect of DNA integrity or the ability to alter the microtubule cytoskeleton as their ultimate targets. These are considered *empirically selected* agents, because the basis for their choice was the empirical evidence of tumor shrinkage, without specific reference to any particular mechanism of action.

Following definition of a schedule yielding efficacy in animal models, usually mice bearing endogenous mouse or xenografted human tumor cells, derivation of a suitable formulation, and definition of dose levels that convey at worst reversible mild toxicity in host animals, such empirically selected agents enter a clinical development path where on a particular schedule of administration Phase I trials define the maximal dose that can be administered with tolerable side effects; Phase II studies define the level of activity at a fixed dose in a particular disease; and Phase III trials define activity in relation to no treatment or a standard comparator therapy. At no point in this process does the biology of the disease or the basis for the drug's action necessarily inform the development path. Molecularly targeted drug discovery and development strategies proceed from a very distinct basis for enthusiasm in their initial discovery and development steps.

Although there is no question that the empirically originated process for chemotherapy development has yielded considerable progress in cancer treatment, seminal discoveries defining the biological basis of tumor development, including oncogenes, tumor suppressor genes, the basis for cell death regulation, and the mechanisms governing invasion and metastasis suggest a distinct paradigm for drug discovery and development in cancer. Hanahan and Weinberg (1) have articulated cogently the notion that successful tumors possess nonoverlapping sets of essential alterations, usually as the result of specific genetic abnormalities.

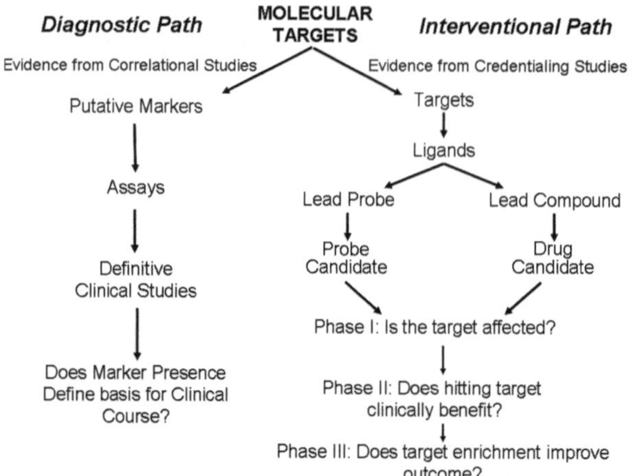

FIGURE 1 Schematic representation of targeted agent therapy development.

These alterations allow autonomy from growth signals, loss of "anti-growth" signals, the ability to evade programmed cell death, indefinite limits on replication potential, and the ability to promote new blood vessel growth and invade tissues. In addition, successful tumors also evade host immunological defenses. Each tumor may utilize different specific mechanisms to achieve each of these outcomes. Thus, one can imagine therapies that are designed to affect each of the common sets of essential alterations of cell physiology in malignancy. The selection of candidate drug molecules would therefore be based not simply on empirical anti-tumor activity, but on modulation of a discrete molecular entity whose activity underlies one or more of the essential alterations sustaining the malignant state.

This pathway for *targeted drug development* in cancer leads to a different development path (Fig. 1) (2). Before entering the familiar Phase I, II, and III progressions, compounds will have been selected on the basis being able to affect target molecules which are "credentialed" in that affecting the target clearly can alter the malignant phenotype. Such information might arise from either clinical epidemiologic evidence pertaining to the target or from actual biological studies with genetically modified animals or cells. Ligands for such targets could either be drug candidates or could serve as imaging probes to inform the presence or function of the target in the tumor. A corollary of this way of proceeding is that a molecular effect of the drug could now be written into early trials as a distinct end point. For example, at the dose and schedule defined at the end of Phase I as suitable for further testing, is the target modified by the agent? In Phase II, does a useful effect of the drug occur in the patient population with the target? Does modulation of the target correlate with any evidence of clinical effect? In Phase III, should the patient populations to be studied be selected on the basis of expressing the target? Figure 1 also makes the point that the same targets that may be candidates for imaging and therapeutic studies could also be the basis for diagnostic assays, through a separate development pathway that will not be considered further here.

Thus, a "targeted" therapy for cancer is one directed at the molecular basis for one or more aspects of a malignancy's biological success in a human host.

Implicit in this definition is the idea that the dose–response relation of a targeted therapy is expected to be *saturable*, in that once the target is fully occupied or affected, no further increment in dose would be expected to add value. From this expectation flows the concept that molecularly targeted agents may require a biological effective dose (BED) to be defined rather than a "maximum tolerated dose," the conventional end point of a Phase I trial. The BED would be the dose at which target function is optimally modulated. In addition, one might imagine clinical trials not actually focused on histologically defined disease, but where patient selection possibly occurs across several different disease types with target expression or function defining a potential basis for clinical study of the new agent. In essence, targeted cancer drug development allows the biology of the tumor to inform the clinical development of its proper treatment.

QUALIFICATION OF CANCER TARGETS

The publicly held databases resulting from sequencing the human genome as well as specialized databases representing the results of sequencing the expressed genes of human tumors (e.g., Cancer Genome Anatomy Project; http://cgap.nci.nih.gov/) allow the definition of hundreds to thousands of targets to be considered as a basis for drug discovery. A target could conceivably be any molecule differentially expressed in tumor as compared to host compartments. How to select the best targets is the subject of much discussion in the academic and pharmaceutical industry communities. One point of view is that evidence of mutational activation of a pathway, or deletion of a tumor suppressor pathway, identifies targets of opportunity by defining a pathway that sustains the tumor's coming into being. Examples of target pathways defined in this way would include the *ras* family of oncoproteins, the *Rb* tumor suppressor pathway particularly as it influences activation of S-phase-related transcripts, the Von Hippel–Lindau tumor suppressor regulation of hypoxia-induced factor (HIF) signaling. The validation of this way of thinking can be pointed to in the obvious clinical success of drugs directed at activated oncoproteins, such as imatinib in *bcr-abl*-driven chronic myelogenous leukemia. These targets have the potential advantage of allowing definition of compounds which function as pharmacological "synthetic lethals," analogous to observations in yeast, where synthetic lethal mutations are defined as mutations assessing import to the organism only in the context of a previously existing mutation (3). By analogy, one can envision drugs that would act only in the context of mutated oncoproteins or deleted tumor suppressor protein function. Mutated oncoprotein targets function in defined pathways which allow the sequential definition of targets ranging from the sites of input into the target pathway and at successive levels of pathway activation. Thus a drug acting as a synthetic lethal could in principle function at any point in the target's own pathway, or in parallel pathways acting in concert with the target.

A contrasting viewpoint is that nonmutated targets may also contribute to a tumor state by sustaining vital functions dispensable to a certain degree in a corresponding normal tissue type, or derive their value as targets owing to the cell's response, e.g., activation of a checkpoint blocking growth or apoptotic pathway causing tumor cell death in response to the drug occupying its target. This latter circumstance is illustrated by the apparent value of tubulin or DNA-directed agents, which are successful only in a tumor milieu that features induction of an apoptotic response after modification of DNA or cytoskeleton structure. Androgen or estrogen receptors are also valuable neoplastic targets in the proper context even without evidence of mutational activation. The point is that real clinical value can be derived from drug interaction with nonmutated targets, in a "correct" intratumoral context.

These considerations prompt a definition of putative molecular targets for cancer treatment as fitting into four general categories. *Pathogenic* targets do in this view actually relate to the causation of a tumor, usually by gene mutation, translocation, or amplification. *Ontogenic* targets relate to the tissue of origin, and may convey cytotoxicity despite lack of mutational activation. *Pharmacological* targets relate to how a tumor accepts, distributes, or metabolizes drugs. *Microenvironmental* targets relate to the stromal environment in which the tumor situates itself, and encompasses new blood vessels, microcirculation, and immune effector cells which live at the interface of the tumor and the host. Each of these target areas have distinct advantages and liabilities, to be highlighted below, in exploiting them for cancer treatment.

AGENT/TARGET DISCOVERY STRATEGIES

How should actual target discovery proceed? How should molecular targets be "qualified?" Clearly, biological approaches, which define mutations and gene activation by amplification, are a potent and proven means of defining pathogenic targets. Proteins resulting from the transcription of genes activated by such translocations have given knowledge of such molecules as *bcr-abl*, *bcl2*, and the leukemia-related fusion proteins such as PML-RARα. The defined target molecule can then be used to develop screens to define small molecules or protein-based modifiers of target function.

Another type of target definition essentially "retrofits" the action of an empirically useful drug to a particular target. Two general approaches to accomplish this end exist. In the first, active molecules are used to define interacting cellular components which are the basis for drug action. This then allows the definition of additional agents affecting the target function. In a second strategy, the patterns of drug action in different cell types can define families of drugs affecting the same target or pathway. A classical example of both approaches would be the tubulin-directed anti-mitotic poisons, including vinca alkaloids and taxanes. These agents have a pattern of action in vitro which allows the facile definition of other microtubule-directed agents (4). More recent agents selected in screens for optimization of anti-mitotic behavior have led to such agents as the epothilones (5) and halichondrin (6). Other targets discovered in this fashion of significance to modern drug development strategies would include a variety of topoisomerase II poisons (7), camptothecins (topoisomerase I) (8), rapamycin (mammalian target of rapamycin) (9), and heat shock protein 90 (binding partner for geldanamycins) (10).

Classical metabolism studies had defined the enzymatic basis for regulation of key biochemical pathways. Medicinal chemistry can then be used to proceed with the straightforward design of inhibitors, aided where possible by target structure studies. There are numerous successful examples in both the classical chemotherapeutic armamentarium [fluoropyrimidines, gemcitabine (11), methotrexate] as well as among more recently approved agents [e.g., pemetrexed (12) and bortezomib (13)].

At a somewhat more preliminary stage of evaluation is the capacity of genetically modified cells or organisms to define compounds which can affect an entire pathway. This approach takes its lead from the observation that yeast mutants can define compounds with distinctive abilities to mediate anti-proliferative effects, presumably by affecting pathways regulated by the mutation (14), akin to the synthetic lethal strategy described above. This concept leads to the definition of particular cell-based screens to detect potential regulators of pathways transcriptionally activated by elements which in the context of the screen regulate reported genes, allowing, e.g., the detection of compounds affecting HIF (15) influenced transcription. Although it is true that successful interpretation of such screening results requires "deconvolution" of the positively selected compounds, such screens allow the definition of hitherto unsuspected activities on the part of screened compounds. They are most valuable in the setting of stringent "counter-screens" to allow discard of compounds affecting processes of lesser interest.

PATHOGENIC TARGETS: ISSUES

Major concerns with pathogenic targets center on when in the context of a disease's evolution a particular target is most relevant. This issue is illustrated by imatinib, which is most successful in treating the chronic phase of chronic myelogenous leukemia (CML), but has more limited real clinical value in the blast crisis phase of the disease. The molecular basis for the resistance in the latter context arises in part from the occurrence of mutations at the adenosine triphosphate binding site (16). This raises the possibility that subsequent generations of inhibitors might be selected with a different mutational spectrum and that combined treatment may retard the emergence of resistance, such that CML therapy of the future may consist of "cocktails of anti-*bcr-abl* inhibitors," a concept for which there is already some preclinical evidence of value (17).

An additional problem with "pathogenic" targets is defining a basis for recognizing critical dependence of a tumor on a target function. The recent elucidation that patients bearing mutations of the endothelial growth factor (EGF) receptor have the greatest susceptibility to EGF-R-directed therapies (18,19) underscores the potential value in defining this dependence prospectively. Recent observations have likewise suggested that PTEN-mutated tumors may have greater susceptibility to rapamycins (20), and B-raf mutations connote great sensitivity to MEK inhibitors (21). It is interesting that in each case, the drug target is actually mutated itself or downstream of the mutated putatively pathogenic entity. In contrast, where the mutation is downstream of the drug target, the resistance would likely be encountered, as seems to be emerging in the case of *ras*-mutated lung cancers exposed to EGF-receptor antagonists.

Although the experience of the *ras*-directed farnesyl transferase antagonists may be taken as an argument against the value of mutational screening of the target population, as, e.g., the activity of model farnesyl transferase inhibitors (FTIs) did not track with mutational status of *ras* alleles (22), this is really not a fair example as the target of drug action, farnesyl transferase, was but indirectly related to *ras* function. It might be argued legitimately that the proper test of the value of *ras* as a target will await the definition of agents that actually can disrupt *ras/raf* interaction.

A more vexing potential problem is how to address evidence of drug resistance by activation of parallel or redundant pathways. For example, evidence has been presented that resistance to trastuzumab may arise by activation of insulin-like growth factor signaling (23), and that *akt* activation status likewise contributes to susceptibility to EGF-receptor antagonists (24). As these relationships are not for the most part predictable a priori, the definition of these potential issues in interpreting clinical data by collection of clinical specimens in the context of a clinical trial should be strongly encouraged.

ONTOGENIC TARGETS: ISSUES

This target class reflects molecules reflecting the tissue of origin of the tumor, or a target acquired adventitiously in the course of tumor's coming into being. In either case, the target has nothing to do with the genetic lesions causing the tumor, but may facilitate cancer cell survival, or serve to deliver an anti-proliferative signal. Tangible examples currently would include the estrogen and androgen receptors (ARs) in breast and prostate cancer, respectively, the I^- transporter in thyroid cancer, or cell surface antigens (e.g., CD20) in lymphomas.

Successful targets of this type must have a relatively tumor-selective distribution, with absence from the stem cell population of normal organs or tissues, and not be critical to the continued existence of the organism. Difficulties in addressing these target categories arise from the dispensability of function of the target from the proliferative activities of the tumor. Thus, estrogen receptor negative tumors arise in the context of breast cancer progression, or there is a functional dissociation of dependence on the target. Lymphomas no longer responding to CD20-directed treatments still express CD20. How to recognize this state would be of great interest in selecting patients for therapies directed at these targets. Recent efforts have raised the possibility in the case of breast cancer that gene expression profiling may define ER+ patients with a greater or lesser susceptibility to hormone receptor antagonists (25). One can envision analogous information of great value to assignment of patients with prostate cancer to different "risk" strata for hormonal therapy.

PHARMACOLOGICAL TARGETS: ISSUES

These target classes affect the handling or uptake of drug in tumors compared to normal tissue. Examples would include drug transport systems (e.g., folate receptor, drug efflux pumps such as pgp, mrp, and bcrp), drug metabolism or activation systems (e.g., nucleoside kinases and diaphorase), or drug retention mechanisms (polyglutamoylation). This target class has been relatively underaddressed in drug discovery efforts, with the possible exception of mdr, and no currently licensed drug addresses these targets in isolation. Recently, the approval of capecitabine for treatment of colon carcinoma illustrates the importance of designing molecules that have favorable handling by these systems. It is intriguing to speculate that cytotoxic molecules of the future may be designable to take advantage of systems that promote selective uptake of the drug into the cancer cell, or avoid uptake into normal cellular compartments.

STROMAL TARGETS: ISSUES

The stroma refers to the interface between the tumor cells and the normal host. It is a heterogeneously populated compartment, with matrix components in various stages of degradation by proteases, sulfatases, and other matrix-degrading enzymes secreted by the tumor; immune effector cells such as lymphocytes and macrophages, components of the neovasculature including new blood vessels formed under the influence of the tumor's angiogenic humors, their supporting pericytes; and a complex mix of cytokines and chemokines derived from both tumor and host cells. Tumor blood vessels do not have the orderly branching pattern associated with parenchymal organ microcirculation. Rather, they are frequently ectatic and tortuous, with very loose junctions between endothelial cells, and indeed in certain tumors with tumor cells actually contiguous with the endothelial cells in direct contact with blood elements in the so-called "vascular channels" rather than true blood vessels (26). In addition to these structural elements, the stroma exists in a physical state defined by the tumor's capacity to alter physical constraints to delivery of nutrients and macromolecules to the tumor cells, resulting in "tumor interstitial hypertension" (27). The latter is the reflection of a permeability-inducing cytokine such as vascular endothelial growth factor (VEGF) coupled with greatly abnormal lymphatic drainage.

This complexity for a long time retarded convincing evidence that the stroma could serve as a useful target for cancer treatment. Initial efforts to utilize bevacizumab, an antibody directed against the VEGF cytokine, were as a single agent problematic, with little evidence of robust antitumor activity. However, data from emerging clinical trials have offered convincing evidence that bevacizumab can by itself retard time to disease progression (in renal carcinoma) and in combination with cytotoxic agents cause in colorectal, lung, and recently breast cancer a marked delay in tumor progression, with some evidence in certain instances of increased response to the cytotoxic agents (28–32).

These findings have validated VEGF signaling as an exceedingly important target for future drug development. One hypothesis explicating the value of bevacizumab in conjunction with cytotoxic agents is that altered VEGF-receptor function may diminish tumor interstitial hypertension and therefore allow optimal delivery of drug to the tumor compartment (28). This mechanism would exist in addition to whatever influences on actual new blood vessel proliferation may exist. In this regard, small molecule VEGF-receptor antagonists that in addition target other receptors mediating stroma function such as platelet derived growth factor (PDGF) and FGF are at advanced stages of development and may offer even more potent and multifaceted approaches to accomplish this end (33,34).

TARGETED THERAPEUTICS: DIFFERENCES IN DEVELOPMENT STRATEGY

Classical cytotoxic agents are designed and screened to disrupt proliferation per se. Therefore, historically they are used at the maximum dose tolerable without bad toxicity to the host. Thus, there is no evidence of saturability of dose and effect in conveying a useful outcome, and indeed often a relatively steep concentration–effect curve in conveying cytotoxicity to the tumor compartment. This is the basis for value of stem cell transplant approaches in certain neoplasms. In contrast, targeted agents in their most pure conception are designed to saturate a receptor molecule, and owing to the altered function of the target, convey a useful antiproliferative effect. Note that this does *not* imply that targeted agents should always be considered cytostatic, or not intrinsically toxic. Most cancer patients present with bulk tumor and therefore the capacity to cause cytoreduction will always be of value. The point is that the useful cytoreductive effect of a targeted agent comes from the agent's ability to alter the downstream functions of its target, and not from the cell's response to physical concomitants of drug-induced damage, as may occur with high doses of "standard" cytotoxics. The best precedent, and indeed a forerunner to many of the issues encountered in targeted therapy, would be the obvious plateau in dose versus antitumor effect encountered with various hormone receptor antagonist strategies, including estrogen receptor antagonists in breast cancer or gonadotropin-releasing hormone agonists in the treatment of prostate cancer.

Thus, targeted agents should have as a prominent part of their development plan a conscientious effort to define an optimal biological dose which will result in occupation of its target. Ideally, there would also be evidence of modulation of downstream effects depending on the target's action. This circumstance has led to prominent efforts to define assays of drug effect in surrogate tissues [e.g., peripheral blood mononuclear cells (35) or buccal mucosa cells (36)] and actually biopsy of tumor in patients participating in early clinical trials of targeted agents. This strategy has been controversial, in that proponents point to the value in going forward with Phase II drug development with the certain knowledge that the drug is likely to have an effect on its target on the proposed schedule. Opponents point to the ethical dilemma in asking patients to submit to invasive procedures of no benefit to themselves, and also the fact that in many, but not all, circumstances the assay of drug effect to be utilized has not been widely applied or "validated" for clinical use (37).

An intermediary position in this set of issues would be to define clearly in animal models the relationship between the area under the concentration (AUC) × time curve of drug at doses conveying a useful anti-proliferative outcome. One then defines an assay applicable to a surrogate compartment, e.g., peripheral blood mononuclear cells, and defines action of the drug at its effective dose in that compartment, and relates that to the degree of effect on the target in the tumor compartment. One is then poised to ask in the human Phase I whether at the recommended Phase II dose one is at the desired AUC, and whether in a human surrogate compartment the same degree of target effect is observed as in the animals. One may then obtain from a very limited sampling, if desired, in patients with easily accessible tumor in the periphery, e.g., cutaneous or node metastases, an assessment of target effect in ways that are minimally invasive. This strategy might even call for a return to animal models after completion of the human Phase I to conscientiously model the human pharmacology, and obtain a more realistic assessment of the likely ability in Phase II to achieve the desired pharmacology and pharmacodynamic effect. A development sequence which closely followed this general approach occurred with the proteosome inhibitor bortezomib (38,39). Indeed, in the latter case, dose escalation during the Phase I was halted at a point defined by biomarker effect, as it was known that obtaining 80% inhibition of proteosome function in the peripheral blood mononuclear compartment was associated with evidence of antitumor effect in animals without severe toxicity.

The interest in targets directly related to tumor blood vessel function described above has introduced the possibility of other types of surrogate marker function which depend on the capacity of the drug to alter the permeability of tumor vessels to imaging agents. Thus, small molecule VEGF-receptor antagonists have recently been demonstrated to alter the distribution of gadolinium tracers using contrast-enhanced magnetic resonance imaging (34), an effect also seen with bevacizumab. These approaches may eliminate the need for biopsy and encourage other types of tracer imaging of drug distribution to tumors, possible in some cases by labeling of drugs with tracers suitable for positron imaging (PET) approaches. Conventional glucose PET may be valuable as well, particularly if the drug is known to affect a target system which directly influences glucose uptake.

An additional opportunity implicit in the development of a targeted agent is the selection of patients for study who possess the target. Although this might seem intuitively obvious in the case of, e.g., immunologic reagents which are specifically and directly targeted toward an expressed cell surface determinant, the application of this concept to small molecules in solid tumors had met with mixed perception of value. Although *bcr-abl* expression was detectable in chronic-phase patients responding to imatinib, and there was evidence of down-modulation of *crkl* phosphorylation, a downstream target, in that case because the clinical response to the drug was so good, the effect on the target really was irrelevant to the subsequent development of the agent. In contrast, preclinical studies with gefitinib really did not have any evidence that EGF-R expression level correlated with response to the agent, and therefore patients were not selected according to the level of expression. Indeed, only a posteriori analysis of responding patients identified EGF-R mutations as a potential correlate of response (17,18). Analysis of patients responding to erlotinib has raised the possibility that EGF-R expression level does indeed correlate with the degree of response, although these data will need to be confirmed in larger studies (40).

The picture thus emerges is that the actual value of patient enrichment by target selection varies. The most cogent argument for such selection exists when preclinical studies clearly indicate that the agent in question has a tight relationship of drug effect to receptor occupancy across a broad range of receptor expression. Where that evidence is lacking, the value of conscientious enrichment in Phase I or early Phase II becomes more dubious, but then the likelihood of a relatively small sample size allowing conclusion of definite value also decreases. The key value of knowing that a Phase I/II population is enriched for target-bearing patients is that an assessment of how "off-target" effects potentially determining therapeutic index becomes more explicitly evident. Good drug target expression, absence of therapeutic effect, acceptable pharmacology or pharmacodynamic effect in a surrogate tissue, and presence of side effects but lack of activity allow a certain basis to not proceed with development, a disappointing outcome but a conclusion better reached after Phase I or early Phase II, rather than after Phase III.

The importance of pharmacology in recognizing these milestones cannot be emphasized enough. Animal models (Fig. 2) allow definition of the AUC causing

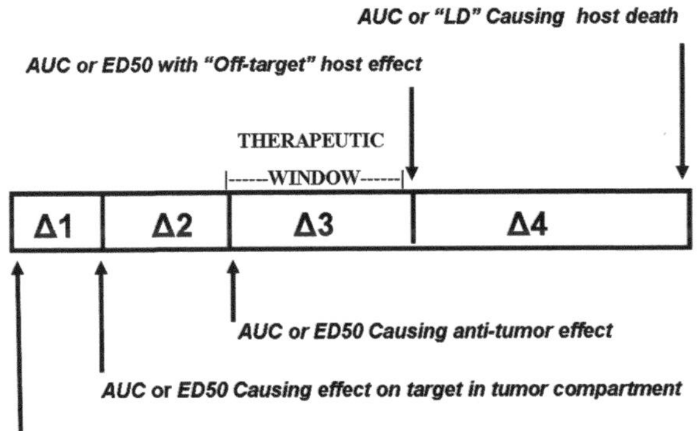

FIGURE 2 Definition of therapeutic window with targeted therapies: use of pharmacokinetic and pharmacodynamic endpoints. *Abbreviation*: AUC, area under the curve.

an effect of the agent on its target in a surrogate compartment, the AUC causing an effect on its target in the tumor compartment, and the AUC associated with useful conventional markers of drug effect. The animal models also allow definition of AUCs causing "off target" effects or dire toxicity. The therapeutic index is the ratio of doses or AUCs between those extremes. What emerges from a human Phase I trial is pharmacology and toxicity information. If augmented by target information from a surrogate or tumor compartment, a likely extrapolation to how closely the animal experience is modeled will emerge, and will aid in decision-making in designing Phase II experiences.

SPECIAL ISSUES WITH PROSTATE CANCER

The preceding discussion was generic and applicable to a variety of drug development scenarios. As this volume is dedicated to a description of the current state of targeted therapy development in prostate carcinoma, one must be cognizant of some unique features, as well as some difficult problems.

The historical importance of manipulation of the AR axis in prostate carcinoma will continue to appropriately dominate therapeutic efforts in this neoplasm. The recognition that in "hormone-refractory" patients evidence persists of continued activity of AR-related transcriptional regulation suggests that additional strategies to influence AR function are desirable even in these advanced cases (41). Specifically, agents that alter AR activator or co-repressor function will be of great interest to consider, or agents which can influence the physical stability of the AR complex. Aromatase inhibitors have proven to be of value in breast cancer considered refractory to estrogen receptor antagonists, yet such strategies have not been embraced by the prostate cancer clinical community. As molecules which can influence the synthesis of androgen-related elements in testis and adrenal gland are defined, these need to be assessed in clinical studies in the so-called hormone-refractory patients (42).

Although the influence of growth factor receptors, oncogenes, and anti-apoptotic proteins are likely to be as important as targets in prostate cancer as in other neoplasms, there really has not emerged a consensus on "prostate-specific" targets. Hopefully the application of genome-wide profiling of clinical specimens will define truly unique prostate cancer targets. The frequent metastasis to bone has encouraged efforts to define bone-microenvironment-altering strategies, such as bisphosphonates. This effort should continue, utilizing a more sophisticated understanding of the bone microenvironment to consider bone remodeling cytokines and matrix-interacting factors as a fertile potential basis for prostate-cancer-directed therapies. The inaccessibility of prostate cancer tissue in the metastatic state owing to its bone and visceral metastasis should encourage functional imaging approaches that might utilize unique metabolic features of prostate tumors, e.g., choline avidity to allow early evidence of treatment effect in metastatic disease that would lessen the need for biopsy procedures (43).

Prostate cancer will become an increasingly important epidemiologic factor in driving cancer therapeutics development, as well as in driving overall cancer mortality, as our population continues to age. The strategies described in this volume describe the promise of several therapeutic strategies that we are on the verge of exploring thoroughly. The principles of targeted therapy development articulated in this chapter will hopefully serve the goals of drug discovery and development in this population, as well as potential principles for design of early clinical trials in prostate cancer patients.

REFERENCES

1. Hanahan D, Weinberg RA. The hallmarks of cancer. Cell 2000; 100(1):57–70.
2. Sausville EA, Feigal E. Evolving approaches to cancer drug discovery and development at the National Cancer Institute, USA. Ann Oncol 1999; 10(11):1287–1291.
3. Kaelin WG Jr. The concept of synthetic lethality in the context of anticancer therapy. Nat Rev Cancer 2005; 5(9):689–698.
4. Paull KD, Lin CM, Malspeis L, Hamel E. Identification of novel antimitotic agents acting at the tubulin level by computer-assisted evaluation of differential cytotoxicity data. Cancer Res 1992; 52(14):3892–3900.
5. Goodin S, Kane MP, Rubin EH. Epothilones: mechanism of action and biologic activity. J Clin Oncol 2004; 22(10):2015–2025.
6. Towle MJ, Salvato KA, Budrow J, et al. In vitro and in vivo anticancer activities of synthetic macrocyclic ketone analogues of halichondrin B. Cancer Res 2001; 61(3):1013–1021.
7. Burden, DA, Osheroff N. Mechanism of action of eukaryotic topoisomerase II and drugs targeted to the enzyme. Biochim Biophys Acta 1998; 1400(1–3):139–154.
8. Liu LF, Desai SD, Li TK, Mao Y, Sun M, Sim SP. Mechanism of action of camptothecin. Ann NY Acad Sci 2000; 922:1–10.
9. Shamji AF, Nghiem P, Schreiber SL. Integration of growth factor and nutrient signaling: implications for cancer biology. Mol Cell 2003; 12(2):271–280.
10. Neckers L. Hsp90 inhibitors as novel cancer chemotherapeutic agents. Trends Mol Med 2002; 8(suppl 4):S55–S61.
11. Obata T, Endo Y, Murata D, Sakamoto K, Sasaki T. The molecular targets of antitumor 2′-deoxycytidine analogues. Curr Drug Targets 2003; 4(4):305–313.
12. Schultz RM. Preclinical development of Alimta (Pemetrexed, LY231514), a multitargeted antifolate. Prog Drug Res 2005; 63:275–300.
13. Chauhan D, Hideshima T, Mitsiades C, Richardson P, Anderson KC. Proteasome inhibitor therapy in multiple myeloma. Mol Cancer Ther 2005; 4(4):686–692.
14. Hughes TR, Marton MJ, Jones AR, et al. Functional discovery via a compendium of expression profiles. Cell 2000; 102(1):109–126.
15. Rapisarda A, Uranchimeg B, Scudiero DA, et al. Identification of small molecule inhibitors of hypoxia-inducible factor 1 transcriptional activation pathway. Cancer Res 2002; 62(15):4316–4324.
16. Shah NP, Tran C, Lee FY, Chen P, Norris D, Sawyers CL. Overriding imatinib resistance with a novel ABL kinase inhibitor. Science 2004; 305(5682):399–401.
17. Burgess MR, Skaggs BJ, Shah NP, Lee FY, Sawyers CL. Comparative analysis of two clinically active BCR-ABL kinase inhibitors reveals the role of conformation-specific binding in resistance. Proc Natl Acad Sci USA 2005; 102(9):3395–3400.
18. Paez JG, Janne PA, Lee JC, et al. EGFR mutations in lung cancer: correlation with clinical response to gefitinib therapy. Science 2004; 304(5676):1497–1500.
19. Lynch TJ, Bell DW, Sordella R, et al. Activating mutations in the epidermal growth factor receptor underlying responsiveness of non-small-cell lung cancer to gefitinib. N Engl J Med 2004; 350(21):2129–2139.
20. Neshat MS, Mellinghoff IK, Tran C, et al. Enhanced sensitivity of PTEN-deficient tumors to inhibition of FRAP/mTOR. Proc Natl Acad Sci USA 2001; 98(18):10314–10319.
21. Solit DB, Garraway LA, Pratilas CA, et al. BRAF mutation predicts sensitivity to MEK inhibition. Nature 2005; 439(7074):274–275.
22. Sepp-Lorenzino L, Ma Z, Rands E, et al. A peptidomimetic inhibitor of farnesyl:protein transferase blocks the anchorage-dependent and -independent growth of human tumor cell lines. Cancer Res 1995; 55(22):5302–5309.
23. Arteaga CL. Interference of the IGF system as a strategy to inhibit breast cancer growth. Breast Cancer Res Treat 1992; 22(1):101–106.
24. Cappuzzo F, Magrini E, Ceresoli GL, et al. Akt phosphorylation and gefitinib efficacy in patients with advanced non-small-cell lung cancer. J Natl Cancer Inst 2004; 96(15):1133–1141.

25. Paik S, Shak S, Tang G, et al. A multigene assay to predict recurrence of tamoxifen-treated, node-negative breast cancer. N Engl J Med 2004; 351(27):2817–2826.
26. Hendrix MJ, Seftor EA, Kirschmann DA, Quaranta V, Seftor RE. Remodeling of the microenvironment by aggressive melanoma tumor cells. Ann NY Acad Sci 2003; 995:151–161.
27. Jain RK. Antiangiogenic therapy for cancer: current and emerging concepts. Oncology 2005; 19(4, suppl 3):7–16.
28. Gerber HP, Ferrara N. Pharmacology and pharmacodynamics of bevacizumab as monotherapy or in combination with cytotoxic therapy in preclinical studies. Cancer Res 2005; 65(3):671–680.
29. Yang JC, Haworth L, Sherry RM, et al. A randomized trial of bevacizumab, an anti-vascular endothelial growth factor antibody, for metastatic renal cancer. N Engl J Med 2003; 349(5):427–434.
30. Hurwitz H, Fehrenbacher L, Novotny W, et al. Bevacizumab plus irinotecan, fluorouracil, and leucovorin for metastatic colorectal cancer. N Engl J Med 2004; 350(23):2335–2342.
31. Tsao AS, Herbst R, Sandler A, et al. Phase I/II trial of bevacizumab plus erlotinib for patients with recurrent non-small cell lung cancer: correlation of treatment response with mutations of the EGFR tyrosine kinase gene. Proc ASCO, 2005. Abstract No. 7092.
32. de Gramont A, Van Cutsem E. Investigating the potential of bevacizumab in other indications: metastatic renal cell, non-small cell lung, pancreatic and breast cancer. Oncology 2005; 69(suppl 3):46–56.
33. Motzer RJ, Michaelson MD, Redman BG, et al. Activity of SU11248, a multitargeted inhibitor of vascular endothelial growth factor receptor and platelet-derived growth factor receptor, in patients with metastatic renal cell carcinoma. J Clin Oncol 2005; 24(1):16–24.
34. Liu G, Rugo HS, Wilding G, et al. Dynamic contrast-enhanced magnetic resonance imaging as a pharmacodynamic measure of response after acute dosing of AG-013736, an oral angiogenesis inhibitor, in patients with advanced solid tumors: results from a phase I study. J Clin Oncol 2005; 23(24):5464–5473.
35. Banerji U, O'Donnell A, Scurr M, et al. Phase I pharmacokinetic and pharmacodynamic study of 17-allylamino, 17-demethoxygeldanamycin in patients with advanced malignancies. J Clin Oncol 2005; 23(18):4152–4161.
36. Adjei AA, Croghan GA, Erlichman C, et al. A Phase I trial of the farnesyl protein transferase inhibitor R115777 in combination with gemcitabine and cisplatin in patients with advanced cancer. Clin Cancer Res 2003; 9(7):2520–2526.
37. Stadler WM, Ratain MJ. Development of target-based antineoplastic agents. Invest New Drugs 2000; 18(1):7–16.
38. Adams J, Palombella VJ, Sausville EA, et al. Proteasome inhibitors: a novel class of potent and effective antitumor agents. Cancer Res 1999; 59(11):2615–2622.
39. Hamilton AL, Eder JP, Pavlick AC, et al. Proteasome inhibition with bortezomib (PS-341): a phase I study with pharmacodynamic end points using a day 1 and day 4 schedule in a 14-day cycle. J Clin Oncol 2005; 23(25):6107–6116.
40. Johnson JR, Cohen M, Sridhara R, et al. Approval summary for erlotinib for treatment of patients with locally advanced or metastatic non-small cell lung cancer after failure of at least one prior chemotherapy regimen. Clin Cancer Res 2005; 11(18):6414–6421.
41. Chen CD, Welsbie DS, Tran C, et al. Molecular determinants of resistance to antiandrogen therapy. Nat Med 2004; 10(1):33–39.
42. Handratta VD, Vasaitis TS, Njar VC, et al. Novel C-17-heteroaryl steroidal CYP17 inhibitors/antiandrogens: synthesis, in vitro biological activity, pharmacokinetics, and antitumor activity in the LAPC4 human prostate cancer xenograft model. J Med Chem 2005; 48(8):2972–2984.
43. Schoder H, Larson SM. Positron emission tomography for prostate, bladder, and renal cancer. Semin Nucl Med 2004; 34(4):274–292.

3 Novel Biomarkers for Disease Diagnosis, Prognosis, and Prediction

James V. Tricoli

Diagnostic Biomarkers and Technology Branch, Division of Cancer Treatment and Diagnosis, Cancer Diagnosis Program, National Cancer Institute, Rockville, Maryland, U.S.A.

INTRODUCTION

Carcinoma of the prostate is the second leading cause of male cancer-related death in the United States. It is estimated that in 2005 there will be approximately 232,090 new cases and 30,350 deaths from this disease (1). Since the introduction of serum prostate-specific antigen (PSA) screening of asymptomatic populations, prostate cancer incidence rates have increased dramatically, as have the number of men undergoing radical prostatectomy and radiation therapy for this disease (1,2). However, false positives for PSA continue to be a significant problem resulting in unnecessary biopsies, and the value of broad-based PSA testing with regard to predicting surgical cures has recently come into question (3).

Currently, there are no markers that differentiate clinically relevant from clinically benign disease. Better indicators of prostate cancer presence and progression are needed in order to avoid unnecessary treatment, predict disease course, and develop more effective therapy. A variety of putative prostate cancer markers have been described in human serum, urine, seminal fluid, and histological specimens. These markers exhibit varying capacities to detect prostate cancer and to predict disease course. In addition to these markers a variety of distinct chromosomal aberrations have been associated with prostate cancer (4).

Determining the diagnostic potential of identified genes and molecules that display loss, mutation, or alteration in expression, between tumor and normal prostate tissues, and during tumor progression, is a major challenge faced by the translational research community. To date few of these markers have achieved widespread clinical utility. If we are to improve upon the treatment of prostate cancer in the 21st century, we must identify and develop markers that are more clinically informative for this disease and that will allow for risk-based individualization of prostate cancer therapy.

A BRIEF HISTORY OF PROSTATE CANCER DIAGNOSTICS

The first documented case of prostate cancer was reported by Langstaff in 1817 (5). One hundred and eighteen years later, in 1935, prostatic acid phosphatase (PAP) levels were identified in the ejaculate of men, thus linking this enzyme to the prostate (6). Subsequent studies showed high PAP concentrations in primary and metastatic prostate cancer tissues, and in human serum, making it the first candidate marker for the diagnosis of prostate cancer (7,8). Reductions in serum PAP levels were found to occur in response to anti-androgen therapy, whereas increasing serum levels were associated with treatment failure and relapse (9,10).

Although serum PAP levels were elevated in a significant number of men with metastatic disease (8), fewer than 20% of men with localized prostate cancer exhibited abnormal enzyme levels (11,12). Meticulous sample collection and preparation were required because both platelets and leukocytes are contaminating sources of acid phosphatases (13), and because PAP activity is rapidly lost at room temperature (14). Development of a radioimmune assay for PAP in 1975 provided some improvement in test sensitivity (15), but the sensitivity levels were still inadequate for detection of early stage disease. Therefore, it was clear that a more sensitive and robust indicator of disease presence would be required in order to detect prostate cancer in its earlier stages, when cure is more likely.

PSA is a kallekrein-like serine protease that was first described in 1971 (16). PSA is secreted from prostate epithelial cells and is encoded by an androgen responsive gene located on chromosome 19q13.3–13.4 (17). The main function of PSA is to liquefy human semen through its proteolytic action (18). PSA was initially thought to be a prostate-specific protein, however subsequent investigations demonstrated that PSA is secreted in small quantities from a number of other normal male, and even some female tissues (19,20). PSA was first detected in the serum of prostate cancer patients in 1980 (19), and a normal PSA serum concentration limit of 4 ng/mL for men was subsequently established (20). A serum level above 4 ng/mL was taken as an indicator of the possible presence of prostate cancer, and served as the trigger for further clinical evaluation. Eventually, a number of studies enrolling large numbers of men over the age of 50 suggested that quantitation of serum PSA was a useful diagnostic tool for detecting the presence of prostate cancer, particularly when combined with digital rectal examination (DRE) (21–24). However, other studies have called into question the sensitivity and specificity of the PSA test (25–28). One problem is that serum PSA levels can be elevated as a result of conditions other than prostate cancer, such as benign prostatic hypertrophy (BPH) and prostatitis. As a result, false positives are a significant problem for the PSA test and can lead to unnecessary biopsies and other interventions. Of greater concern, 20–30% of men with prostate cancer have serum PSA levels in the normal range, resulting in undiagnosed disease (22–24). A recent study by Stamey et al. has concluded that pre-operative serum PSA levels do not correlate with cancer volume or the Gleason grade of radical prostatectomy specimens (3). This study also showed a poor correlation between pre-operative serum PSA levels in the 2–9 ng/mL range and prostate cancer cure rates. Thus, in general the weaknesses of PSA as a prostate cancer biomarker are (1) that it can be elevated as a result of BPH or prostatitis (2), PSA exhibits poor sensitivity and specificity, particularly in 4–10 ng/mL range, and (3) pre-operative PSA levels fail to correlate with tumor grade or volume. In addition, PSA is not a diagnostic marker and yet is being used to trigger an ever-increasing number of prostate needle biopsies and other invasive procedures.

However, despite the drawbacks and criticisms cited against it, PSA is currently the best clinical biomarker available for prostate cancer, and the only one approved by the U.S. Food and Drug Administration (FDA) for both posttreatment monitoring of disease recurrence, and when combined with DRE, for evaluation of asymptomatic men (29,30).

GENES AND PROTEINS CORRELATING WITH PROSTATE CANCER

At the direction of the United States Congress, and spearheaded by the National Cancer Institute (NCI), support for basic and translational research in prostate cancer has expanded dramatically since 1992. This has resulted in an avalanche of data, much of it attempting to correlate various gene and protein biomarkers with prostate cancer presence, progression, or disease-free survival. Some of these markers have also been proposed as potential therapeutic targets for prostate cancer treatment. The identification of potential biomarkers has been further accelerated by the advent of cDNA microarray and proteomic techniques that can potentially identify cDNA and protein signatures that will better inform us about disease progression and patient outcome. The recent association of micro-RNA gene expression profiles with the developmental origins of certain tumors and the utilization of phage display methodologies for detecting autoantibody signatures has opened up novel areas of biomarker investigation for prostate cancer. However, despite the wealth of candidate biomarkers available, none have been adequately validated for clinical use, and no replacement for PSA is currently available.

The array of potential biomarkers available for prostate cancer detection, diagnosis, and prognosis represent a wide spectrum of biochemical and cellular functions. Table 1 provides information on 94 genes and their encoded proteins, each of which has been reported to have a potential role in prostate cancer development, detection, progression, cancer recurrence, disease-free survival, and/or prediction of response to therapy. Information on these markers was accumulated through literature searches using PubMed, and from the GeneCards database of human genes, their products, and their involvement in diseases (31). These potential biomarkers include transcription factors, proteases, kinases, phosphatases, protease inhibitors, CDK inhibitors, cytokines, reverse transcriptase, racemases, reductases, synthases, hydrolases, RNAse, molecular chaperones, nuclear matrix proteins, membrane scaffolding proteins, and an assortment of other binding and permeability control proteins. The potential biomarkers also include chromosomal regions and gene loci that are deleted, duplicated, mutated, or hypermethylated. This provides a large and varied landscape of biomarkers to choose from for developing clinically useful tools for prostate cancer diagnosis and prognosis. However, how do we determine which of these potential biomarkers are the best candidates for advancement "from the laboratory bench to the clinic?" " Several issues to consider in addressing this problem are, on what basis do we select from this growing list of candidate biomarkers, how should the selected biomarkers be validated, what evidence is required to demonstrate that a new marker provides a defined "value added" to the existing methods of prostate cancer detection, and for determining the likelihood of disease progression and recurrence, and/or response to a given therapy? These are all questions that must frame our approach to selecting biomarkers for further study.

CRITERIA FOR BIOMARKER SELECTION

There are several important criteria to consider when selecting one or more of these potential biomarkers for development as a clinical tool. One of the most important items regarding the selection of a candidate biomarker is the quality of scientific and clinical data supporting its potential utility. These include scientific studies relating the functional role of the gene/protein to the biology of the disease, and clinical data linking the candidate marker with disease presence, alterations in stage, response to therapy, and/or overall survival. Another important criterion is that the biomarker should be measurable by a robust, reproducible, widely available assay that provides useful information that is readily interpretable by the

TABLE 1 Potential Prostate Cancer Biomarkers

Marker	Ch. locus	M_r (kDa)	Subcellular location	Biochemical function	Biological/cellular function
A2M	12p13.3–12	163	Secreted	Protease inhibitor	Protein carrier
Akt-1	14q32.32	56	Nucleus/cytoplasm	Protein kinase	Apoptotic inhibition
AMACR[b]	5p13.2–q11	42	Mitochondria/peroxisome	Racemase	Stereoisomerization
Annexin 2	1q21	11	Plasma membrane	Calcium and lipid binding	Membrane trafficking
Bax	19q13.3–.4	21	Cytoplasm/membrane	Bcl-2 binding	Apoptosis
Bcl-2	18q21.3	26	Mitochondrial membrane	Membrane permeability	Apoptosis
Cadherin-1	16q22.1	97	Plasma membrane	Catenin/integrin binding	Cell adhesion
Caspase 8	2q33–34	55	Cytoplasm	Protease	Apoptosis
Catenin	5q31	100	Cytoskeleton	Cadherin binding	Cell adhesion
Cav-1	7q31.1	20	Plasma membrane	Scaffolding	Endocytosis/signaling
CD34	1q32	41	Plasma membrane	Scaffolding	Cell adhesion
CD44	11p13	82	Plasma membrane	Hyaluronate binding	Cell adhesion
Clar1	19q13.3–.4	34	Nucleus	SH3 binding	Unknown
Cox-2	1q25.2–.3	69	Microsomal membrane	Prostaglandin synthase	Inflammatory response
CTSB	8p23.1	38	Lysosome	Protease	Protein turnover
Cyclin D1	11q13	34	Nucleus	CDX regulation	Cell cycle
DD3	9q21–22	0	Nucleus/cytoplasm	Noncoding	Unknown
DRG-1	22q12.2	43	Cytoplasm	Unknown	Cell growth/differentiation
EGFR	7p12	134	Plasma membrane	EGF binding	Signaling
EphA2	1p36	11	Plasma membrane	Tyrosine kinase	Signaling
ERG	21q22.3	52	Nucleus	Transcription factor	Chromatin modification
ERGL	15q22–23	57	Plasma membrane	Lectin	Unknown
ETK/BMK	Xp22.2	78	Cytoplasm	Tyrosine kinase	Signaling
ETV1	7p21.3	55	Nucleus	Transcription factor	Gene regulation
EZH2	7q36.1	85	Nucleus	Transcription repressor	Homeotic gene regulation
Fas	11q13.3	23	Plasma membrane	Caspase recruitment	Apoptosis
GDEP	4q21.1	4[a]	Unknown	Unknown	Unknown
GRN-A	14q32	50	Secretory granules	Statin	Endocrine function
GRP78	9q33.3	72	Endoplasmic reticulum	Multimeric protein assembly	Cell stress response
GSTP1[b]	11q13	23	Cytoplasm	Glutathione reduction	DNA protection
Hepsin	19q11–13.2	45	Plasma membrane	Serine protease	Cell growth/morphology

(*Continued*)

TABLE 1 Potential Prostate Cancer Biomarkers (*Continued*)

Marker	Ch. locus	M_r (kDa)	Subcellular location	Biochemical function	Biological/cellular function
Her-2/Neu	17q21.1	138	Plasma membrane	Tyrosine kinase	Signaling
HSP27	7q11.23	23	Cytoplasm	Chaperone	Cell stress response
HSP70	6p21.3	70	Cytoplasm	Chaperone	Cell stress response
HSP90	11q13	63	Cytoplasm	Chaperone	Cell stress response
IGF-1	12q22–23	17	Secreted	IGFR ligand	Signaling
IGF-2	11p15.5	20	Secreted	IGFR ligand	Signaling
IGFBP-2	2q33–34	35	Secreted	IGF binding	Signaling
IGFBP-3	7p13–12	32	Secreted	IGF binding	Signaling/apoptosis
IL-6	7p15–3	24	Secreted	Cytokine	B-cell differentiation
IL-8	4q13.3	11	Secreted	Cytokine	Neutrophil activation
KAI1	11p11.2	30	Plasma membrane	CD4/CD8 binding	Signaling
KAi67	10q25-ter	358	Nucleus	Nuclear matrix associated	Cell proliferation
KLF6	10q15	32	Nucleus	Transcription factor	B-cell development
KLK2	19q13.41	29	Secreted	Protease	Met-lys/ser arg cleavage
Maspin	18q21.3	42	Extracellular	Protease inhibitor	Cell invasion suppressor
MSR1	8p22	50	Plasma membrane	LDL receptor	Endocytosis
MXI1	10q25.2	26	Nucleus	Transcription factor	Myc suppression
MYC	8q24.12–.13	49	Nucleus	Transcription factor	Cell proliferation
NF-kappa8	10q24	97	Nucleus	Transcription factor	Immune response
NKX3.1	8p21	26	Nucleus	Transcription factor	Cell proliferation
OPN	4q22.1	35	Secreted	Integrin binding	Cell-matrix interaction
p16	9p21	17	Nucleus	CDK inhibitor	Cell cycle
p21	6p21.2	18	Nucleus	CDK inhibitor	Cell cycle
p27	12p13.1–12	22	Nucleus	CDK inhibitor	Cell cycle
p53	17p13.1	44	Nucleus	Transcription factor	Growth arrest/apoptosis
PAP	3q21–23	45	Secreted	Tyrosine phosphatase	Unknown
PART1	5q12.1	7	Nucleus/cytoplasm	Unknown	Unknown
PATE	11q24.2	14	Plasma membrane	Phospholipase	Lipid catabolism
PC-1	5q35	32	Nucleus	RNA binding	Ribosome transport
PCGEM1	2q32	0	Nucleus/cytoplasm	Noncoding	Cell proliferation/survival
PCTA1	1q42–43	36	Cytoplasm	Suger binding	Cell adhesion

(*Continued*)

TABLE 1 Potential Prostate Cancer Biomarkers (*Continued*)

Marker	Ch. locus	M_r (kDa)	Subcellular location	Biochemical function	Biological/cellular function
PDEF	6p21.31	38	Nucleus	Transcription factor	PSA promoter binding
PI3K p85	5q12–13	84	Cytoplasm	Lipid kinase	Signaling
P13K p110	1p36.2	120	Cytoplasm	Lipid kinase	Signaling
PIM-1	6p21.2	36	Cytoplasm	Protein kinase	Cell differentiation/survival
PMEPA1	20q13.31–33	32	Plasma membrane	Unknown	Unknown
PRAC	17q21.3	6	Nucleus	Choline/Ethanolamine Kinase	Unknown
Prostase	19q13.3–.4	27	Secreted	Serine protease	ECM degradation
Prostasin	16p11.2	36	Plasma membrane	Serine protease	Cell invasion suppressor
Prostein	1q32.1	60[a]	Plasma membrane	Unknown	Unknown
PSA	19q13.3–.4	71	Secreted	Protease	Semen liquification
PSCA[b]	8q24.2	13	Plasma membrane	Unknown	Unknown
PSDR1	14q23–24.3	35[a]	Nucleus/cytoplasm	Dehydrogenase reductase	Steroid metabolism
PSGR	11p15	35	Plasma membrane	Odorant receptor	Signaling
PSMA[b]	11p11.2	84	Plasma membrane	Folate hydrolase	Cell stress response
PSP94	10q11.23	13	Secreted	FSH inhibitor	Growth inhibition
PTEN	10q23.3	47	Cytoplasm	Protein/lipid phopatase	Signaling
RASSF1	3p21.31	33	Cytoplasm	Ras binding	Cell cycle
RB1	13q14.2	106	Nucleus	E2F-1 inactivation	Cell cycle
RNAseL	1q25.3	84	Cytoplasm/mitochondria	RNAse	Viral resistance
RTVP1	12q21.1	30	Plasma membrane	Unknown	Immune response
SHH[b]	7q36.3	50	Secreted	Patched ligand	Signaling
ST7	7q31.2	60/85	Plasma membrane	Unknown	Cell proliferation
STEAP	7q21.23	40	Plasma membrane	Unknown	Unknown
TERT[b]	5p15.33	127	Nucleus	Reverse transcriptase	Telomere synthesis
TIMP 1	Xp11.3–.23	23	Secreted	Protease inhibitor	Cell adhesion
TIMP 2	17q25	24	Secreted	Protease inhibitor	Cell adhesion
TMPRSS2	21q22.3	54	Plasma membrane	Serine protease	Unknown
TRPM2	8p21–12	52	Plasma membrane	Calcium channel	Ion flux
Trp-p8	2q37.1	120	Plasma membrane	Calcium channel	Ion flux
UROC28	6q23.3	17	Nucleus/cytoplasm	Choline/ethanolamine Kinase	Unknown
VEGF	6p12	27	Secreted	VEGFR binding	Angiogenesis

[a]Molecular weight estimated from amino acid data.
[b]Discussed at length in chapter.
Source: From Ref. 31.

clinician. The ideal candidate for an early detection or disease monitoring marker would be one that is prostate-specific, detectable in an easily accessible biological fluid such as human serum, urine, or prostatic fluid and able to distinguish between normal, BPH, prostatic intraepithelial neoplasia (PIN), and cancerous prostate tissues. In addition, the marker should have sufficiently convincing clinical correlation data from several different laboratories before it is brought forward for large-scale evaluation.

For a marker to be useful for diagnosis and monitoring of disease it must address certain clinical issues. These include early detection of prostate cancer, the accurate diagnosis at disease presentation, predicting disease course after the initial diagnosis, the determination of an appropriate course of treatment (or nontreatment), or the monitoring of treatment outcomes.

Data analyses should be multivariate and show that the biomarker predicts the outcome of interest independently of the usually available characteristics, such as stage or grade. These assessments should be conducted on a set of cases with adequate outcome data and a sufficient number of events to allow statistical significance to be evaluated. In the absence of these supportive data even the most promising marker will not convince either the clinical or pharmaceutical communities that it is worth substantial investment for further evaluation. There are several potential biomarkers listed in Table 1 that fulfill a number of the above criteria, and upon further investigation provide the promise of adding to the armamentarium of molecular markers for this disease.

PROSTATE CANCER BIOMARKERS OF INTEREST

There are a number of proteins listed in Table 1 with extensive supportive data regarding their role in this disease, and their potential as practical prostate cancer biomarkers. However, several of these proteins either have extensive supportive data of the nature cited above, or point toward new paradigms in either the etiology of this disease, or in prostate cancer diagnosis/prognosis. These include glutathione-S-transferase-pi 1 (GSTP1), prostate stem cell antigen (PSCA), prostate-specific membrane antigen (PSMA), telomerase reverse-transcriptase (TERT), alpha-methyl-CoA racemase (AMACR), and sonic hedgehog (SHH). What follows is a brief description of each of these potential biomarkers and a discussion of their strengths and weaknesses.

Glutathione-S-Transferase pi 1

GSTP1 is a member of a large family of glutathione transferases that function to protect cells from oxidative insult (32), thus, the biologic rationale for discussing this prostate cancer biomarker is its role in preventing damage to cells by neutralizing free radicals. This biomarker is also unique in its capacity to provide a facile methylation-based detection method for an important epigenetic phenomenon. GSTP1 has been extensively studied in prostate cancer and its reduced expression, due predominantly to promoter hypermethylation, represents the most common epigenetic alteration associated with this disease. One study has shown that in prostate cancer cells methylation of the GSTP1 gene is not confined to the promoter, but is extensive throughout the CpG islands (33). Several studies have shown a high sensitivity for this marker to detect the presence of both PIN and prostate cancer, an ability to distinguish these from BPH, and a prevalence of methylation in the range of 60–80% in prostate cancer (33–43). In addition, several GSTP1 polymorphisms have shown a correlation with increased risk of disease development, although data regarding this ability is conflicting (44–49). Among the strengths of GSTP1 as a clinical marker are the ability to quantitate this gene's methylation status in biopsy/prostatectomy tissues, in cells derived from serum, urine, and seminal plasma, and its high prevalence in this disease. Recent studies utilizing quantitative real-time methylation-sensitive polymerase chain reaction (PCR) demonstrate that GSTP1 methylation could be a sensitive marker for prostate cancer in men with clinically localized disease (33). In addition, there is no correlation between GSTP1 methylation status and PSA levels, making GSTP1 a potential early and independent marker for the disease. The ability of GSTP1 hypermethylation to distinguish between BPH and prostate cancer is well documented, and one recent study correlated methylation status with poor prognosis in 101 patients diagnosed with prostate cancer (50). Although these results are statistically significant, they were not tested by multivariate analysis. Reversal of GSTP1 CpG island hypermethylation and gene reactivation in LNCaP prostate carcinoma cells can be achieved by procainamide treatment, however no effect on tumor cell growth was observed in these studies (51). The strengths of GSTP1 methylation status as cited earlier and the possible availability in the near future of drugs that can reverse hypermethylation, make it a good candidate for further evaluation as an early detection biomarker. If successfully validated, GSTP1 methylation testing of cells derived from serum and urine samples may have clinical usefulness for both early detection of prostate cancer and posttreatment monitoring of disease.

Prostate Stem-Cell Antigen

PSCA is a glycosylphosphatidylinositol anchored cell surface antigen that is found predominantly in prostate and may play a role in stem-cell functions such as proliferation or signal transduction (52). Although the biological role of PSCA in prostate cancer is unclear, the marker is expressed predominantly in the prostate and has potential as a therapeutic target. Other strengths of PSCA as a prostate cancer biomarker include elevated PSCA expression levels in the majority of prostate cancers, and a correlation between this elevation and higher Gleason grade and more advanced tumor stage (53–56). Published studies also show a high correlation (64–94%) between increased PSCA expression and the presence of prostate cancer, with protein expression localized to both the basal and secretory cells (53–57). PSCA has been assayed by a variety of methods including in situ hybridization, quantitative reverse transcriptase polymerase chain reaction (RT-PCR) and immunohistochemistry (IHC) demonstrating a prevalence of 48–94% for prostate cancer (53,54,58). One IHC study demonstrated an association between increased PSCA expression and higher Gleason score, more advanced tumor stage, and progression to androgen-independent prostate cancer (AIPC) (54). However, extensive multivariate analysis to confirm these findings has yet to be performed. PSCA expression is maintained in AIPC and is highly expressed in metastatic disease (53–58). Although most of the studies performed to date have been on prostate tissue samples, there is at least one report of PSCA detection in peripheral blood (55). An additional strength of this marker is its potential as a therapeutic target. Anti-PSCA monoclonal antibodies have been shown to inhibit tumor growth and metastasis formation of human xenografts grown in *scid* mice (58).

This opens up the possibility for therapeutic treatment of human prostate cancers, or pre-cancers, using immunotherapeutic regimens (58–60). In addition, PSCA is co-amplified with the tumor progression factor and the oncogene c-myc in locally advanced prostate cancers, suggesting a role for PSCA in the progression of this disease (56,61). Three weaknesses of PSCA as a candidate for further development are the limited number of published studies supporting its value as a biomarker, a need for better quantitation methods, and uncertainty as to whether analysis of PSCA levels adds information to the results of PSA testing. However, based on the available data, and the value of PSCA as a therapeutic target, further evaluation of PSCA as a clinical prostate cancer marker should be performed to determine its utility.

Prostate-Specific Membrane Antigen

Discovered in 1987, PSMA is a cell-surface membrane protein and one of the most extensively studied prostate cancer markers cited in Table 1 (62). PSMA is a type II integral membrane protein that displays multiple enzymatic activities (63,64). The protein translocates from the cytosol in normal prostate to the plasma membrane in prostate cancer (65). The exact biological role of PSMA in the disease mechanism is unclear at this time, however extensive data exists on its utility as a biomarker and therapeutic target. Numerous studies have shown that PSMA serum levels are elevated in primary prostate cancer and metastatic disease, that PSMA demonstrates a >90% prevalence in the disease, and that levels can be detected in both tumor tissue and serum using several antibodies (66–73). PSMA has been detected in prostate tissues using IHC and Western analysis, in circulating prostate cancer cells by RT-PCR, and in serum using ELISA assays. One study using western analysis demonstrated that in post-prostatectomy patients PSMA values are elevated in hormone-refractory tumors, suggesting that PSMA levels may correspond with poor clinical outcome (67). In another study, PSMA serum levels were found to increase with age and were significantly elevated in men over 50 years of age (74). To date however increased PSMA serum levels have not been convincingly linked to disease aggressiveness, and perhaps due to tumor differentiation status, some studies have shown that levels actually decrease in advanced disease (75). PSMA protein has also been shown to be up-regulated in prostate cancer patients after androgen deprivation therapy (76). Recent technological advances have allowed for the high throughput assay of this marker in human serum using a protein chip, mass spectrometry platform (77). The study demonstrated significantly greater PSMA levels in men with prostate cancer than those with BPH or with no evidence of disease. PSMA is moderately prostate-specific and has been investigated as a target for immunotherapy using autologous dendritic cells (78). Efforts are also underway using the PSMA gene promoter to pursue gene therapy strategies by introducing cytotoxic agents into prostate cancer cells (79). A weakness of PSMA as a clinical marker for early diagnosis is that elevated serum levels have been observed in healthy males and females, and in the serum of breast cancer patients (80). Another is that serum levels of PSMA have been shown to increase with increasing age, which could be a confounding factor in a disease that most often occurs late in life. However, there is an abundance of data supporting the ability of PSMA to detect the presence of prostate cancer, and new technologies are being developed that allow quantitative high throughput analysis of biological fluids. This argues in favor of further evaluation of this marker to determine whether or not it has clinical utility for prostate cancer detection, treatment monitoring, or as a treatment target.

Telomerase Reverse-Transcriptase

The TERT gene encodes the reverse-transcriptase component of telomerase that maintains the telomeric ends of chromosomes and has been associated with senescence and cancer (81). The TERT component is expressed in cells that exhibit telomerase activity and is undetectable in most benign tissues (82). TERT has the ability to confer cellular immortalization, a major step in the process of malignant transformation. Thus, this marker may provide a very sensitive means for detecting infiltrating cancer cells in benign tissue. A significant number of studies have been conducted to evaluate TERT or telomerase activity as a marker for prostate cancer (83–101). Published reports demonstrate TERT activity levels exhibit a prevalence range of 63–94% for prostate cancer, and activity has been detected in some cases of high-grade PIN (HGPIN) (82–93). TERT has been most often assayed by IHC or the telomeric repeat amplification protocol (TRAP) assay. Most studies find this biomarker consistently absent from normal prostate and the majority of BPH tissues. The highest TERT activity appears to correlate with poorly differentiated disease, and there is some evidence for a correlation with tumor stage and grade, and patient mortality and disease recurrence (82,86,89–91). Although statistical significance has been demonstrated in some of these studies the correlations have not been tested by multivariate analysis. TERT activity does not correlate with PSA level making it a potential independent marker for prostate cancer. One study suggests that telomere length in tumor tissues correlates with survival and recurrence in prostate cancer patients (102). However, TERT also displays several weaknesses as a clinical biomarker for prostate cancer detection. TERT is not prostate-specific, and in most studies assays were conducted in prostate tissues, and thus required biopsy material prior to marker assay. However, several studies have now successfully utilized human urine, seminal fluid, and prostatic fluid to detect TERT activity (95,96,103). Although TERT activity levels appear to be independent of PSA, the "value added" of TERT for early detection, staging or prognosis, and its overall clinical utility remains to be fully uncovered. Further evaluation of TERT may reveal a niche for its use as a supplement to PSA testing.

Alpha-Methyl-CoA Racemase

AMACR is a peroxisomal and mitochondrial enzyme that is involved with branched chain fatty acid beta-oxidation (104). It is responsible for the interconversion of $R \rightarrow S$ stereoisomers of 2-methyl branched chain fatty acids. It has been suggested that the elevation of AMACR reflects a general metabolic change that may favor prostate cell transformation (105). Enhanced expression of AMACR is detectable in tissues, needle biopsies, PIN, and in tumor cells isolated from the urine of prostate cancer patients, and AMACR appears to be independent of PSA (106–112). Some evidence suggests that the specificity of AMACR as a biomarker can be enhanced by combining it with the basal cell markers cytokeratin, p63, or other markers, and that this may be of value in distinguishing PIN from cancer in AMACR positive needle biopsies (109,112,113). However, another report finds that a combination of AMACR and p63 is no better in diagnosing prostate cancer in needle biopsies than the use of each antibody separately (114).

One study suggests that AMACR is higher in normal prostate tissue from men less than 45 years of age than in older men (115). This may make the detection of elevated AMACR in prostate cancer more effective as levels appear to fall off with age in normal prostate tissue and this disease is most commonly detected in men of more advanced age. Although AMACR levels do not appear to correlate with Gleason score tumor stage or tumor volume, recent evidence suggests that decreased levels of AMACR in localized prostate cancer may correlate with an increased biochemical failure rate and greater incidence of cancer-specific death (116). This is consistent with a previous study showing that AMACR levels were lower in metastatic disease than in localized prostate cancer (106). Thus, AMACR may be a useful predictor of prostate cancer progression.

However, AMACR displays a number of weaknesses as a potential prostate cancer biomarker including relatively low expression levels in atrophic lesions, a lower specificity when assayed in post-prostatectomy urine samples, poor expression in hormone-refractory and foamy gland prostate cancers, and the fact that to date AMACR levels do not correlate with Gleason score, tumor stage, or tumor volume. However, AMACR does show significant promise as a supplement to PSA for diagnosing this disease, reducing the need for re-biopsy of patients and as a possible indicator of tumor progression.

Sonic Hedgehog

SHH is a signaling protein associated with body pattern formation in Drosophila melanogaster and is essential to cephalic formation in higher organisms (117,118). The SHH pathway activates target genes involved in cell proliferation, differentiation, extra-cellular matrix interactions and angiogenesis (119). SHH is also critical for the process of normal ductal morphogenesis in the developing prostate and it is required for the regeneration of prostate epithelium (120,121). In the mouse, over expression of SHH has been shown to accelerate the growth of prostate tumor xenografts (122). SHH expression has been detected at significantly greater levels in some prostate cancers and increased activity of the SHH pathway appears to be associated with prostate cancer metastasis (123–125). SHH expression is greater in prostate tumors than in control tissues, is detectable as a secreted protein in the glandular lumen, and correlates with increased cell proliferation (126). SHH appears not only to be a potential biomarker for prostate cancer, but a possible therapeutic target for the pathway antagonist cyclopamine and anti-SHH antibodies (125,127). Cyclopamine is a plant alkaloid derived from a poisonous herb of the genus Veratrum (128). SHH normally functions by binding to its receptor protein called patched that in turn activates a protein called smoothened which triggers the signaling cascade (129,130). Cyclopamine functions by binding to smoothened and keeping it in the inactive form (131). In prostate cancer cell lines cyclopamine was found to suppress SHH signaling, down-regulate cell invasiveness and induce apoptosis (132). In addition, a recent study has shown that a combination of cyclopamine and the EGFR inhibitor gefitinib was more effective at suppressing the invasiveness of PC-3 cells than either drug alone (133). However, SHH displays several weaknesses as a prostate cancer biomarker in that so far it is only detectable in tumor tissue and glandular luminal secretions not in serum or urine, and SHH expression levels do not correlate with Gleason score and expression levels exhibit a high variability in prostate cancer with increases ranging from 1.5- to 300-fold (125). However, SHH has the potential to predict those prostate tumors that are more likely to spread from those that will remain confined to the prostate capsule, and shows significant promise as a therapeutic target in this disease.

FUTURE DIRECTIONS

The development of novel and clinically relevant markers for prostate cancer diagnosis, prognosis and prediction is essential to the optimal identification and treatment of this disease. Ultimately, our ability to develop better biomarkers and identify therapeutic targets for prostate cancer will depend upon our understanding of the basic biology of the prostate and the molecular mechanisms underlying the development of this disease. Therefore, recent studies linking pathways important in prostate development with prostate cancer progression are pertinent as developmental pathways are often reinitiated in the malignant state, abrogating the checks and balances put in place once early development of the organism is complete. The role of stromal–epithelial interactions will also be important to our understanding of the complexities of prostate biology and malignancy because epithelial cells do not exist in isolation, but are constantly interacting with their surroundings.

With the advent of DNA expression analysis, tissue microarrays, and proteomic analysis the list of potential prostate cancer markers grows daily. These technologies have provided some preliminary yet exciting prostate cancer biomarker candidates. Among these are Hepsin, a serine protease associated with cell growth and morphology (134–136), RNAse L, a ribonuclease involved in viral resistance and a candidate for the HPC1 gene (137,138), ST7, a protein of unknown function (139–141), and EZH2, a homeotic protein that participates in the repression of gene expression (142,143). In addition, proteomic analysis of serum from prostate cancer patients has shown promise for diagnostic and prognostic use for this disease (144). Recently, a chromosomal rearrangement that places the androgen-responsive promoter element of the TMPRSS2 gene in the 5′-region of either the ERG or ETV1 gene in prostate cancer has sparked new interest in the importance of chromosomal rearrangements in this disease (145). The rearrangement causes the ERG and ETV1 to become androgen responsive and thus may provide valuable markers for monitoring or predicting the onset of androgen independence in human prostate cancer.

Candidate biomarkers identified by these new technologies will require confirmation, and correlation with disease formation or progression, or with patient survival or response to therapy, in additional human samples before they can be considered for validation studies. Sorting through these potential biomarkers and bringing them from the laboratory environment into clinical use at the patient bedside will require a comprehensive pursuit and rigorous analysis. Many of the molecules cited in Table 1 have languished for years in a "gray zone" between usefulness as a clinical biomarker for prostate cancer, and elimination from further consideration. Thus, the challenge to the prostate cancer biomarker community is three-fold. First, discover novel and more informative biomarkers that can supplement PSA and perhaps eventually replace it as the biomarker of choice for prostate cancer. Second, begin working to move the current collection of prostate cancer biomarkers out of the "gray zone" between utility and elimination. Third, make a concerted effort to provide the validation data that will convince the clinical community to adopt novel biomarkers for use in making medical decisions. As a research community it is incumbent upon us to devise approaches that will accomplish this, and that will pave the way towards the next generation of clinically relevant prostate cancer biomarkers.

REFERENCES

1. Jemal A, Murray T, Ward E, et al. Cancer Statistics 2005. CA Cancer J Clin 2005; 55:10–30.
2. Stamey TA, Donaldson AN, Yemoto CE, et al. Histological and clinical findings in 896 consecutive prostates treated only with radical retropubic prostatectomy: epidemiologic significance of annual changes. J Urol 1998; 160:2412–2417.
3. Stamey TA, Johnstone IM, Mcneal JE. Preoperative serum prostate specific antigen levels between 2 and 22 ng/ml correlate poorly with post-radical prostatectomy cancer morphology: prostate specific antigen cure rates appear constant between 2 and 9 ng/ml. J Urol 2002; 167:103–111.
4. Brothman A. Cytogenetics and molecular genetics of cancer of the prostate. Am J Med Genet 2002; 115:150–156.
5. Langstaff HRH, Polskey HJ. Prostatic malignancy. In: Ballenger EG, Fontz WA, Hamer HG, Lewis B, eds. History of Urology. Vol. 2. Baltimore: Wilkins & Wilkins Co., 1933:187.
6. Kutscher W, Wolbergs H. Prostata phosphatase. Hoppes-Seylers Z Physiol Chem 1935; 236:237.
7. Gutman EB, Sproul EE, Gutman AB. Significance of increased phosphatase activity of bone at the site of osteoplastic metastases secondary to carcinoma of the prostate gland. Am J Cancer 1936; 28:485–495.
8. Gutman AB, Gutman EB. An acid phosphatase occurring in the serum of patients with metastasizing carcinoma of the prostate gland. J Clin Invest 1938; 17:473–478.
9. Huggins C, Hodges CV. Studies on prostatic cancer. I. The effect of castration, of estrogen and of androgen injection on serum phosphatases in metastatic carcinoma of the prostate. Cancer Res 1941; 1:293–297.
10. Schacht MJ, Garnett JE, Grayhack JT. Biochemical markers in prostatic cancer. Urol Clin North Am 1984; 11:253–267.
11. Sullivan TJ, Gutman EB, Gutman AB. Theory and application of the serum "acid" phosphatase determination in metastasizing prostatic carcinoma: early effects of castration. J Urol 1942; 48:426.
12. Nesbit RM, Baum WB. Serum phosphatase determination in diagnosis of prostatic cancer. A review of 1,150 cases. JAMA 1951; 145:1321.
13. King EJ, Jegatheesan KA. A method of the determination of tartrate-labile prostatic acid phosphatase in serum. J Clin Pathol 1959; 12:85.
14. Ladenson JH. Nonanalytical sources of variation in clinical chemistry results. In: Sonnenwirth AC, Jarett L, eds. Gradwohl's Clinical Laboratory Methods and Diagnosis. 8th ed. St. Louis: CV Mosby, 1980:149–192.
15. Foti AG, Cooper JF, Herschman H, et al. Detection of prostatic cancer by solid-phase radioimmunoassay of serum prostatic acid phosphatase. N Engl J Med 1975; 297:1357–1361.
16. Hara M, Koyanagi Y, Inoue T. Physico-chemical characteristics of "y-seminoprotein," an antigenic component specific for human seminal plasma. Jpn J Legal Med 1971; 25:322–324.
17. Riegman PH, Vlietstra RJ, Klaassen P, et al. The prostate-specific antigen gene and the human glandular kallikrein-1 gene are tandemly located on chromosome 19. FEBS Lett 1989; 247:123–126.
18. Dawson NA, Vogelzang NJ, eds. Prostate cancer. New York: Wiley-Liss, Inc., 1994.
19. Papsidero LD, Wang MC, Valenzuela LA, et al. A prostate antigen in sera of prostatic cancer patients. Cancer Res 1980; 40:2428–2432.
20. Myrtle JF, Klimley PG, Ivor LP, et al. Clinical utility of prostate specific antigen (PSA) in the management of prostate cancer. In: Advances in Cancer Diagnostics. San Diego: Hybritech, Inc., 1986:1–4.

21. Brawer MK, Chetner MP, Beatie J, et al. Screening for prostatic carcinoma with prostate specific antigen. J Urol 1992; 147:841–845.
22. Labrie F, Dupont A, Suburu R, et al. Serum prostate specific antigen as pre-screening test for prostate cancer [comment]. J Urol 1992; 147:846–851.
23. Catalona WJ, Smith DS, Ratliff TL, et al. Measurement of prostate-specific antigen in serum as a screening test for prostate cancer [comment] [erratum appears in N Engl J Med 1991; 325(18):1324]. N Engl J Med 1991; 324:1156–1161.
24. Cooner WH, Mosley BR, Rutherford CL, et al. Prostate cancer detection in a clinical urological practice by ultrasonography, digital rectal examination and prostate specific antigen. J Urol 1990; 143:1146–1152; discussion:1144–1152.
25. Wang TY, Kawaguchi TP. Preliminary evaluation of measurement of serum prostate-specific antigen level in detection of prostate cancer. Ann Clin Lab Sci 1986; 16:461–466.
26. Guinan P, Bhatti R, Ray P. An evaluation of prostate specific antigen in prostatic cancer. J Urol 1987; 137:686–689.
27. Stamey TA, Yang N, Hay AR, et al. Prostate-specific antigen as a serum marker for adenocarcinoma of the prostate. N Engl J Med 1987; 317:909–916.
28. Stamey TA. Prostate specific antigen in the diagnosis and treatment of adenocarcinoma of the prostate. Monogr Urol 1989; 10:50.
29. FDA Approval Document P850048. Use of PSA for Disease Monitoring. 1986.
30. FDA Approval Document P94–16. Use of PSA for Prostate Cancer Screening. 1994.
31. Rebhan M, Chalifa-Caspi V, Prilusky J, et al. GeneCards: Encyclopedia for Genes, Proteins and Diseases. 1997.
32. Hayes JD, Pulford DJ. The glutathione S-transferase supergene family: regulation of GST and the contribution of the isoenzymes to cancer chemoprotection and drug resistance. Crit Rev Biochem Mol Biol 1995; 30:445–600.
33. Jeronimo C, Usadel H, Henrique R, et al. Quantitation of GSTP1 methylation in non-neoplastic prostatic tissue and organ-confined prostate adenocarcinoma. J Natl Cancer Inst 2001; 93:1747–1752.
34. Chu DC, Chuang CK, Fu JB, et al. The use of real-time quantitative polymerase chain reaction to detect hypermethylation of the CpG islands in the promoter region flanking the GSTP1 gene to diagnose prostate carcinoma. J Urol 2002; 167:1854–1858.
35. Brooks JD, Weinstein M, Lin X, et al. CG island methylation changes near the GSTP1 gene in prostatic intraepithelial neoplasia. Cancer Epidemiol Biomarkers Prev 1998; 7:531–536.
36. Cairns P, Esteller M, Herman, JG, et al. Molecular detection of prostate cancer in urine by GSTP1 hypermethylation. Clin Cancer Res 2001; 7:2727–2730.
37. Lin X, Tascilar M, Lee WH, et al. GSTP1 CpG island hypermethylation is responsible for the absence of GSTP1 expression in human prostate cancer cells. Am J Pathol 2001; 159:1815–1826.
38. Lee WH, Morton RA, Epstein JI, et al. Cytidine methylation of regulatory sequences near the pi-class glutathione S-transferase gene accompanies human prostatic carcinogenesis. In: Proceedings of the National Academy of Sciences of the United States of America 1994; 91:11733–11737.
39. Lee WH, Isaacs WB, Bova GS, et al. CG island methylation changes near the GSTP1 gene in prostatic carcinoma cells detected using the polymerase chain reaction: a new prostate cancer biomarker. Cancer Epidemiol Biomarkers Prev 1997; 6:443–450.
40. Goessl C, Muller M, Heicappell R, et al. DNA-based detection of prostate cancer in urine after prostatic massage. Urology 2001; 58:335–338.
41. Millar DS, Ow KK, Paul CL, et al. Detailed methylation analysis of the glutathione S-transferase pi (GSTP1) gene in prostate cancer. Oncogene 1999; 18:1313–1324.
42. Cookson MS, Reuter VE, Linkov I, et al. Glutathione-S-Transferase P1 (GST-pi) class expression by immunohistochemistry in benign and malignant prostate tissue. J Urol 1997; 157:673–676.
43. Moskaluk CA, Durray PH, Cowan KH, et al. Immunohistochemical expression of pi-class glutathione-S-transferase is down regulated in adenocarcinoma of the prostate. Cancer 1997; 79:1595–1599.

44. Jeronimo C, Varzim G, Henrique R, et al. 1105V polymorphism and promoter methylation of the GSTP1 gene in prostate adenocarcinoma. Cancer Epidemiol Biomarkers Prev 2002; 11:445–450.
45. Kote-Jarai Z, Easton D, Edwards SM, et al. Relationship between glutathione S-transferase M1, P1 and T1 polymorphisms and early onset prostate cancer. Pharmacogenetics 2001; 11:325–330.
46. Gsur A, Haidinger G, Hinteregger S, et al. Polymorphisms of glutathione-S-transferase genes (GSTP1, GSTM1 and GSTT1) and prostate-cancer risk. Int J Cancer 2001; 95: 152–155.
47. Wadelius M, Autrup JL, Stubbins MJ, et al. Polymorphisms in NAT2, CYP2D6, CYP2C19 and GSTP1 and their association with prostate cancer. Pharmacogenetics 1999; 9:333–340.
48. Steinhoff C, Franke KH, Golka K, et al. Glutathione transferase isozyme genotypes in patients with prostate and bladder carcinoma. Arch Toxicol 2000; 74:521–526.
49. Ho GY, Knapp M, Freije D, et al. Transmission/disequilibrium tests of androgen receptor and glutathione S-transferase pi variants in prostate cancer families. Int J Cancer 2002; 98:938–942.
50. Maruyama R, Toyooka S, Toyooka KO, et al. Aberrant promoter methylation profile of prostate cancers and its relationship to clinicopathological features. Clin Cancer Res 2002; 8:514–519.
51. Lin X, Asgari K, Putzi MJ, et al. Reversal of GSTP1 CpG island hypermethylation and reactivation of pi-class glutathione S-transferase (GSTP1) expression in human prostate cancer cells by treatment with procainamide. Cancer Res 2001; 61:8611–8616.
52. Reiter RE, Gu Z, Watabe T, et al. Prostate stem cell antigen: a cell surface marker overexpressed in prostate cancer. Proc Natl Acad Sci USA 1998; 95:1735–1740.
53. Reiter RE, Magi-Galluzzi C, Hemmati H, et al. Two genes upregulated in androgen-independent prostate cancer are also selectively expressed in the basal cells of normal prostate epithelium. J Urol 1997; 157:269A.
54. Gu Z, Thomas G, Yamashiro J, et al. Prostate stem cell antigen (PSCA) expression increases with high gleason score, advanced stage and bone metastasis in prostate cancer. Oncogene 2000; 19:1288–1296.
55. Hara N, Kasahara T, Kawasaki T, et al. Reverse transcription-polymerase chain reaction detection of prostate-specific antigen, prostate-specific membrane antigen, and prostate stem cell antigen in one milliliter of peripheral blood: value for the staging of prostate cancer. Clin Cancer Res 2002; 8:1794–1799.
56. Jalkut MW, Reiter RE. Role of prostate stem cell antigen in prostate cancer research. Curr Opin Urol 2002; 12:401–406.
57. Christiansen JJ, Rajasekaran SA, Moy P, et al. Polarity of prostate specific membrane antigen, prostate stem cell antigen, and prostate specific antigen in prostate tissue and in a cultured epithelial cell line. Prostate 2003; 55:9–19.
58. Ross S, Spencer SD, Holcomb I, et al. Prostate stem cell antigen as therapy target: tissue expression and in vivo efficacy of an immunoconjugate. Cancer Res 2002; 62:2546–2553.
59. Saffran DC, Raitano AB, Hubert RS, et al. Anti-PSCA mAbs inhibit tumor growth and metastasis formation and prolong the survival of mice bearing human prostate cancer xenografts. Proc Natl Acad Sci USA 2001; 98:2658–2663.
60. Dannull J, Diener PA, Prikler L, et al. Prostate stem cell antigen is a promising candidate for immunotherapy of advanced prostate cancer. Cancer Res 2000; 60:5522–5528.
61. Reiter RE, Sato I, Thomas G, et al. Coamplification of prostate stem cell antigen (PSCA) and MYC in locally advanced prostate cancer. Genes Chromos Cancer 2000; 27:95–103.
62. Horoszewicz JS, Kawinski E, Murphy GP. Monoclonal antibodies to a new antigenic marker in epithelial prostatic cells and serum of prostatic cancer patients. Anticancer Res 1987; 7:927–935.
63. Israeli RS, Powell CT, Corr JG, et al. Expression of the prostate-specific membrane antigen. Cancer Res 1994; 54:1807–1811.
64. Pinto JT, Suffoletto BP, Berzin TM, et al. Prostate-specific membrane antigen: a novel folate hydrolase in human prostatic carcinoma cells. Clin Cancer Res 1996; 2:1445–1451.

65. Chung LWK, Isaacs W, Simons JW, eds. Prostate Cancer: Biology, Genetics, and the New Therapeutics. Totowa: Humana Press, 2001.
66. Silver DA, Pellicer I, Fair WR, et al. Prostate-specific membrane antigen expression in normal and malignant human tissues. Clin Cancer Res 1997; 3:81–85.
67. Murphy GP, Kenny GM, Ragde H, et al. Measurement of serum prostate-specific membrane antigen, a new prognostic marker for prostate cancer. Urology 1998; 51:89–97.
68. Bostwick DG, Pacelli A, Blute M, et al. Prostate specific membrane antigen expression in prostatic intraepithelial neoplasia and adenocarcinoma. Cancer 1998; 83:2256–2261.
69. Sweat SD, Pacelli A, Murphy GP, et al. Prostate-specific membrane antigen expression is greatest in prostate adenocarcinoma and lymph node metastases. Urology 1998; 52:637–640.
70. Murphy GP, Tino WT, Holmes EH, et al. Measurement of prostate-specific membrane antigen in the serum with a new antibody. Prostate 1996; 28:266–271.
71. Murphy GP, Maguire RT, Rogers B, et al. Comparison of serum PSMA, PSA levels with results of Cytogen-356 ProstaScint scanning in prostatic cancer patients. Prostate 1997; 33:281–285.
72. Troyer JK, Beckett ML, Wright GL Jr. Detection and characterization of the prostate-specific membrane antigen (PSMA) in tissue extracts and body fluids. Int J Cancer 1995; 62:552–558.
73. Murphy G, Ragde H, Kenny G, et al. Comparison of prostate specific membrane antigen, and prostate specific antigen levels in prostatic cancer patients. Anticancer Res 1995; 15:1473–1479.
74. Beckett ML, Cazares LH, Vlahou A, et al. Prostate-specific membrane antigen levels in sera from healthy men and patients with benign prostate hyperplasia or prostate cancer. Clin Cancer Res 1999; 5:4034–4040.
75. Douglas TH, Morgan TO, McLeod DG, et al. Comparison of serum prostate specific membrane antigen, prostate specific antigen, and free prostate specific antigen levels in radical prostatectomy patients. Cancer 1997; 80:107–114.
76. Wright GL Jr., Grob BM, Haley C, et al. Upregulation of prostate-specific membrane antigen after androgen-deprivation therapy. Urology 1996; 48:326–334.
77. Xiao Z, Adam BL, Cazares LH, et al. Quantitation of serum prostate-specific membrane antigen by a novel protein biochip immunoassay discriminates benign from malignant prostate disease. Cancer Res 2001; 61:6029–6033.
78. Tjoa B, Boynton A, Kenny G, et al. Presentation of prostate tumor antigens by dendritic cells stimulates T-cell proliferation and cytotoxicity. Prostate 1996; 28:65–69.
79. O'Keefe DS, Uchida A, Bacich DJ, et al. Prostate-specific suicide gene therapy using the prostate-specific membrane antigen promoter and enhancer. Prostate 2000; 45:149–157.
80. Uria JA, Velasco G, Santamaria I, et al. Prostate-specific membrane antigen in breast carcinoma. Lancet 1997; 349:1601.
81. Shay JW, Werbin H, Wright WE. Telomere shortening may contribute to aging and cancer: a perspective. Mol Cell Diff 1994; 2:1–22.
82. Iczkowski KA, Pantazis CG, McGregor DH, et al. Telomerase reverse transcriptase subunit immunoreactivity: a marker for high-grade prostate carcinoma. Cancer 2002; 95:2487–2493.
83. Sommerfeld HJ, Meeker AK, Piatyszek MA, et al. Telomerase activity: a prevalent marker of malignant human prostate tissue. Cancer Res 1996; 56:218–222.
84. Orlando C, Gelmini S, Selli C, et al. Telomerase in urological malignancy. J Urol 2001; 166:666–673.
85. Lin Y, Uemura H, Fujinami K, et al. Telomerase activity in primary prostate cancer. J Urol 1997; 157:1161–1165.
86. Wang Z, Ramin SA, Tsai C, et al. Telomerase activity in prostate sextant needle cores from radical prostatectomy specimens. Urol Oncol 2001; 6:57–62.
87. Latil A, Vidaud D, Valeri A, et al. htert expression correlates with MYC overexpression in human prostate cancer. Int J Cancer 2000; 89:172–176.
88. Liu BC, LaRose I, Weinstein LJ, et al. Expression of telomerase subunits in normal and neoplastic prostate epithelial cells isolated by laser capture microdissection. Cancer 2001; 92:1943–1948.

89. Wullich B, Rohde V, Oehlenschlager B, et al. Focal intratumoral heterogeneity for telomerase activity in human prostate cancer. J Urol 1999; 161:1997–2001.
90. Koeneman KS, Pan CX, Jin JK, et al. Telomerase activity, telomere length, and DNA ploidy in prostatic intraepithelial neoplasia (PIN). J Urol 1998; 160:1533–1539.
91. Chieco P, Bertaccini A, Giovannini C, et al. Telomerase activity in touch-imprint cell preparations from fresh prostate needle biopsy specimens. Eur Urol 2001; 40:666–672.
92. Zhang W, Kapusta LR, Slingerland JM, et al. Telomerase activity in prostate cancer, prostatic intraepithelial neoplasia, and benign prostatic epithelium. Cancer Res 1998; 58:619–621.
93. Paradis V, Dargere D, Laurendeau I, et al. Expression of the RNA component of human telomerase (hTR) in prostate cancer, prostatic intraepithelial neoplasia, and normal prostate tissue. J Pathol 1999; 189:213–218.
94. Straub B, Muller M, Krause H, et al. Molecular staging of surgical margins after radical prostatectomy by detection of telomerase activity. Prostate 2001; 49:140–144.
95. Ohyashiki K, Yahata N, Ohyashiki JH, et al. A combination of semiquantitative telomerase assay and in-cell telomerase activity measurement using exfoliated urothelial cells for the detection of urothelial neoplasia. Cancer 1998; 83:2554–2560.
96. Wang Z, Ramin SA, Tsai C, et al. Detection of telomerase activity in prostatic fluid specimens. Urol Oncol 2000; 6:4–9.
97. Kallakury BV, Brien TP, Lowry CV, et al. Telomerase activity in human benign prostate tissue and prostatic adenocarcinomas. Diagn Mol Pathol 1997; 6:192–198.
98. Scates DK, Muir GH, Venitt S, et al. Detection of telomerase activity in human prostate: a diagnostic marker for prostatic cancer? Br J Urol 1997; 80:263–268.
99. Takahashi C, Miyagawa I, Kumano S, et al. Detection of telomerase activity in prostate cancer by needle biopsy. Eur Urol 1997; 32:494–498.
100. Lin Y, Uemura H, Fujinami K, et al. Detection of telomerase activity in prostate needle-biopsy samples. Prostate 1998; 36:121–128.
101. Caldarera E, Crooks NH, Muir GH, et al. An appraisal of telomerase activity in benign prostatic hyperplasia. Prostate 2000; 45:267–270.
102. Donaldson L, Fordyce C, Gilliland F, et al. Association between outcome and telomere DNA content in prostate cancer. J Urol 1999; 162:1788–1792.
103. Meid FH, Gygi CM, Leisinger HJ, et al. The use of telomerase activity for the detection of prostatic cancer cells after prostatic massage. J Urol 2001; 165:1802–1805.
104. Ferdinandusse S, Denis S, IJlst W, et al. Subcellular localization and physiological role of α-methylacyl-CoA racemase. Lipid Res 2000; 41:1890–1896.
105. Zha S, Ferdinandusse S, Hicks JL, et al. Peroxisomal branched chain fatty acid β-oxidation pathway is upregulated in prostate cancer. Prostate 2005; 63:316–323.
106. Rubin MA, Zhou M, Dhanasekaran SM, et al. α-Methylacyl-Coenzyme A racemase as a tissue biomarker for prostate cancer. JAMA 2002; 287:1662–1670.
107. Luo J, Zha S, Gage WR, et al. α-Methylacyl-Coenzyme A Racemase: A new molecular marker for prostate cancer. Cancer Res 2002; 62:2220–2226.
108. Magi-Galluzzi C, Luo J, Isaacs WB, et al. α-Methylacyl-Coenzyme A Racemase: A variably sensitive immunohistochemical marker for the diagnosis of small prostate cancer foci on needle biopsy. Am J Surg Pathol 2003; 27:1128–1133.
109. Browne T-J, Hirsch MS, Brodsky G, et al. Prospective evaluation of AMACR (P504S) and basal cell markers in the assessment of routine prostate needle biopsy specimens. Hum Pathol 2004; 35:1462–1468.
110. Sreekumar A, Laxman B, Rhodes DR, et al. Humoral immune response to α-Methylacyl-Coenzyme A racemase and prostate cancer. J Natl Cancer Inst 2004; 96:834–843.
111. Anathanarayanan V, Deaton RJ, Yang XJ, et al. α-Methylacyl-Coenzyme A racemase (AMACR) in normal prostatic glands and high grade prostatic intraepithelial neoplasis (HGPIN): Association with diagnosis of prostate cancer. Prostate 2005; 63:341–346.
112. Sanderson SO, Sebo TJ, Murphy LM, et al. An analysis of p63/α-Methylacyl-Coenzyme A racemase immunohistochemical cocktail stain in prostate needle biopsy specimens and tissue micro arrays. Anatomic Pathol 2004; 121:220–225.
113. Jiang Z, Li C, Fischer A, et al. Using an AMACR (P504S)/34betaE12/p63 cocktail for the detection of small focal prostate carcinoma in needle biopsy specimens. Am J Clin Pathol 2005; 123:231–236.

114. Hameed O, Sublett J, Humphrey PA. Immunohistochemical staining for p63 and α-methylacyl-coenzyme A racemase, versus a cocktail containing both, in the diagnosis of prostate cancer. Am J Surg Pathol 2005; 29:579–587.
115. Gologan A, Bastacky S, McHale T, et al. Age associated changes in α-methylacyl-coenzyme A racemase (AMACR) expression in nonneoplastic prostatic tissues. Am J Surg Pathol 2005; 29:1435–1441.
116. Rubin MA, Bismar TA, Adren O, et al. Decreased α-Methylacyl-Coenzyme A racemase expression in localized prostate cancer is associated with an increased rate of biochemical recurrence and cancer-specific death. Cancer Epid Biomarkers Prev 2005: 14:1424–1432.
117. Chiang C, Litingtun Y, Lee E, et al. Cyclopia and defective axial patterning in mice lacking sonic hedgehog gene function. Nature 1996; 383:407–413.
118. Roessler E, Belloni E, Gudenz K, et al. Mutations in the human sonic hedgehog gene cause holoprocencephaly. Nat Genet 1996; 14:357–360.
119. Ingham PW, McMahon AP. Hedgehog signaling in animal development: paradigms and principles. Genes Dev 2001; 15:3059–3087.
120. Lamm MLG, Catbagan WS, Laciak RJ, et al. Sonic hedgehog activates mesenchymal GLI1 expression during prostate ductal bud formation. Dev Biol 2002; 249: 349–366.
121. Freestone SH, Marker P, Grace OC, et al. Sonic hedgehog regulates prostatic growth and epithelial differentiation. Dev Biol 2003; 264:352–362.
122. Berman DM, Desai N, Wang X, et al. Roles for hedgehog signaling in androgen production and prostate ductal morphogenesis. Dev Biol 2004; 267:387–398.
123. Fan L, Pepicelli CV, Dibble CC, et al. Hedgehog signaling promotes prostate xenograft tumor growth. Endocrinology 2004; 145:3961–3970.
124. Karhadkar SS, Bova GS, Abdallah N, et al. Hedgehog signaling in prostate regeneration, neoplasia and metastasis. Nature 2004; 431:707–712.
125. Sanchez P, Hernandez AM, Stecca B, et al. Inhibition of prostate cancer proliferation by interference with sonic hedgehog-GLI1 signaling. Proc Natl Acad Sci 2004; 101:12561–12566.
126. Sanchez P, Clement V, Altaba AR. Therapeutic targeting of the hedgehog-GLI pathway in prostate cancer. Cancer Res 2005; 65:2990–2992.
127. Chen JK, Taipale J, Cooper MK, et al. Inhibition of hedgehog signaling by direct binding of cyclopamine to smoothened. Genes Dev 2002; 16:2743–2748.
128. Fried J, Klingsberg A. The structure of jervine III. Degradation to nitrogen-free derivatives. J Am Chem Soc 1953; 75:4929–4938.
129. Marigo V, Davey RA, Zuo Y, et al. Biochemical evidence that patched is the hedgehog receptor. Nature 1996; 384:176–179.
130. Stone DM, Hynes M, Armanini M, et al. The tumor suppressor gene patched encodes a candidate receptor for sonic hedgehog. Nature 1996; 384:129–134.
131. Taipale J, Chen JK, Cooper MK, et al. Effects of oncogenic mutations in smoothened and patched can be reversed by cyclopamine. Nature 2000; 406:1005–1009.
132. Tao S, Li C, Zhang X, et al. Activation of the hedgehog pathway in advanced prostate cancer. Mol Cancer 2004; 3:29.
133. Mimeault M, Moore E, Moniaux N, et al. Cytotoxic effects induced by a combination of cyclopamine and gefitinib, the selective hedgehog and epidermal growth factor receptor signaling inhibitors, in prostate cancer cells. Int J Cancer 2006; 118:1022–1031.
134. Magee JA, Araki T, Patil S, et al. Expression profiling reveals hepsin overexpression in prostate cancer. Cancer Res 2001; 61:5692–5696.
135. Dhanasekaran SM, Barrette TR, Ghosh D, et al. Delineation of prognostic biomarkers in prostate cancer. Nature 2001; 412:822–826.
136. Srikantan V, Valladares M, Rhim JS, et al. HEPSIN inhibits cell growth/invasion in prostate cancer cells. Cancer Res 2002; 62:6812–6816.
137. Carpten J, Nupponen N, Isaacs S, et al. Germline mutations in the ribonuclease L gene in families showing linkage with HPC1. Nat Genet 2002; 30:181–184.
138. Casey G, Neville PJ, Plummer SJ, et al. RNASEL Arg462Gln variant is implicated in up to 13% of prostate cancer cases. Nat Genet 2002; 32: 581–583.

139. Qing J, Wei D, Maher VM, et al. Cloning and characterization of a novel gene encoding a putative transmembrane protein with altered expression in some human transformed and tumor-derived cell lines. Oncogene 1999; 18:335–342.
140. Zenklusen JC, Conti CJ, Green ED. Mutational and functional analyses reveal that ST7 is a highly conserved tumor-suppressor gene on human chromosome 7q31. Nat Genet 2001; 27:392–398.
141. Dong SM, Sidransky D. Absence of ST7 gene alterations in human cancer. Clin Cancer Res 2002; 8:2939–2941.
142. Varambally S, Dhanasekaran SM, Zhou M, et al. The polycomb group protein EZH2 is involved in progression of prostate cancer. Nature 2002; 419:624–629.
143. Rhodes DR, Sanda MG, Otte AP, et al. Multiplex biomarker approach for determining risk of prostate-specific antigen-defined recurrence of prostate cancer. J Natl Cancer Inst 2003; 95:661–668.
144. Petricoin EF, Ornstein DK, Paweletz CP, et al. Serum proteomic patterns for detection of prostate cancer. J Natl Cancer Inst 2002; 94:1576–1578.
145. Tomlins SA, Rhodes DR, Perner S, et al. Recurrent fusion of TMPRSS2 and ETS transcription factor genes in prostate cancer. Science 2005; 310:644–648.

4 The Endothelin Pathway and its Modulation in Prostate Cancer

Antonio Jimeno and Michael Carducci

The Sidney Kimmel Comprehensive Cancer Center, The Johns Hopkins University School of Medicine, Baltimore, Maryland, U.S.A.

INTRODUCTION

Recent advances in the understanding of prostate cancer biology have led to the development of drugs directed against precise molecular alterations in the prostate tumor cell. Targeting specific pathways to stop cancer growth is generally less toxic to normal cells and improves tolerability, and thus anticancer drug discovery has shifted from an empiric random screening approach to a more rational and mechanistic, target-directed approach, where specific abnormalities in cell functioning are modulated in a classic drug-receptor fashion (1). Endothelins (ETs) and their receptor have emerged as a potential target in prostate cancer and will be discussed in detail in this chapter.

THE ENDOTHELIN AXIS

Endothelins and Their Receptors

The ETs constitute a family of three 21-amino-acid peptides (ET-1, ET-2, and ET-3) that are synthesized as pro-peptides and are transformed to their active forms by sequential endopeptidase- and ET-converting enzyme-mediated cleavage. ET-1 is the most common circulating form of ET, has a median half-life of 7 min (2), and is cleared by a double mechanism consisting in ET receptor B (ET_B)-mediated uptake and degradation by neutral endopeptidase (NEP) (3). Each of the three ETs has a unique pattern of distribution; ET-1 is not organ-specific and is expressed primarily by endothelial cells, whereas ET-2 is mainly present in the intestine and kidney, and ET-3 is mainly localized in the brain and to a lesser extent in gastrointestinal stromal cells and lung epithelial cells (4). ETs exert their effect by binding to two different membrane receptors, ET_A and ET_B. ET_B has a similar affinity for the three peptides and functions primarily as a decoy receptor and modulator of ET-1 (5,6). ET_A preferentially binds ET-1 and is considered the major effector of the ET axis. Therefore, it has been the main focus of research and also the main target in the development of pharmacologic strategies to modulate the ET axis. However, evidence is mounting of the increasing relevance of ET_B in cancer pathophysiology.

Intracellular Pathways

Upon activation by ET-1, ET_A interacts with and activates a pertussis-insensitive G-protein that triggers a parallel activation of several signal-transducing pathways. These include phospholipase C activity with a consequent increase in intracellular

Ca^{2+} levels, protein kinase C (PKC) (7), epidermal growth factor receptor (EGFR) (8), phosphatidylinositol 3-kinase (9), and ras/raf/mitogen-activated protein kinase (MAPK) pathways (Fig. 1) (10,11). This cascade of events ultimately induces nuclear transcription of several protooncogenes, including *c-myc*, *c-fos*, and *c-jun*, that have the capability of influencing cell growth and proliferation. The complexity of these interactions, the still-to-be-determined cross-talking phenomena, and the potential for altering key elements in the cell machinery emphasize the relevance of ET-1 in maintaining the signal transduction homeostasis.

Physiologic Actions

ET-1 is one of the most potent endogenous vasoconstrictors known and is characterized by its long action suggesting that it may be involved in the long-term regulation of vascular tone (12). ET-1 production is stimulated by cytokines [interleukin-1β (IL-1β)], growth factors [tumor necrosis factor-α (TNF-α), transforming growth factor-β (TGF-β), platelet-derived growth factor (PDGF)], and major signals of cardiovascular stress, such as vocative agents (angiogenesis II, norepinephrine, vasopressin, and bradykinin), thrombin, mechanical stress, and hypoxia.

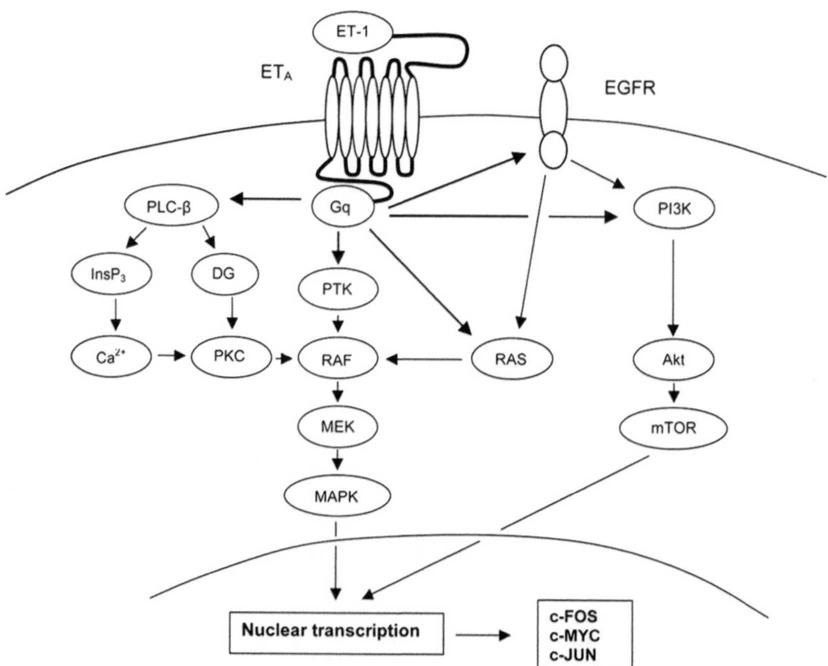

FIGURE 1 Endothelin 1 binding to endothelin receptor A activates a pertussis-insensitive G-protein (Gq) that triggers a parallel activation of multiple signal-transducing pathways, including phospholipase C and diacylglycerol-mediated protein kinase C activation, protein tyrosine kinase and RAS-mediated activation of the RAF/MEK/MAPK axis, phosphatidylinositol-3 kinase-mediated Akt activation, and epidermal growth factor receptor trans activation. *Abbreviations*: DG, diacylglycerol; EGFR, epidermal growth factor receptor; ET_A, endothelin receptor A; ET-1, endothelin 1; InsP3, inositol 1,4,5 triphosphate; MAPK, mitogen-activated protein kinase; MEK, MAPK kinase; PKC, protein kinase C; PLC, phospholipase C; PTK, protein tyrosine kinase.

Prostacyclin, nitric oxide, and atrial natriuretic peptide are the predominant effectors of negative feedback loops (13). ET-1 is secreted by a wide array of normal cells, including endothelial cells, vascular smooth myocytes, and bronchial, mammary, endometrial, and prostatic epithelial cells. ET-1 acts as a potent vasoconstrictor and is a putative factor in vascular lesion development. In addition, it exerts a mitogenic stimulus on vascular and bronchial myocytes, fibroblasts, melanocytes, osteoblasts, mesangial cells, and endometrial cells, among others. ET-1 has been implicated in hypertension, heart failure, atherosclerosis, and pulmonary hypertension. In all of these conditions, plasma immunoreactive and tissue ET-1 levels are elevated (14). Consequently, pharmacologic strategies directed at modulating ET-1-induced vascular changes have been developed, and a nonselective ET_{A-B} antagonist, bosentan (Tracleer, Actelion Pharmaceuticals Ltd, Allschwil, Switzerland) was recently approved by the U.S. Food and Drug Administration for use in pulmonary hypertension (13,15).

Pathophysiology of ET-1 in Cancer

ET-1 is produced by several epithelial tumors, where it acts as an autocrine and/or paracrine growth factor (11). Extensive research has revealed that the ET axis is relevant in cancer development and progression at several stages. The majority of these studies have been developed in prostate and ovarian cancer models where several findings are overlapping, indicating that they are not model-dependent and constitute general and consistent mechanisms for the cancer cell to acquire beneficial features (16).

ET-1 Deregulation

In the normal prostate ET-1 is produced by epithelial cells, and the highest body concentrations of ET-1 are found in the seminal fluid with concentrations 500-fold superior to those found in plasma (17). ET_A receptors are present in the prostate gland, and their expression is directly proportional to tumor grade and stage in prostate carcinoma (17). In prostate cancer specimens, ET-1 clearance mechanisms such as ET_B binding capacity and NEP activity are decreased (18,19). ET_B expression is reduced or abolished, presumably by a promoter methylation-mediated mechanism; the functionality of the remaining receptors is also abnormal, due to an absence of active ET-1-binding sites (20). The other major mechanism of ET-1 clearance, NEP-mediated degradation, is also diminished in the prostate cancer's environment (21). ET-1 is overexpressed in ovarian cancer tissue and is present at high concentrations in ovarian cancer ascites, suggesting a potential role in the progression and metastasis of ovarian carcinoma (22).

Proliferation

ET-1 stimulates DNA synthesis and proliferation in several normal cell types, such as vascular smooth muscle, osteoblasts, glomerular mesangial cells, melanocytes, and fibroblasts. It also prompts division and growth in malignant cell types, such as prostate, cervical, and ovarian cancer models. ET_A has been shown to be the primary mediator of ET-1-induced mitogenesis in prostate cancer models, and its effect is impeded following pharmacologic ET_A inhibition (18). However, the effect of ET-1 is modest per se and seems to be enhanced when acting in parallel with other growth factors, such as basic fibroblastic growth factor, insulin growth factors (IGFs) I and II, epidermal growth factor (EGF), and PDGF (10). Considering the abovementioned cross-talk events between the pathways activated by these ligands, it could be hypothesized that distinct combinations of ET-1 and other ligands elicit different levels of mitogenic response, in diverse cell strains. A higher expression of ET_A has been documented in increasingly aggressive prostate cancer cell lines (23).

Apoptosis

Programmed cell death, or apoptosis, is a natural defence against aberrant or uncontrolled growing cells, and short-circuiting pre-established apoptotic mechanisms is one of the most consistent features characterizing tumor cells. This is especially relevant in tumors with low proliferative rates, such as prostate cancer, where clinical growth is mainly because of decreased apoptosis rather than increased cell proliferation (24). The ET-1 axis suppresses paclitaxel-induced apoptosis in colon and ovarian carcinoma cells, a process mediated by the anti-apoptotic Bcl-2 and Akt pathways and reversed by ET_A inhibition (11,25). Wortmannin-mediated inhibition of PI3K prevented ET-1-induced Akt activation in the ovarian model (26). This has also been observed in prostate cancer cells, where the anti-apoptotic effects of ET-1 are mediated, at least in part, through the Bcl-2 family (27). Although no significant changes in Bcl-2 expression occurred with ET-1, the proapoptotic family members Bad, Bax, and Bak all significantly decreased. Further analysis of the survival pathway demonstrated that ET-1 causes phosphorylation of Akt in a time- and dose-dependent manner through phosphatidylinositol 3-kinase activation. This action seems to be selectively mediated by the ET_A, as demonstrated by its reversal using the selective ET_A inhibitor BQ123, but not after administration of a selective ET_B inhibitor, BQ788 (28).

Invasion

ET-1 facilitates the abnormal migration of tumor cells by several mechanisms. First, ET-1-mediated activation of ET_A induces overexpression and activation of a panel of proteinases [matrix metalloproteinase (MMP) 2 and 9, urokinase-type plasminogen activator, and plasminogen activator inhibitor type-1 and type-2] associated with invasiveness and metastatic potential in ovarian cancer cells; to further support this concept, the inhibition of ET_A using a specific antagonist (BQ123) reverses tumor protease activity (29,30). A similar mechanism has been described in Kaposi's sarcoma models (31). In addition, ET-1 enhances the secretion of two tissue inhibitors of MMPs (TIMP-1 and -2), increasing the net MMP/TIMP ratio and the lytic capacity that results in rapid degradation of the extracellular matrix. In melanoma cells ET-1 and ET-3 activation of ET_B leads to loss of expression of the cell adhesion molecule E-cadherin and associated catenin proteins and gain of N-cadherin expression (32). Loss of gap junctional intercellular communication is critical for tumor progression by allowing the cells to escape growth control; the addition of ET-1 to ovarian cancer cells provokes a 50–75% inhibition in intercellular communication and a decrease in the connexin 43 (Cx43)-based gap junction plaques, an action thought to be mediated by the Src tyrosine kinase pathway (33). BQ123, a selective (ET_A) antagonist, blocked the ET-1-induced Cx43 phosphorylation and cellular uncoupling.

Angiogenesis

ET_B mediates endothelial cell mitogenesis, whereas ET_A mediates mitogenic stimuli in vascular smooth muscle cells and pericytes. ET-1 induces angiogenic responses through ET_B in cultured endothelial cells stimulating neovascularization in vivo in concert with vascular endothelial growth factor (VEGF) (34). In ovarian cancer cells, ET-1 increases VEGF mRNA expression and induces VEGF protein levels in a time- and dose-dependent fashion, which is greater under hypoxic conditions (35). ET-1 also increases hypoxia-inducible factor-1alpha (HIF-1alpha) accumulation and activates the HIF-1 transcription complex under both normoxic and hypoxic conditions, suggesting a role for HIF-1 in the induction of VEGF expression, effects that were inhibited by selective ET_A targeting. In ovarian cancer specimens high levels of ET-1 were detected in the majority of ascitic fluids of patients with ovarian carcinoma and significantly correlated with VEGF ascitic concentration; in addition, ET-1 expression correlated with neovascularization (measured as microvessel density) and with VEGF expression, and exposure to ascitic fluid increased endothelial cell migration in an in vitro model (22).

In ovarian cancer models, ET-1 increases the expression of cyclooxygenases (COX)-1 and COX-2 both at the mRNA and protein level, by MAPK- and EGFR-mediated trans activation. The inhibition of the ET_A significantly decreased COX-1 and COX-2 expressions (36). There is increasing evidence that PGE_2 induces tumor progression also by stimulating angiogenesis and that this effect is mediated by VEGF. COX-2 axis activation is considered one of the main pathogenic events in prostate cancer; COX-2 is overexpressed in the vast majority of human prostate cancer specimens (37) and its selective inhibition has evidenced biologic activity in a clinical setting (38). The potential connection between ET-1 and COX-2 in prostate cancer is still undetermined.

Osteogenesis

ET-1 is associated with the osteoblastic nature of breast and prostate cancer bone metastasis, as it is the basis of a unique interaction between the in-transit metastatic cell and the local environment. It was postulated that ET-1 production by metastatic prostate and breast cancer cells located in the bone is stimulated by osteoblast- and endothelial cell-secreted IL-1, TNF-α, and TGF-β. ET-1 in turn, closing this paracrine loop, would stimulate mitotic activity in osteoblasts, decreasing both osteoclastic bone resorption and motility (39). This was demonstrated in a series of elegant experiments where co-culture of human prostate cancer cell lines with bone slices increased the level of ET-1 mRNA, osteoclastic bone resorption was significantly blocked by the presence of both prostate cancer cells and ET-1 in a dose-dependent manner. This inhibition was neutralized by a specifically directed anti-ET-1 antibody (40). In another series of experiments, tumor-produced ET-1 stimulated new bone formation in vitro and osteoblastic metastases in vivo via ET_A (41). These findings explain in part the characteristic blastic nature of prostate and breast cancer bone metastases. It may well be that more than a true osseous tropism of prostate cancer cells, this ET-1-secreting capability and the resulting environment favoring disorganized bone growth explain the preponderance of bone disease and its devastating clinical consequences in prostate cancer patients. In prostate and breast cancer models selective ET_A inhibition, but not ET_B modulation, abrogated ET-1-induced osteoblastic response (42).

Nociception

ET-1 is thought to play a pathogenic role in pain elicitation and control. ET-1 is found in high concentrations in dorsal root ganglion neurons and ET_A receptors are found on small- to medium-sized root ganglion neurons and their axons (43).

ET-1 enhances pain states in various models of acute chemical- and inflammation-induced pain and in chronic pain types such as neuropathic pain, where selective ET_A inhibition with atrasentan shows preclinical efficacy (44). The key relevance of ET-1 and the effectiveness of ET_A inhibition have also been demonstrated in acute pain models, both irritant-induced and prostate cancer-related (45). In the latter experiments, ET-1 axis inhibition both with atrasentan and YM598 resulted in significant pain control. ET-1-mediated enhancement of pain responses in a prostate cancer inoculation-induced pain model is mediated through ET_A (the selective ET_B agonist sarafotoxin failed to elicit pain), and this effect is reversed by selective ET_A inhibition with atrasentan (46). Recently, a compensatory analgesic action has been proposed, which is initiated by ET-1 upon binding to ET_B and is mediated through the release of β-endorphin (47). Thus, ET_A selective inhibition might theoretically abrogate ET-1-initiated nociceptive response while preserving the analgesic effect In a murine osteolytic 2472 sarcoma model of bone cancer pain, the 2472 sarcoma cells expressed high levels of ET-1, but expressed low or undetectable levels of ET_A or ET_B whereas a subpopulation of sensory neurons express the ET_A and nonmyelinating Schwann cells express the ET_B (48). Acute (10 mg/kg, i.p.) or chronic (10 mg/kg/day, p.o.) administration of the ET_A selective antagonist atrasentan significantly attenuated ongoing and movement-evoked bone cancer pain and chronic administration of atrasentan reduced several neurochemical indices of peripheral and central sensitization without influencing tumor growth or bone destruction.

Rationale for Targeting the Endothelin Axis in Prostate Cancer

By activating ET_A, ET-1 is pathogenically involved in facilitating several aspects of prostate cancer progression including proliferation, escape from apoptosis, invasion, and new vessel formation, processes which are general to many malignancies. Notwithstanding, there are a number of features specifically driven by the ET axis in prostate cancer, such as creating and perpetuating a unique interaction between the metastatic prostate cancer cell and the bone microenvironment (osteoblast, osteoclast, and stroma), or altering the equilibrium in pain modulation. These features have led to the preferential clinical evaluation of atrasentan as a biological therapy in prostate carcinoma, first in hormone-refractory prostate cancer (HRPC) patients.

LEADING COMPOUND IN CANCER: ATRASENTAN

Pharmacology

Chemical Name, Structure, and Properties

Atrasentan ([2*R*,3*R*,4*S*]-4-(1,3-benzodioxol-5-yl)-1-[2-(dibutylamino)-2-oxoethyl]-2-(4-methoxyphenyl)-3-pyrrolidinecarboxylic acid, monohydrochloride; A-147627.1; ABT-627;) is a crystalline, nonhygroscopic ($<2\%$ weight gain when exposed to relative humidity up to 90%), and readily soluble in water, with a molecular weight of 547.09 g/mol (Fig. 2). Atrasentan is the (+) enantiomer, hydrochloride salt of the racemate A-127722, and is approximately twice as active as the racemate in bioactivity assays. The solubility of the hydrochloride salt in water is approximately

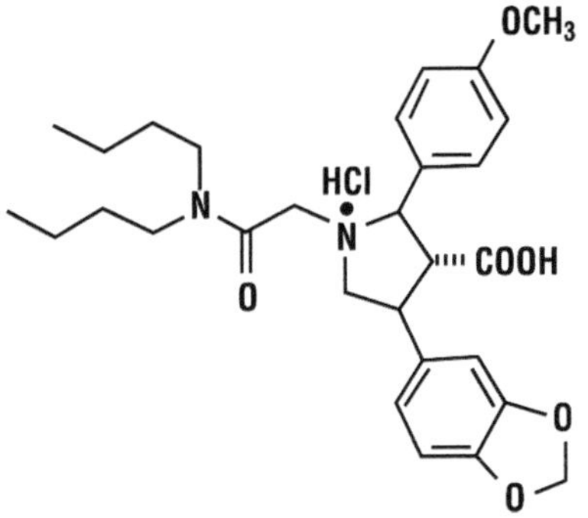

FIGURE 2 Chemical structure of atrasentan.

1 mg/mL at 37°C. The drug substance is stable and shows minimal degradation over a 3-yr period.

Mechanism of Action

Atrasentan exerts its activity by selective inhibition of the ET_A. Competition and saturation binding studies were performed using membranes prepared from either Chinese hamster ovary (CHO) cells that were permanently transfected to express either human ET_A or ET_B, rat pituitary (MMQ) cells (ET_A), and porcine cerebellum tissue (ET_B). Atrasentan effectively inhibited specific [^{125}I]ET-1 binding to ET_A in both the CHO cells and membranes from MMQ cells (49). Atrasentan was much less effective inhibiting specific [^{125}I]ET-3 binding to ET_B in the CHO cells and porcine cerebellum membranes. In membranes from transfected CHO cells, the inhibitor constant, K_i, of unlabeled atrasentan was 0.034 nM for ET_A and 63.3 nM for ET_B. In saturation binding assays, atrasentan effected a change in the equilibrium dissociation constant of ET-1 binding, but did not have a significant effect on the B_{max} (maximal [^{125}I]ET-1 binding). Atrasentan decreases the binding affinity of ET-1 without affecting the receptor density, indicating that it is a potent, competitive inhibitor of ET-1 binding, with 1800-fold superior selectivity for ET_A compared with ET_B.

Distribution and Metabolism

The in vitro plasma protein binding of ^{14}C-labeled atrasentan was determined in mouse, rat, dog, and human, showing extensive (98.8–99.0%) plasma protein binding across all species at drug concentrations between 0.05 and 50 mcg/mL. Additional in vitro binding studies indicated that atrasentan was extensively bound to both human serum albumin and human α1-acid glycoprotein. However, competitive binding studies showed that concentrations of atrasentan from 0.05 to 0.5 μg/mL had no effect on the plasma protein binding of either warfarin or phenytoin. Metabolism and disposition studies of ^{14}C indicate that atrasentan is cleared almost exclusively by metabolism. In the animal studies, the predominant pathway was glucuronidation of the carboxylic acid moiety of atrasentan, while oxidative metabolism via *O*-demethylation and *N*-debutylation were minor pathways. Results in humans indicated that the metabolism of atrasentan was about equally distributed between oxidation and glucuronidation. In all species, $>90\%$ of the radioactive dose was eliminated in the feces while $<5\%$ was in urine. Bile cannulation studies in animals demonstrated that the glucuronic acid conjugate of atrasentan was extensively secreted in bile and underwent hydrolysis in the gut, suggesting that atrasentan may undergo enterohepatic recirculation. Unchanged parent drug was the predominant circulating component in all species, including human, while the *O*-demethyl and *N*-debutyl metabolites were found only in the feces.

Food and Drug Interaction Studies

A series of studies in healthy volunteers evaluated atrasentan absorption, metabolism, and interaction with other drugs. In a trial that compared the effect of a high-fat meal versus fasting, food did not appear to affect the extent of atrasentan absorption, but induced a delay in the time to maximum concentration (T_{max}) and a 65% lower maximum concentration (C_{max}). Two studies designed to evaluate the impact of CYP3A modulation showed that co-administration of the inhibitor ketoconazole delayed atrasentan metabolism (increasing AUC_{∞} by 90% with no effect on C_{max}) (50), whereas co-administration of the inducer rifampin increased atrasentan C_{max} 2.7-fold, decreased half-life ($t_{1/2}$) from 22 to 5 hr, but had no effect on T_{max} or AUC (51). Co-administration of atrasentan with a *P*-glycoprotein (Pgp) substrate (fexofenadine) suggested that atrasentan moderately inhibited Pgp efflux intestinally but not systemically, when the drugs were co-administered (52).

Pharmacogenomic Studies

A pharmacogenetic joint analysis of single-dose pharmacokinetic parameters from three clinical studies ($n=44$) and steady-state pharmacokinetic parameters from two clinical studies ($n=38$) was performed to assess the influence of gene polymorphisms of drug metabolizing enzymes or drug transporters in atrasentan pharmacokinetics (53). Genotypes in *CYP3A5, UGT1A1, UGT2B4, UGT2B15, ABCB1, SLC21A6,* and *SLC22A2* were assessed. Exposure and apparent volume of distribution were correlated with organic anion transport protein C (OATP-C, a mediator of drug uptake into hepatocytes now renamed OATP1B1) activity predicted by the *SLC21A6* genotype ($p=0.0034$ and 0.03, respectively), suggesting that atrasentan is an OATP-C substrate.

Clinical Development of Atrasentan

Pharmacokinetics

The pharmacokinetics of single oral doses (1, 10, 23.25, and 139.5 mg) of atrasentan was assessed in a placebo-controlled, double-blind study in 24 healthy male subjects (54). Atrasentan pharmacokinetics was linear in the 1–23.25 mg dose range, with relative dose dependency in the highest dose group. However, $t_{1/2}$ was similar across all dose groups (20–25 hr), and the apparent volume of distribution was consistent with extensive tissue distribution (6 L/kg). Three Phase I studies have been conducted in 31, 39, and 35 patients with solid tumors (55–57). Two of the trials predominantly accrued prostate cancer patients [14 out of 31 (55) and 30 out of 39 (56)], whereas the third treated subjects with diverse solid tumors. All three trials explored identical route (oral), dosing schedule (uninterrupted daily), and dose levels [10, 20, 30, 45, 60, and 75 mg/day; one of the studies explored an additional dose level of 95 mg/day (56)] and all three obtained highly consistent pharmacokinetic and clinical results. Atrasentan was rapidly absorbed, with T_{max} of approximately 1.5 hr. The $t_{1/2}$ ranged from 21 to 24 hr, a volume of distribution of 726–790 L was documented, and steady-state plasma concentrations were achieved within 5–7 days. There was no significant trend for a change with dose for several pharmacokinetic variables tested on days 1 and 28. Pharmacokinetics was approximately dose-proportional (especially at doses <45 mg/day) and time-independent across doses. It is noteworthy that the free (not protein-bound) plasma concentrations achieved at doses of 2.5 mg and above exceeded the human ET_A K_i (0.034 nM) for atrasentan and corresponded to biologically active concentrations achieved in vivo in animal studies.

Toxicity

In a placebo-controlled healthy volunteer study, headache, rhinitis, and nausea were more frequent in the atrasentan group, whereas no other clinically significant differences in vital signs or laboratory parameters were observed between groups. In all three reported continuous-dosing Phase I studies in cancer patients, the most common adverse events were rhinitis, headache, asthenia, and peripheral edema; they were reversible on drug discontinuation and responded to symptom-specific treatment. Reversible hemodilution was apparent in laboratory findings, as was weight gain. In both U.S.-based trials, the maximum-tolerated dose was 60 mg/day, and the occurrence of headache (55), and hyponatremia and hypotension (57) were the dose-limiting adverse events at 75 mg/day in those trials. In the third Phase I trial conducted in The Netherlands, no dose-limiting adverse events were observed up to 95 mg/day (56).

The toxicity profile documented during the clinical development of atrasentan Phases I to III has shown a high level of consistency and appears to be mainly related to ET_A inhibition, which results in fluid retention and/or vasodilation. Taking the preliminary results of the completed Phase III trial as a reference, the main (incidence ≥5%) adverse events associated with atrasentan compared with placebo were peripheral edema (40% vs. 12%, $p < 0.001$), rhinitis (36% vs. 14%, $p < 0.001$), dyspnea (9% vs. 4%, $p = 0.005$), headache (21% vs. 14%, $p = 0.013$), infection (13% vs. 8%, $p = 0.019$), dry mouth (6% vs. 2%, $p = 0.009$), and edema (5% vs. 2%, $p = 0.033$). Over 96% of these events were rated as Grade 1 or 2 and few resulted in discontinuation of study drug. Over a third of the atrasentan recipients reporting peripheral edema experienced resolution of peripheral edema during the treatment period, both with and without diuretics. Although less prevalent, there was an increased incidence of heart failure in the atrasentan group (4% vs. 1%, $p = 0.002$). Subjects developing heart failure tended to be older (mean age: 78 yr), had larger metastatic tumor burden, and presented with pre-existing cardiovascular disorders; some patients resumed atrasentan therapy after treatment with diuretics and/or angiotensin-converting enzyme inhibitors.

Efficacy

Phase I and II Data

In one of the abovementioned Phase I trials, early hints of clinical activity were documented, as evidenced by a decrease in cancer-related pain in 5 of 15 subjects and in PSA in 5 of 11 subjects with HRPC (55). The disease-specific activity of atrasentan was evaluated in a double-blind, randomized, placebo-controlled Phase II trial conducted in 288 asymptomatic patients with HRPC and evidence of metastatic disease. Patients were randomly assigned to one of three study groups consisting in daily oral placebo, 2.5 mg atrasentan, or 10 mg atrasentan (58).

Median time to progression (TTP) in intent-to-treat (ITT) patients ($n = 288$) was nonsignificantly longer in the 10-mg atrasentan group compared with the placebo group (183 days vs. 137 days, respectively; $p = 0.13$). A subset analysis was planned in patients who met classification criteria defined prior to breaking the study blind; this analysis excluded patients not meeting disease classification ($n = 15$), receiving $< 50\%$ of the doses of study drug or fewer than 20 doses ($n = 10$), noncomplying ($n = 8$), with insufficient anti-androgen withdrawal ($n = 7$), or taking excluded medications ($n = 4$). Median TTP in this assessable patient population ($n = 244$) was significantly prolonged in patients treated with atrasentan 10 mg from 129 to 196 days ($p = 0.021$) compared with placebo. For both ITT and per-protocol assessable populations in the 10-mg atrasentan group, median time to PSA progression was twice that of the placebo group (155 vs. 71 days; $p = 0.002$). Patients who received placebo continued to have significant increases from baseline in serum lactate dehydrogenase (LDH), a marker of disease burden; elevations in LDH were uniformly attenuated by atrasentan in the ITT population.

In a separate pharmacodynamic analysis of biologic end points in this trial, changes in bone deposition markers [total alkaline phosphatase (TAP) and bone alkaline phosphatase (BAP)] and bone resorption markers (N-telopeptides, C-telopeptides, and deoxypyridinoline) were assessed (59). Baseline 1.5- to 2.7-fold elevations above respective upper limits of normal in markers of bone deposition and resorption were demonstrated. Subjects receiving placebo experienced a 58% elevation in mean TAP and a 99% elevation in mean BAP, whereas subjects receiving 10-mg atrasentan maintained stable mean TAP and BAP values compared with baseline. TAP, BAP, and deoxypyridinoline mean changes from baseline were consistently lower in patients receiving 10-mg atrasentan compared with placebo (all $p < 0.05$); N-telopeptides and C-telopeptides showed nonsignificant decreases in treated subjects. Changes in clinical bone scan studies paralleled bone marker changes, adding to the robustness of these findings.

Phase III Data

In a randomized, double-blind, placebo-controlled Phase III study of 10-mg atrasentan that enrolled 809 (401 placebo and 408 atrasentan) subjects with metastatic HRPC, TTP (a composite of radiographic and clinical measures), time to BAP progression (TTBAP, $> 50\%$ increase from nadir), quality of life (QoL), and changes from baseline to final value in PSA, BAP, and TAP were compared (60). This study was closed early by an Independent Data Safety Monitoring Committee upon review of the unexpectedly large number of early events that suggested the trial results would not be different from control outcomes. Once all of the events were accounted for, on ITT analysis, atrasentan compared with placebo nonsignificantly delayed TTP [log-rank $p = 0.091$; hazard ratio (HR) $= 1.14$, 95% CI $= 0.98$–1.34]. As mentioned, the rate of progression was unexpectedly rapid, with $> 50\%$ of subjects achieving end point within 100 days, the majority through bone scan progression. In order to evaluate the differences on median TTP, a $G^{1,1}$ analysis was used per protocol. Although the study statistics were based on the progression rates in the earlier Phase II study, the Phase II study did not mandate bone scans at a 12-wk frequency. The mandated bone scans demonstrated early radiographic progression in the absence of clinical symptoms in the majority of patients. The significance of early radiographic progression without clinical symptoms remains controversial.

On evaluation of secondary end points, atrasentan delayed TTBAP (254 days vs. 505 days; log-rank $p < 0.001$; HR = 1.78, 95% CI = 1.34–2.37), and significantly preserved prostate cancer-specific QoL measured by the FACT-P prostate cancer subscore ($p = 0.032$). Time to PSA progression was longer in patients taking atrasentan, but not significantly (log-rank p = 0.056). The atrasentan group showed smaller mean increases from baseline to final value than the placebo group in PSA ($p = 0.025$), BAP ($p = 0.001$), and TAP ($p < 0.001$). A protocol-specified analysis was conducted on a subset of 671 patients (329 placebo and 342 atrasentan) who met classification criteria defined prior to breaking the study blind, showing that atrasentan significantly delayed TTP (log-rank $p = 0.007$; HR = 1.26, 95% CI = 1.06–1.50) and TTBAP (log-rank $p < 0.001$), and resulted in smaller mean changes from baseline to final in the three biological markers.

To assess the hypothesis that atrasentan efficacy would be more evident in men who had metastases confined to bone at baseline [474 out of 809 patients (59%)] an exploratory analysis was conducted. Atrasentan-treated subjects in this subgroup experienced a significant delay in time to disease progression ($p = 0.002$) further emphasizing the targeted effect of this drug on the ET_A receptor in the bone microenvironment.

Based on the large unmet need for therapies for this patient population, the biologic rationale of the ET_A target in prostate cancer, as well as consistent trends in the clinical trial results, a solicitation for approval of atrasentan for patients with metastatic HRPC was reviewed by the Food and Drug Administration's Oncologic Drugs Advisory Committee. The committee did not recommend approval of atrasentan, citing that more definitive data of clinical benefit were required from additional studies in the metastatic hormone-refractory patient population. Results from the maturing study of atrasentan in nonmetastatic hormone-refractory disease are anticipated in late 2006.

OTHER COMPOUNDS UNDERGOING EVALUATION IN CANCER: ZD4054

ZD4054 is an orally active, specific ET_A antagonist in clinical development. In receptor-binding studies, ZD4054 specifically bound to ET_A with high affinity and no binding with ET_B was detected. In a randomized placebo-controlled trial in eight healthy volunteers, a single oral dose of ZD4054 reduced forearm vasoconstriction in response to brachial artery infusion of ET-1, thus providing clinical evidence of ET_A blockade (61). ET_B blockade was assessed in an ascending, single-dose, placebo-controlled trial in 28 volunteers. The authors used ET-1 plasma levels as a surrogate for ET_B blockade (a rise in ET-1 would indicate ET_B blockade) and concluded that mean plasma ET-1 concentrations measured at 4 and 24 hr were within the placebo reference range and that there was no evidence of dose-related changes. They conclude that as a result of this specificity, ZD4054 has the potential to block multiple ET_A-induced pathological processes, while allowing beneficial ET_B-mediated processes to continue.

CONCLUSIONS

The ET-1/ET_A receptor is a pathway that is profoundly dysregulated in prostate cancer and which is involved in key tumorigenic cellular events such as proliferation, invasion, escape from programmed cell death, new vessel formation, abnormal osteogenesis, and alteration of nociceptive stimuli. Atrasentan is a novel agent that effectively targets this pathway. Biologic activity in patients with prostate cancer has been demonstrated by the suppression of biochemical markers of prostate cancer progression in bone, and clinical activity is evidenced by a consistent trend demonstrating a delay in time to disease progression when compared with placebo, especially in patients with bone metastases. In addition, this success demonstrates that agents targeting resistance to apoptosis are especially relevant to slow growing tumors, such as prostate cancer, whose growth is due to increased apoptosis rather than to increased cell proliferation.

The ET paradigm shows that the interaction of the tumor cell with the microenviroment at the different organ systems ultimately dictates the biologic pattern of disease progression. It may well be that more than a true osseous tropism of prostate cancer cells, their ET-1-secreting capability and the favorable environment that results create a welcoming atmosphere that promotes tumor growth not only by direct, active invasion, but by cooperation with the host organ. This collaboration, together with the disorganized bone growth help explain the preponderance of bone disease with its devastating clinical consequences in prostate and breast cancer patients. Therefore, as is the case in similar interactions such as sepsis, it may be worthwhile and pathogenically relevant to aim therapy at rationally modulating the host's response (e.g., TNF-α secretion or osteoblastic reaction) rather than just targeting the triggering factor (Gram-negative germs or prostate tumor cells, respectively).

The treatment of patients with asymptomatic prostate cancer showing early signs of disease progression while on hormone therapy is one of the most controversial therapeutic scenarios encountered in the management of prostate cancer. This subset of patients represents both a challenge and an opportunity at the same time. The challenge is efficiently and safely delaying the initiation of therapies that may potentially deteriorate QoL such as taxane-based chemotherapy. The opportunity is having an optimal setting to first develop and then employ agents rationally designed to target biologically relevant tumorigenic pathways, with the ultimate goal of stabilizing and controlling the course of the disease. One of the pitfalls usually encountered in cancer management has been the difficulty in evidencing QoL benefits in the context of active treatment strategies, usually due to therapy-related adverse events blunting QoL benefit. The significant maintenance of QoL observed in the above-mentioned atrasentan trials highlights the good tolerability of this agent.

As the rationale for targeting the ET axis appears reasonable and the drug demonstrates clinical activity in prostate cancer, and bearing in mind that it theoretically seems better suited to act in the early Phases of the cell–bone interaction, it is particularly appealing to assess atrasentan in patients with a low disease burden. The first evidence of metastatic spread in prostate cancer patients is the occurrence of bone disease, and atrasentan is under investigation in a further Phase III study in more than 900 men with nonmetastatic HRPC to test the hypothesis that it delays the onset of metastatic disease. This would test the biologic principle that the disruption of the initial cancer cell–bone microenvironment interaction would prevent or delay the initiation of the mutual stimulation processes. In addition, Phase III studies of atrasentan in combination with docetaxel are planned in advanced stage prostate cancer patients through the Southwest Oncology Group.

We are entering a new era of cancer treatment where a shift in the way drugs are developed, clinical studies are designed, and efficacy end points are evaluated is likely to occur, following the paradigm of cancer as a chronic disease for which control rather than cure is the main goal. This is particularly promising in a disease such as prostate cancer that generally occurs in older patients, and where a significant delay in disease progression would, in turn, decrease cancer-related deaths.

SUMMARY

Prostate cancer is an increasingly prevalent tumor in Western societies due to increasing life expectancy. There is a lack of therapeutic options besides cytotoxic chemotherapy for asymptomatic patients that show signs of biochemical failure after hormone therapy. Dysregulation of the ET axis triggers a series of events that ultimately activate proliferation, invasion, escape from programmed cell death, new vessel formation, abnormal osteogenesis, and alteration of nociceptive stimuli. ET receptor antagonists, such as atrasentan and ZD4054, are novel and selective oral agents that effectively target the ET axis and are able to inhibit and/or reverse several of those events. Atrasentan is characterized by dose-proportional pharmacokinetics, which is time-independent across doses, with a moderately rapid absortion, extensive tissue accumulation, metabolism about equally distributed between oxidation and glucuronidation, and an intermediate half-life (21–24 h) that allows a single-daily dosing schedule. The toxicity profile of atrasentan is consistent and manageable, and includes rhinitis, peripheral edema, headache, and asthenia. Atrasentan has demonstrated clinical and biologic activity in patients with metastatic HRPC in a Phase III, placebo-controlled setting. Atrasentan may represent a potential new therapeutic option in the management of prostate cancer, but its precise role in this disease is yet to be defined.

REFERENCES

1. Fox E, Curt GA, Balis FM. Clinical trial design for target-based therapy. Oncologist 2002; 7:401–409.
2. Rubin SA, Levin ER. Clinical review 53: The endocrinology of vasoactive peptides: synthesis to function. J Clin Endocrinol Metab 1994; 78:6–10.
3. Bremnes T, Paasche JD, Mehlum A, Sandberg C, Bremnes B, Attramadal H. Regulation and intracellular trafficking pathways of the endothelin receptors. J Biol Chem 2000; 275:17596–17604.
4. Levin ER. Endothelins. N Engl J Med 1995; 333:356–363.
5. Gray GA, Webb DJ. The endothelin system and its potential as a therapeutic target in cardiovascular disease. Pharmacol Ther 1996; 72:109–148.
6. Bagnato A, Natali PG. Endothelin receptors as novel targets in tumor therapy. J Transl Med 2004; 2:16.
7. Obara K, Koide M, Ishikawa T, Tanabe Y, Nakayama K. Protein kinase C delta but not PKC epsilon activity is involved in contractile potentiation by endothelin-1 in the porcine coronary artery. J Cardiovasc Pharmacol 2000; 36:S120–S121.
8. Daub H, Weiss FU, Wallasch C, Ullrich A. Role of trans activation of the EGF receptor in signalling by G-protein-coupled receptors. Nature 1996; 379:557–560.
9. Jiang ZY, Zhou QL, Chatterjee A, et al. Endothelin-1 modulates insulin signaling through phosphatidylinositol 3-kinase pathway in vascular smooth muscle cells. Diabetes 1999; 48:1120–1130.
10. Battistini B, Chailler P, D'Orleans-Juste P, Briere N, Sirois P. Growth regulatory properties of endothelins. Peptides 1993; 14:385–399.
11. Vacca F, Bagnato A, Catt KJ, Tecce R. Trans activation of the epidermal growth factor receptor in endothelin-1-induced mitogenic signaling in human ovarian carcinoma cells. Cancer Res 2000; 60:5310–5317.

12. Clarke JG, Benjamin N, Larkin SW, Webb DJ, Davies GJ, Maseri A. Endothelin is a potent long-lasting vasoconstrictor in men. Am J Physiol 1989; 257:H2033–H2035.
13. Remuzzi G, Perico N, Benigni A. New therapeutics that antagonize endothelin: promises and frustrations. Nat Rev Drug Discov 2002; 1:986–1001.
14. Touyz RM, Schiffrin EL. Role of endothelin in human hypertension. Can J Physiol Pharmacol 2003; 81:533–541.
15. Nelson J, Bagnato A, Battistini B, Nisen P. The endothelin axis: emerging role in cancer. Nat Rev Cancer 2003; 3:110–116.
16. Bagnato A, Spinella F, Rosano L. Emerging role of the endothelin axis in ovarian tumor progression. Endocr Relat Cancer 2005; 12:761–772.
17. Nelson JB, Hedican SP, George DJ, et al. Identification of endothelin-1 in the pathophysiology of metastatic adenocarcinoma of the prostate. Nat Med 1995; 1:944–949.
18. Nelson JB, Chan-Tack K, Hedican SP, et al. Endothelin-1 production and decreased endothelin B receptor expression in advanced prostate cancer. Cancer Res 1996; 56:663–668.
19. Papandreou CN, Usmani B, Geng Y, et al. Neutral endopeptidase 24.11 loss in metastatic human prostate cancer contributes to androgen-independent progression. Nat Med 1998; 4:50–57.
20. Nelson JB, Lee WH, Nguyen SH, et al. Methylation of the 5′ CpG island of the endothelin B receptor gene is common in human prostate cancer. Cancer Res 1997; 57:35–37.
21. Usmani BA, Harden B, Maitland NJ, Turner AJ. Differential expression of neutral endopeptidase-24.11 (neprilysin) and endothelin-converting enzyme in human prostate cancer cell lines. Clin Sci (Lond) 2002; 103(suppl 48):314S–317S.
22. Salani D, Di Castro V, Nicotra MR, et al. Role of endothelin-1 in neovascularization of ovarian carcinoma. Am J Pathol 2000; 157:1537–1547.
23. Godara G, Cannon GW, Cannon GM Jr., Bies RR, Nelson JB, Pflug BR. Role of endothelin axis in progression to aggressive phenotype of prostate adenocarcinoma. Prostate 2005; 65:27–34.
24. Kopetz ES, Nelson JB, Carducci MA. Endothelin-1 as a target for therapeutic intervention in prostate cancer. Invest New Drugs 2002; 20:173–182.
25. Eberl LP, Valdenaire O, Saintgiorgio V, Jeannin JF, Juillerat-Jeanneret L. Endothelin receptor blockade potentiates FasL-induced apoptosis in rat colon carcinoma cells. Int J Cancer 2000; 86:182–187.
26. Del Bufalo D, Di Castro V, Biroccio A, et al. Endothelin-1 protects ovarian carcinoma cells against paclitaxel-induced apoptosis: requirement for Akt activation. Mol Pharmacol 2002; 61:524–532.
27. Nelson JB, Udan MS, Guruli G, Pflug BR. Endothelin-1 inhibits apoptosis in prostate cancer. Neoplasia 2005; 7:631–637.
28. Del Bufalo D, Di Castro V, Biroccio A, et al. Endothelin-1 acts as a survival factor in ovarian carcinoma cells. Clin Sci (Lond) 2002; 103(suppl 48):302S–305S.
29. Rosano L, Varmi M, Salani D, et al. Endothelin-1 induces tumor proteinase activation and invasiveness of ovarian carcinoma cells. Cancer Res 2001; 61:8340–8346.
30. Rosano L, Salani D, Di Castro V, Spinella F, Natali PG, Bagnato A. Endothelin-1 promotes proteolytic activity of ovarian carcinoma. Clin Sci (Lond) 2002; 103(suppl 48):306S–309S.
31. Rosano L, Spinella F, Di Castro V, et al. Endothelin receptor blockade inhibits molecular effectors of Kaposi's sarcoma cell invasion and tumor growth in vivo. Am J Pathol 2003; 163:753–762.
32. Bagnato A, Rosano L, Spinella F, Di Castro V, Tecce R, Natali PG. Endothelin B receptor blockade inhibits dynamics of cell interactions and communications in melanoma cell progression. Cancer Res 2004; 64:1436–1443.
33. Spinella F, Rosano L, Di Castro V, Nicotra MR, Natali PG, Bagnato A. Endothelin-1 decreases gap junctional intercellular communication by inducing phosphorylation of connexin 43 in human ovarian carcinoma cells. J Biol Chem 2003; 278:41294–41301.
34. Salani D, Taraboletti G, Rosano L, et al. Endothelin-1 induces an angiogenic phenotype in cultured endothelial cells and stimulates neovascularization in vivo. Am J Pathol 2000; 157:1703–1711.

35. Spinella F, Rosano L, Di Castro V, Natali PG, Bagnato A. Endothelin-1 induces vascular endothelial growth factor by increasing hypoxia-inducible factor-1alpha in ovarian carcinoma cells. J Biol Chem 2002; 277:27850–27855.
36. Spinella F, Rosano L, Di Castro V, Nicotra MR, Natali PG, Bagnato A. Inhibition of cyclooxygenase-1 and -2 expression by targeting the endothelin a receptor in human ovarian carcinoma cells. Clin Cancer Res 2004; 10:4670–4679.
37. Gupta S, Srivastava M, Ahmad N, Bostwick DG, Mukhtar H. Over-expression of cyclooxygenase-2 in human prostate adenocarcinoma. Prostate 2000; 42:73–78.
38. Pruthi RS, Derksen JE, Moore D. A pilot study of use of the cyclooxygenase-2 inhibitor celecoxib in recurrent prostate cancer after definitive radiation therapy or radical prostatectomy. BJU Int 2004; 93:275–278.
39. Nelson JB, Nguyen SH, Wu-Wong JR, et al. New bone formation in an osteoblastic tumor model is increased by endothelin-1 overexpression and decreased by endothelin A receptor blockade. Urology 1999; 53:1063–1069.
40. Chiao JW, Moonga BS, Yang YM, et al. Endothelin-1 from prostate cancer cells is enhanced by bone contact which blocks osteoclastic bone resorption. Br J Cancer 2000; 83:360–365.
41. Yin JJ, Mohammad KS, Kakonen SM, et al. A causal role for endothelin-1 in the pathogenesis of osteoblastic bone metastases. Proc Natl Acad Sci USA 2003; 100:10954–10959.
42. Guise TA, Yin JJ, Mohammad KS. Role of endothelin-1 in osteoblastic bone metastases. Cancer 2003; 97:779–784.
43. Pomonis JD, Rogers SD, Peters CM, Ghilardi JR, Mantyh PW. Expression and localization of endothelin receptors: implications for the involvement of peripheral glia in nociception. J Neurosci 2001; 21:999–1006.
44. Jarvis MF, Wessale JL, Zhu CZ, et al. ABT-627, an endothelin ET(A) receptor-selective antagonist, attenuates tactile allodynia in a diabetic rat model of neuropathic pain. Eur J Pharmacol 2000; 388:29–35.
45. Yuyama H, Koakutsu A, Fujiyasu N, et al. Inhibitory effects of a selective endothelin-A receptor antagonist YM598 on endothelin-1-induced potentiation of nociception in formalin-induced and prostate cancer-induced pain models in mice. J Cardiovasc Pharmacol 2004; 44(suppl 1):S479–482.
46. Yuyama H, Koakutsu A, Fujiyasu N, et al. Effects of selective endothelin ET(A) receptor antagonists on endothelin-1-induced potentiation of cancer pain. Eur J Pharmacol 2004; 492:177–182.
47. Khodorova A, Navarro B, Jouaville LS, et al. Endothelin-B receptor activation triggers an endogenous analgesic cascade at sites of peripheral injury. Nat Med 2003; 9: 1055–1061.
48. Peters CM, Lindsay TH, Pomonis JD, et al. Endothelin and the tumorigenic component of bone cancer pain. Neuroscience 2004; 126:1043–1052.
49. Wu-Wong JR, Dixon DB, Chiou WJ, et al. Pharmacology of endothelin receptor antagonists ABT-627, ABT-546, A-182086 and A-192621: in vitro studies. Clin Sci (Lond) 2002; 103(suppl 48):107S–111S.
50. Zhu T, Andre A, Facey I, et al. Effect of ketoconazole (KET) on the pharmacokinetics (PK) of atrasentan (ABT-627, ATN). In: Proceedings of the 40th American Society of Clinical Oncology Annual Meeting, New Orleans, LA, USA, 2004.
51. Xiong H, Jankowski J, Ashbrenner E, et al. Effect of rifampin (RIF) on the pharmacokinetics (PK) of atrasentan (ABT-627, ATN). In: Proceedings of the 40th American Society of Clinical Oncology Annual Meeting, New Orleans, LA, USA, 2004.
52. Klein CE, Schroeder MC, Facey I, et al. Effect of atrasentan (ABT-627, ATN) on the pharmacokinetics (PK) of fexofenadine (FEX). In: Proceedings of the 40th American Society of Clinical Oncology Annual Meeting, New Orleans, LA, USA, 2004.
53. Katz DA, Grimm DR, Carr R, et al. Pharmacogenetic meta-analysis suggests that atrasentan is an organic anion transport protein C substrate. Clin Pharm Ther 2004; 75:94.
54. Samara E, Dutta S, Cao G, Granneman GR, Dordal MS, Padley RJ. Single-dose pharmacokinetics of atrasentan, an endothelin-A receptor antagonist. J Clin Pharmacol 2001; 41:397–403.

55. Carducci MA, Nelson JB, Bowling MK, et al. Atrasentan, an endothelin-receptor antagonist for refractory adenocarcinomas: safety and pharmacokinetics. J Clin Oncol 2002; 20:2171–2180.
56. Zonnenberg BA, Groenewegen G, Janus TJ, et al. Phase I dose-escalation study of the safety and pharmacokinetics of atrasentan: an endothelin receptor antagonist for refractory prostate cancer. Clin Cancer Res 2003; 9:2965–2972.
57. Ryan CW, Vogelzang NJ, Vokes EE, et al. Dose-ranging study of the safety and pharmacokinetics of atrasentan in patients with refractory malignancies. Clin Cancer Res 2004; 10:4406–4411.
58. Carducci MA, Padley RJ, Breul J, et al. Effect of endothelin-A receptor blockade with atrasentan on tumor progression in men with hormone-refractory prostate cancer: a randomized, Phase II, placebo-controlled trial. J Clin Oncol 2003; 21:679–689.
59. Nelson JB, Nabulsi AA, Vogelzang NJ, et al. Suppression of prostate cancer induced bone remodeling by the endothelin receptor A antagonist atrasentan. J Urol 2003; 69:1143–1149.
60. Carducci MA, Nelson JB, Saad F, et al. Effects of atrasentan on disease progression and biological markers in men with metastatic hormone-refractory prostate cancer: Phase 3 study. In: Proceedings of the 40th American Society of Clinical Oncology Annual Meeting, New Orleans, LA, USA, 2004.
61. Morris CD, Rose A, Curwen J, Hughes AM, Wilson DJ, Webb DJ. Specific inhibition of the endothelin A receptor with ZD4054: Clinical and pre-clinical evidence. Br J Cancer 2005; 92:2148–2152.

5 Targeting Extracellular Molecules in Prostate Cancer—Mechanisms to Inhibit Entry into the Cell-Signaling Abyss

Susan F. Slovin

Genitourinary Oncology Service, Department of Medicine, Memorial Sloan-Kettering Cancer Center, New York, New York, U.S.A.

INTRODUCTION

Rationale for Targeted Investigation

The rationale for the development of drugs which target extracellular and intracellular pathways has been predicated on the observation that there are a variety of overexpressed and underglycosylated molecules on the cell surface to which ligands bind or somehow interact causing a cascade of events that lead to intracellular signaling modulation and/or interference with cell growth (Tables 1 and 2). However, while some extracellular molecules can serve as potential targets for drug development, one of the major concerns is that they may not always be in contact with intracellular pathways to affect cellular function; their expression on the cell surface may also be variable because of a wide variety of host factors. Despite targeting receptor-like molecules such as the epidermal growth factor receptor (EGFR), human epidermal growth factor receptor-2 (HER-2)/neu, and BCL-2 pathways which can stimulate intracellular signaling pathways, the cell can develop "collateral" signaling and survival pathways. Although target activation can be blocked using "small" molecules or monoclonal antibodies, the cell can still overcome blockade via multiple mechanisms rendering treatment markedly inadequate. There are multiple cell surface molecules which can serve as targets for immunologic approaches including those on the cell surface such as mucins [MUC-1 (1–3), MUC-2 (3–5), and MUC-18 (6)], glycolipids [Globo H (7–9) and GM2 (10)], and glycoproteins [prostate-specific antigen (PSA) (11,12), prostate-specific membrane antigen (PSMA) (Figs. 1 and 2) (13,14), and prostate stem-cell antigen (PSCA) (15)], in addition to the androgen receptor (16,17), EGFR (18–20), insulin growth factor receptor (21), laminin receptor (22), granulocyte-macrophage colony-stimulating factor (GM-CSF) receptor (23), Platelet-derived growth factor receptor (PDGFR) (24) and checkpoint molecules such as cytotoxic T lymphocyte-associated antigen 4 (CTLA-4) (25–27). Agents which target-specific intracellular sites have included calcitriol (28,29) for the vitamin D receptor; Hsp90 via the ansamycins, e.g., 17-AAG (30,31); the proteasome via PS-341, i.e., Velcade™ (32–34), histone deacetylase (HDACs) via suberoylanilide hydroxamic acid (35–37), as well as the relationship of all of these molecules to stroma and neovasculature. The interactions between the binding of cell surface molecules to their respective ligands leading to a cascade of intracellular events have become extraordinarily complex with multiple interactions occurring synchronously. The article will highlight some of the many extracellular surface molecules to which novel drugs can be

TABLE 1 Rationale for Targeted Intervention

Pro	Con
Overexpression and underglycosylation of cell surface molecules	Strictly extracellular, no contact with intercellular pathways; expression varies
Can target receptor-like molecules which can stimulate intracellular signaling pathways	Cell can develop "collateral" signaling/survival pathways
Can prevent target activation	Cell can overcome via multiple mechanisms rendering treatment inadequate

targeted with the idea that there remains a stunning diversity of other mechanisms by which cell growth can be modulated.

POTENTIAL ROLE OF CLUSTER-DEFINED MOLECULES

Attempts to target-specific cell surface molecules have been limited by a variety of problems (Table 1). First, cell surface expression of a particular molecule may be inconsistent given the fact that multiple factors can alter cell surface expression such as the cell's nutritional status, duration of the cells in a particular phase of the cell cycle, and environmental insults such as changes temperature or pH. A second issue is that prostate tumor growth is heterogeneous such that it is difficult to identify earlier those malignant cells which have the potential for aggressive behavior and will impact on the patient's longevity, while other populations remain indolent. Crucial to the identification of these more aggressive cell types is the need to identify markers which can be used to isolate these cells for study. Liu (38–41) and others reported the presence of specific cell surface molecules as defined by flow cytometry using monoclonal antibodies. These "cluster-defined" or differentiation/designation antigens, CD57 and CD44 (38,39) could be used to identify two prostate cancer cell types as well as identify and define cell functionality. As expression of CD molecules is linked to the physiologic state of cells, these molecules can be used to study not only cell function but also cellular differentiation. The integrin family is one such example of complexes and their ligands which are well characterized and may be a target for small molecules. CD49a/CD29 ($\alpha_1\beta_1$) (37), whose ligand is laminin is present only on stromal cells. Recent work with small molecules such as PCK3145 (42), a 15mer synthetic peptide bearing homology to prostate secretory protein 94 (PSP^{94}) (amino acids 31–45), is one

TABLE 2 Have We Succeeded or Failed in Our Treatments for Prostate Cancer?

Success	Failure
Docetaxel: new standard of care	Few approved Ph III drugs
Multiple targeting pathways	Which is the "one" to stop growth?
New drugs in the pipeline	Too many approved too fast or too few reaching approval status
Responses after first-line CAB	Disease moves too fast, less response to second-line combined androgen blockade
Bone-seeking drugs: improved toxicity profile	No impact on important measures
Immune therapies: vaccines, MoAbs, cytokines	End points: biologic, therapeutic?

Abbreviations: MoAb, monoclonal antibody.

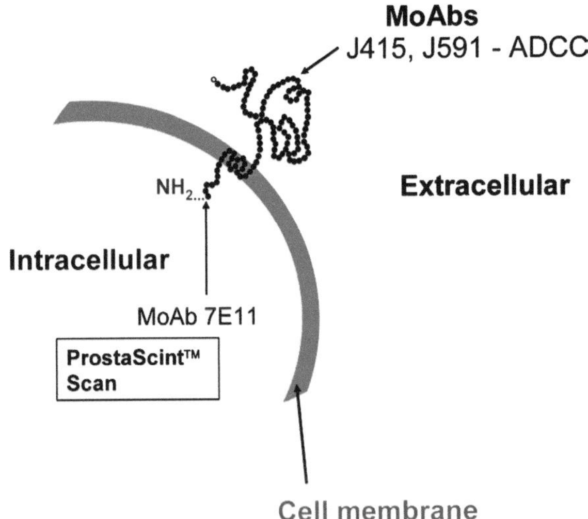

FIGURE 1 Cartoon depicting the type II integral transmembrane nature of prostate-specific membrane antigen. *Source*: Courtesy of Dr. Peter Smith-Jones.

such agent in clinical trials which may not only interact with the laminin receptor but also function at multiple levels to inhibit growth pathways via inhibition of angiogenesis and matrix metalloproteinases 4 and 9. CD44 (37,38) represents an advanced cancer cell type as it was found less frequently in primary tumors and more prominently in soft tissue metastases. Normal luminal cells are positive for CD57 whereas basal cells are positive for CD55. A total of 119 CD specificities were screened for reactivity to several prostate cancer cells lines including LNCaP, PC3, and DU145 (37). The expression phenotypes for cell lines derived from metastasis-derived metastatic cell lines such as DU145 and PC3 are similar as these two lines are biologically alike in behavior. Whereas LNCaP retained the differentiated functions of prostate secretory cells in the synthesis of PSA and response to androgen

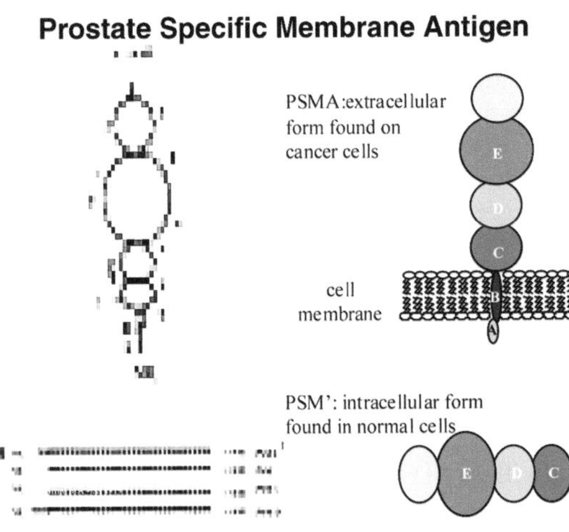

FIGURE 2 (*See color insert*) Prostate-specific membrane antigen as a globular molecule with demonstration of the extracellular, transmembrane, and intracellular domains. *Abbreviations*: PSMA, prostate-specific membrane antigen. *Source*: Courtesy of the Cancer Information Group, I.P.

regulation, PC3 and DU145 have not. Neither of these cell lines stain positively for CD57, a luminal cell marker found in a majority of cancer cells in primary tumor as and a marker of well-differentiated cancer. However, they expressed basal cell markers such as CD49b (integrin α_2), CD49f (α_6), CD55 (colony-accelerating factor), CD59 (membrane attack complex-inhibitory factor), CD99R, CD104 (integrin β_4), and CD44. CD49b/CD29 ($\alpha_2\beta_1$), whose ligand is collagen, is present only on basal cells. This complex has been shown to promote adhesion of prostatic cells to bone cell matrix and are another site for potential drug development. Along similar lines, work by Luo et al. (43), showed that human CD66 protein, a molecule which has been shown to mediate homotypic cell adhesion, when expressed in DU145 prostate cancer cells, could reduce the ability of these cells to form tumors in a xenograft animal model, suggesting that human CD661 has tumor-suppressive activity. CD66a, like its rat homolog cell–cell adhesion molecule is a cell adhesion molecule when expressed in vitro and may function in maintain communication between prostate epithelial cells.

PSCA—WHAT ROLE DOES IT PLAY AS A CELL SURFACE MOLECULE?

PSCA, a 123 amino acid cell surface glycoprotein is highly expressed in both local and metastatic prostate cancers as well as in a high percentage of bladder and pancreatic cancers. It is a member of the Thy-1/Ly-6 family of glycosylphosphatidylinositol-anchored cell surface antigens with its expression regulated by androgens (15,44,45). Its overexpression correlates with a high risk of recurrence after primary therapy for prostate cancer, high tumor grade, advanced stage, extracapsular invasion, and androgen-independent progression (46). PSCA is co-amplified by MYC, an independent predictor of progression and death (47). While it remains unclear as to the cause of PSCA overexpression, the gene is localized on chromosome 8q24.2, distal to the MCY gene. MYC overexpression has also been shown to be an independent predictor of progression and death in men with locally advanced prostate cancer. Reiter et al. (15) demonstrated that MYC and PSCA were co-amplified in 25% of tumors and that PSCA gene amplification correlated with PSCA protein expression suggesting that amplification was one mechanism by which PSCA was overexpressed in advanced tumors. PSCA was therefore viewed as a potential cell surface marker for further investigation.

While there are many molecules which are highly overexpressed on the cell surface of localized and metastatic prostate cancers, PSCA has been evaluated as a potential diagnostic and therapeutic target for the development of prostate cancer therapies (48,49). Dannull et al. (50) demonstrated that cytotoxic T cell from patients with metastatic prostate cancer could be generated against PSCA. Not only did the T cells peptide-pulsed targets but were also capable of recognizing prostate cancer cell lines by chromium release assays. An anti-PSCA monoclonal antibody, 1G8 (51), was developed and shown to inhibit tumor growth, prevent metastasis, and prolong survival of mice inoculated with human prostate cancer cell lines and xenografts (LAPC-9). More recently, Gu et al. (51) demonstrated that 1G8 worked by an Fc-independent mechanism to inhibit tumor growth both in vitro and in vivo. This is in contradistinction to other antitumor antibodies such as Rituxan and Herceptin which require the presence of function FcγRIII (52) receptor on macrophages and natural killer cells for their preclinical activity. PSCA as a clinical target has been further studied by Ross et al. (53) who showed that established xenograft tumors could be successfully eradicated by a passive immunotherapy approach. Several anti-PSCA monoclonal antibodies (MoAbs) were generated which recognized PSCA on the surface of live cells and were efficiently internalized after antigen recognition. When given alone or when conjugated with DM1, a maytansinoid toxin, the authors were able to demonstrate in vitro cytotoxicity in an antigen-specific manner and in vivo efficacy with complete tumor eradication in a majority of treated animals (53). Similar approaches are now being translated into the clinical arena.

MEDIATORS OF RECEPTOR TYROSINE KINASE PATHWAYS

The HER family of receptor tyrosine kinases (TKs) is one of multiple pathways involved in the development and progression of prostate cancer. HER-kinase receptors include the family of EGFRs, HER2, HER3, and HER4, which can homodimerize or heterodimerize to affect signaling (20). There are multiple mechanisms which can lead to increased or inappropriate EGFR TK activity including altered expression of EGFR, its ligand, or interacting molecules; decreased deactivation through phosphatases or down-regulation, or possible mutation of the EGFR protein (20,54). Different combinations of receptors produce different qualities and levels of pathway activation. Among HER-family receptors, HER2 activation is particularly important in breast cancer, as HER2 gene amplification is associated with a distinct clinical course and response to treatment with a HER2-directed therapy (trastuzumab).

EGF has also been shown to induce vascular endothelial growth factor (VEGF) gene expression in DU145 and PC3 prostate cell lines in a dose-dependent manner (55,56). Given that autocrine production of TGF-α and over-expression of EGFR may contribute to the androgen-independent state at both primary and metastatic sites, one monoclonal antibody previously studied, C225, has also been shown to inhibit growth of DU145 prostate cancer cell line by inducing G1 arrest with a marked decrease in CDK2-, cyclin A- and cyclin E-associated histone H1 kinase activities in concert with a sustained increase in cell cycle inhibitor p27KIP1 (57). EGFR activation did not appear to play a functional role in androgen-stimulated growth of LNCaP cells in vitro (58).

Unlike Herceptin, the inhibitory MoAb that blocks HER-2 requires that the tumor express high levels of EGFR for optimal response to second-line therapy, this was not the case with a combination trial of chemotherapy and C225 in colon cancer, where response to drug was 22% irrespective of levels of receptor expression in biopsy tissue from patients' tumors (59,60). Innovative therapies have been aimed at inhibiting increased EGFR TK activity include antibodies that block the extracellular ligand-binding site, antibody or ligand fusion proteins that specifically target toxins or chemotherapeutic drugs to the tumor cells, or small-molecule TK inhibitors that act intracellularly to block downstream signal transduction from EGFR. Studies have shown that blockade can lead to reduced cellular proliferation, inhibition of survival signals, and inhibition of tumor metastasis and to a limited degree, angiogenesis. Additional agents, including EGFR antibodies and TK inhibitors such as C225 have been shown to be effective against various human solid tumors in preclinical models (61) and have shown activity in advanced nonsmall cell lung cancer, colon, head and neck, breast, renal, prostate, and pancreatic cancers.

TK inhibitors, such as gefitinib (Iressa, ZD1839), block the EGFR (62). As a result, there is inhibition of cellular proliferation, promotion of apoptosis, and inhibition of anti-angiogenesis. Gefitinib, combined with flutamide, produced an additive growth inhibition in prostate cancer. The antitumor activity of PD168393 (62), an irreversible EGFR inhibitor, with or without chemotherapeutic agents for the treatment of androgen-independent prostate cancer has also been studied. Both the androgen-independent cell lines PC-3 and DU145 expressed higher levels of EGFR than the androgen-dependent MDA PCa 2b and androgen-responsive LNCaP cells by Western blotting. DU145 was much more sensitive to PD168393 and ZD1839 than MDA PCa 2b. PD168393, but not ZD1839, significantly potentiated paclitaxel cytotoxicity against DU145 by MTT assay and median-effect analysis. The combination of PD168393 or ZD1839 with other cytotoxic agents including docetaxel and 5-fluorouracil, however, was either additive or antagonistic. Compared with paclitaxel alone, PD168393 significantly enhanced paclitaxel-induced DNA fragmentation, sub-G1 fraction accumulation, mitochondrial membrane dysfunction, cytochrome C release, caspase-3 activation, and eventually apoptosis (62). The combination of paclitaxel and PD168393 produced a profound synergistic growth inhibition of AIPC cells. Combining PD168393 with paclitaxel may have clinical benefits and may warrant further investigation.

Recently, Veeramani et al. (63) found that in addition to the secreted form of prostatic acid phosphatase which has been used as a surrogate serologic marker in lieu of PSA, the cellular form of prostatic acid phosphatase (cPAcP) functioned as a neutral protein tyrosine phosphatase in prostate cancer cells and dephosphorylated HER-2/ErbB-2/Neu at the phosphotyrosine (p-Tyr) residues. By dephosphorylating HER-2 at its p-Tyr residues, there was a down-regulation of its specific activity, which led to decreases in growth and tumorigenicity of cancer cells. Conversely, decreased cPAcP expression correlated with hyperphosphorylation of HER-2 at tyrosine residues and activation of downstream extracellular signal-regulated kinase (ERK)/mitogen-activated protein kinase signaling, which resulted in prostate cancer progression as well as androgen-independent growth of prostate cancer cells. These in vitro results on the effect of cPAcP on androgen-independent growth of prostate cancer cells appeared to correlate with the clinical observations that cPAcP level was greatly decreased in androgen-independent disease and may impact on prostate cancer progression.

While the EGFR system has been well-studied, a second distinct class of receptor, the urokinase-type plasminogen activator (uPAR) has also been shown to be upregulated in aggressive prostate cancers (64). uPAR can promote tumor invasion not only by cellular signaling of migration via surface receptors such as EGFR, but also by matrix degradation by its protease ligand, uPA. The interest in this pathway has widened due to part of the cellular signaling from uPAR occurring in part via EGFR trans activation (65,66). Inhibition of EGFR kinase activity blocks uPAR-initiated activation of ERK MAP kinase but not of the small rho-GTPases. ERK is required for EGFR induction of both motility and proliferation; inhibition of this secondary function leads to blockade of cell motility and proliferation otherwise induced by uPAR (64,65). The EGFR appears to be a needed constituent for uPAR-mediated tumor progression based on tumor model systems which demonstrated that abrogation of EGFR signaling blocks uPAR-associated invasiveness through an extracellular matrix. Mamouone et al. (66) demonstrated for the first time that EGFR signaling increased uPAR-mediated phenotypic cell behavior in prostate tumor cells and that this increase in uPAR activity was downstream from the phospholipase C-γ (PLCγ) signaling. The authors concluded that the uPAR–uPA complex contributed to invasion of prostate cancer cells but only in the presence of the EGFR/PLCγ signaling cascade.

Preclinical work in mice using C225, an anti-EGFR MoAb developed by Mendelsohn (59), in combination with cisplatin suggested a synergistic antitumor effect (61). Recent studies (67,68) in mice receiving the gefitinib–trastuzumab combination, the reduction in tumor volume was inferior to that predicted by the observed impact of the agents alone. Clinical trials in prostate cancer (14) have not been as promising as those in other diseases probably because of subtherapeutic dosing and drugs which at the time of testing were inferior to the current taxanes. The idea that two monoclonal antibodies against EGFR might be synergistic was studied by Formento et al. (67,68) using prostate cancer cell lines. Data from DU-145 cells suggested that dual targeting of EGFR and HER-2 may be inappropriate for the treatment of hormone-refractory prostate cancer, especially in the context of their combination with radiation. The application of ZD1839 led to a marked elevation in the level of p27, a negative regulator of cell division, p27. The ZD1839–trastuzumab combination was inferior on p27 expression compared with the effect of ZD1839 alone. A diminished expression of Bax, an apoptotic-related protein, was observed in the presence of the drug combination. There was a significant synergy between radiation and either ZD1839 or trastuzumab treatments. In contrast, the drug combination with radiation resulted in antagonistic cytotoxic effects. These data suggested that multiple other molecular mechanisms might be involved in these results. Despite these results, there has been renewed interest in re-assessing the combination of C225 and similar agents with novel drugs.

PLATELET-DERIVED GROWTH FACTOR AS A TARGET FOR THERAPY

The platelet-derived growth factor (PDGF) is a diverse family of peptide growth factors that signal through cell surface, TK receptors (PDGFR) and stimulate growth, proliferation, transformation, and differentiation. While initially thought to exist as three dimeric polypeptides (homodimers AA and BB, and the heterodimer, AB), recently PDGF-C and -D chains were discovered. Increased expression of PDGF-D has been found in several tumors including ovarian, lung, renal, and glioma-derived cell lines suggesting a correlation between increased PDGF-D expression and human cancer (69,70). Ustach et al. (70) studied the possible relationship between PDGF-B, thought to be critical for prostate cancer progression, and PDGF-D, a specific ligand for PDGFR-β. The authors showed that human prostate cancer cells, LNCaP processes latent PDGF DD into an active form under serum-free conditions, resulting in the promotion of LNCaP growth. PDGF DD expression also was shown to enhance the prostate carcinoma cell interaction with the surrounding stromal layer in a SCID mouse model suggesting some potential form of oncogenic activity. As in the case of EGFR, PDGFR is expressed on a diversity of solid tumors including prostate cancers where it is expressed in up to 88% of primary prostate cancers (71) and in 80% of prostate metastases (71). It also functions via autocrine and paracrine stimulations impacting both the adjacent stroma and vasculature (72). Compounds such as imatinib mesylate (STI571) or Gleevec which has been used to block Bcr-Abl in hematologic tumors, and has been studied in prostate cancer based on its potent inhibition of PDGFR autophosphorylation. Given the sometimes limited potential of single agent therapy, Kubler et al. (69) examined the cytotoxic effects of imatinib in combination with estramustine phosphate and 4-hydroperoxy-cyclophosphamide in LNCaP, PC-3, and DU145 prostate cell lines. The authors found that imatinib produced additive effects with estramustine phosphate and 4-hydroperoxy-cyclophosphamide in all three cell lines with etoposide producing additive effects in two of the three lines, and docetaxel causing antagonistic effects in PC-3. Because of the variability of expression of PDGFR-β on prostate cancer, strategies have been developed to detect which patients might likely benefit from imatinib using a cDNA expression array from 10,000 transcripts for PDGFR expression and divided tumors in groups based on the PDGFR expression level (73). A set of genes was identified whose expression was associated with PDGFR-β status including early growth response 1 (Egr1), an upstream effector of PDGF, α-methylacyl-CoA racemase, and v-Maf and neuroblastoma suppressor of tumorigenicity. This data supported the idea that a small subset of prostate cancers may be sensitive to TK inhibitors specific for PDGF.

INHIBITORS OF PDGFR

PDGFR inhibitors such as SU101 was studied in a multi-institutional Phase II trial of 44 hormone-refractory patients (71). SU101 was administered intravenously at $400\,mg/m^2$ as a loading dose for 4 days followed by 10 weekly infusions at $400\,mg/m^2$ with the primary end points of the study being a decline in PSA and decrease in measurable tumor. Of the 39 assessable patients, three patients had a PSA decline of $>50\%$ from baseline and a median time to progression of 90 days. Of 19 patients evaluated for measurable disease, only one patient had a partial response with nine patients have significant improvement in pain control. Although the response was modest, the authors felt that its significant expression profile on prostate cancer warranted further investigation. Another study by Roa et al. (74) studied 21 patients with androgen sensitive disease in a Phase II trial with patients receiving 400 mg of imatinib orally twice daily for 24 wk. Immunohistochemistry on the corresponding tumor samples of four patients confirmed PDGFR-α and -β. Of 16 assessable patients, nine demonstrated a stable PSA and seven patients had PSA progression. Grade 3 and 4 toxicity included rash, hematuria, diarrhea, and neutropenia. While safe, activity was again modest in this small series of androgen sensitive patients. Recent data (75) have suggested that calcitriol, a hormonal form of vitamin D, could regulate the expression of PDGFR and PDGF-BB isoform mediated growth. Calcitriol was found to downregulate PDGFR-β expression and negatively regulate PDGF-mediated cell growth without affecting PDGFR-α and -β mRNA expression. The authors suggested that inhibition of PDGFR-β expression by calcitriol might be able to reduce responsiveness of prostate cells to mitogenic action of PDGF-BB.

TARGETS OF IMMUNOLOGIC RECOGNITION: ENHANCING IMMUNOGENICITY THROUGH VACCINES BY ENHANCING T CELL FUNCTION

Recombinant approaches have afforded the opportunity to test the hypothesis that immunologic tolerance can be disturbed with vaccines which target molecules such as PSMA (Figs. 1,2) and PSA. Plasmids which encode the sequence of molecules such as PSMA and DNA have been used (13,14,76,77). The main effectors in antitumor immunity after DNA immunizations are $CD8^+$ cytotoxic T cells that recognize tumor or tumor-associated antigen-derived peptides or proteins expressed in the context of the class I major histocompatibility molecules (MHC). The benefits of a DNA vaccine are many and include: (1) it is relatively inexpensive and simple to purify in large quantities (2), avoids complex ex vivo expansion and manipulation of patients cell (3), antigen of interest is cloned into a bacterial expression plasmid with a constitutively active promoter (4), the bacterial plasmid DNA contains immunostimulatory sequences (cpG motifs) which act as an immunologic adjuvant, and (5) direct entry of the antigen into the intracellular MHC class I pathway.

Mincheff et al. (77) studied two plasmid DNA vaccines encoding either produces that are retained in the cytosol and degraded in the proteasome (TVacs and HPSMAT, respectively), or secreted proteins (sVacs and hPSMAs). Immunization with both vectors given in combination with the cytokine GM-CSF led to the generation of T cell-mediated cytotoxicity in preclinical studies supported the use of a strategy which could induce a strong cellular cytotoxic response. The authors demonstrated that priming with tVacs and boosting with protein could induce antibody formation; antibodies were of the cytotoxic Th1 isotype. Therefore this model seemed to suggest that the best strategy in gene-based vaccination was to prime with the xenogeneic and boost with the autologous constructs. This has also shown to be feasible in patients (13).

STUDIES IN MEN

A study by Todorova et al. (76) immunized prostate patients with plasmid and adenoviral vectors, each encoding for the extracellular portion of human PSMA, then tested for anti-PSMA antibodies by Western blot. PSMA-producing LNCaP cells were used as a control. Using these multiple gene-based vaccinations induced an anti-PSMA humoral immune response. Specific anti-PSMA antibodies were detected in the immunized patients' sera, mainly against the PSMA protein core.

An alternative strategy has been shown by Dunphy and McNeel (78) who identified prostate-associated antigens which were immunologically recognized in 13 prostate patients treated with multiple cycles of a potent growth and differentiation factor for dendritic cells, flt3 ligand. Flt3 ligand has been shown in murine tumor models to induce dendritic cells systemically which can lead to the eradication of established solid tumors such a murine melanoma and lymphoma. A prior vaccine, E75 HLA-A2 epitope from HER-2/neu, was given with flt3 ligand as a systemic vaccine adjuvant for a peptide vaccine to patients with advanced hormone resistant prostate cancer (79). Using a normal prostate cDNA expression library and sera from subjects before and after treatment with flt3 ligand, a modified SEREX approach was used to identify six proteins to which IgG antibody responses were augmented posttreatment versus pretreatment with flt3. The results of this technology resulted in a novel prostate-associated antigen, MAD-CaP-5 now the target of increased interest. This molecule was found to encode a protein of unknown function (KIAA1404) that has also been identified in other tumor types.

One of the issues in using PSMA as a target has been based on the observation that PSMA is normally targeted directly to the apical plasma membrane, thereby suggesting than any therapeutic antibodies to PSM would only be able to bind to highly transformed and poorly differentiated tumor cells. While metastatic cells are generally considered highly transformed and nonpolarized, Christiansen et al. (80), found that within an occult metastatic lesion, populations of prostatic carcinoma cells maintain a well-differentiated epithelial morphology. The authors postulated that while PSMA-directed immunotherapy would be effective at combating highly transformed prostate cancer cell, such an approach would not be equally effective for treatment of well-differentiated tumors. They recommend that therapeutic strategies are needed which could reduce the obstructive influence of epithelial barriers. Their data supports this by demonstrating that treating polarized epithelial cells with the microtubule-targeting agents of the class of *Vinca* alkaloids results in increased binding and endocytosis of PSMA-specific antibodies from the basolateral surface in an in vitro system. This suggests that chemotherapeutic agents may more effectively target PSMA by directing therapy to intrinsic protein trafficking machinery to reverse the apical polarity of an antigen to the basolateral plasma membrane.

PSA still remains a target of interest for immune therapy through multidisciplinary approaches. A recent report by Miller et al. (11) studied six patients with advanced hormone-refractory prostate cancer for their ability to elicit PSA-specific cytotoxic T cell responses following a pVAX/PSA DNA vaccine given at doses of 100 and 900 μg, respectively. The vaccine was produced from a gene coding for the full-length human PSA protein which was inserted into the pVAX1 vector. The pVAX/PSA vaccine was administered together with GM-CSF and IL-2 as vaccine adjuvants. While initial studies with this construct was safe, preliminary results suggested that 900 μg dose of the vaccine could induce cellular and humoral immune responses against PSA protein. Additional analyses suggested that a cellular immune response could be induced using ELISPOT analyses demonstrating production of interferon-γ as well as IL-4 and IL-6.

MANIPULATION OF THE T CELL—CAN CHANGING EXPRESSION OF CELL SURFACE MOLECULES AFFECT FUNCTION?

Allison's group (25–27,81–83) has identified a protein on the T cell surface, CTLA-4 that can suppress their ability to attack cancer cells. While attempts at manipulating T cells as a major component of immune responses to a wide-range of immunologic therapies, the rationale for less than optimal results has been felt to be due to technical difficulties in assessing T cell responses in the laboratory as well as limitations in understanding the normal regulatory processes that limit T cells responses in order to avoid autoimmunity. While T cell responses are initiated by T cell antigen receptor signaling in the context of an antigen within the pocket of MHC on the cell surface, multiple cell surface molecules also participate in a complex interplay with cytokines which can act in a stimulatory or inhibitory manner. Our understanding of the complexity of these regulatory pathways was increased by the demonstration by several groups that B7.1 and B7.2, whose expression is limited to "professional" antigen presenting cells (APCs):fsfc (Fig. 3), can also interact with another molecule, CTLA-4 (84) (Fig. 3). while initially thought to be another co-stimulatory molecule, Allison's group showed that it was an inhibitory molecule which functioned as a "checkpoint" that limits T cell activation and expansion. It also has been shown to play a critical role in preventing or enhance autoimmunity in several animal systems. Prior studies using multiple experimental tumors in mice showed that CTLA-4 blockade could

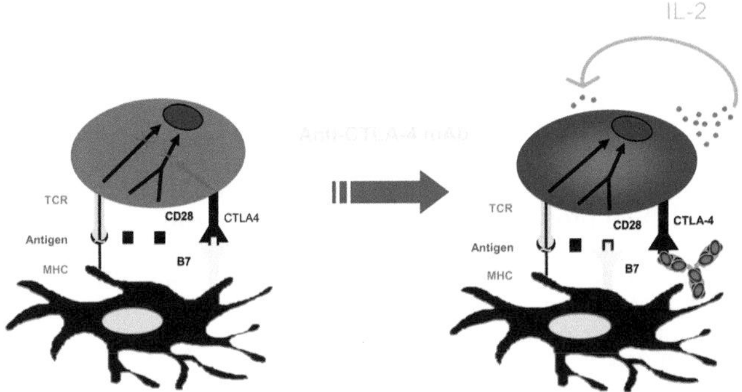

FIGURE 3 Interaction of cytotoxic T lymphocyte-associated antigen 4 on the cell surface with monoclonal antibody, MDX-010. Note engagement of the T cell receptor with antigen on the dendritic cell along with engagement of B7.1, B7.2 with CD28 leading to activation of cytokines and

enhance antitumor responses either as a single agent or in combination with a vaccine (85–87) CTLA-4 blockade could synergize with conventional cytotoxic therapies including vaccines in patients with prostate cancer, melanoma, renal carcinoma and ovarian cancers. One study demonstrated significant synergism when given with G-Vax™ to a patient with recurrent ovarian cancer (88). Rechallenge of the patient with CTLA-4 after receiving prior vaccine resulted in decline in CA-125 for over two years with stabilization of disease. While there have been instances of "autoimmune breakthrough events," characterized in rare instances by hypophysitis, colitis, and pancreatitis, they have been seen mainly in what are thought to be immunologically-driven malignancies such as melanoma and renal cell carcinoma. Clinical trials are currently underway in patients with metastatic prostate cancer. While CTLA-4 is the prototype of checkpoint blockade, there are other molecules that may offer additional targets for blockade. While there are at least seven members of the extended B7 family of molecules, at least three of these, B7-H1, B7-H3, and B7x (the latter identified by Allison's group), also inhibit T cells response but do so at later stages than CTLA-4.

CONCLUSIONS

Like the intracellular milieu, the extracellular domain remains an appealing area of research and discovery. Those molecules discussed here are only a small representation of the heterogeneous population of molecules which impact in some capacity on prostate cancer growth. While the interactions between cell surface molecules and the intracellular pathways governing cell growth remain highly complex and interactive, nevertheless, novel drugs should continue to be evaluated which may impact at some level of the signaling hierarchy thereby leading to complete growth arrest and/or cell death.

REFERENCES

1. Slovin SF, Livingston P, Keeperman K, et al. Targeted therapy in prostate cancer: vaccination with glycoprotein, MUC-1-KLH-QS21 peptide conjugate [abstr 620]. J Urol 1997; 157:160.

2. Slovin SF, Livingston P, Zhang S, et al. Targeted therapy in prostate cancer (PC): Vaccination with a glycoprotein, MUC-1-KLH-QS21 peptide conjugate [abstr 1107]. Proc Am Soc Clin Onc 1997; 16:311a.
3. Ragupathi G, Adluri R, Amaravathi R, et al. Specificity analysis of sera from breast and prostate cancer patients vaccinated with MUC1-KLH and MUC-2-KLH conjugate vaccines [abstr 2070]. Proc Am Assoc Cancer Res 1999; 40:312.
4. Slovin SF, Ragupathi G, Donaldson C, et al. MUC-2-KLH conjugate vaccine: Immunogenicity in patients with relapsed prostate cancer [abstr 2071]. Proc Am Assoc Cancer Res 1999; 40:312.
5. Slovin SF, Ragupathi G, Fernandez C, et al. A bivalent conjugate vaccine in the treatment of biochemically relapsed prostate cancer: A study of glycosylated MUC-2-KLH and Globo H-KLH conjugate vaccines given with the new semi-synthetic saponin immunological adjuvant GPI-0100 or QS-21. Vaccine 2005; 23:3114–3122.
6. Wu GJ, Varma VA, Wu MW, et al. Expression of a human cell adhesion molecule, MUC18, in prostate cancer cell lines and tissues. Prostate 2001; 48:305–315.
7. Ragupathi R, Slovin SF, Adluri S, et al. A fully synthetic globo H carbohydrate vaccine induces a focused humoral response to prostate cancer patients: A proof of principle. Angew Chem Int Ed 1999; 38:563–566.
8. Slovin SF, Ragupathi G, Adluri S, et al. Carbohydrate vaccines in cancer: Immunogenicity of a fully synthetic globo hexasaccharide conjugate in man. Proc Natl Acad Sci USA 1999; 96:5710–5715.
9. Wang ZG, Williams LJ, Zhang XF, et al. Polyclonal antibodies from patients immunized with a globo H-keyhole limpet hemocyanin vaccine: Isolation, quantification, and characterization of immune responses by using totally synthetic immobilized tumor antigens. Proc Natl Acad Sci USA 2000; 97:2719–2724.
10. Slovin S, Ragupathi G, Israel R, et al. Ganglioside vaccines in relapsed prostate cancer (PC): Experience with GM2–KLH conjugate plus the immunologic adjuvant, QS21-A trial comparing QS21 doses [abstr 1214]. Proc Am Soc Clin Onc 1999; 18:316Aa.
11. Miller AM, Ozenci V, Kiessling R, Pisa P. Immune monitoring in a phase I trial of a PSA DNA vaccine in patients with hormone-refractory prostate cancer. J Immunother 2005; 28:389–395.
12. Pavlenko M, Roos AK, Lundquist A, et al. A phase I trial of DNA vaccination with a plasmid expressing prostate-specific antigen in patients with hormone-refractory prostate cancer. Br J Cancer 2004; 91:68–694.
13. Wolchok JD, Gregor PD, Nordquist LT, Slovin SF, Scher HI. DNA vaccines: An active immunization strategy for prostate cancer. Sem Onc 2003; 30:659–666.
14. Slovin SF. PSMA vaccines: Naked DNA and protein approaches. Clin Prostate Cancer 2005; 4:1–6.
15. Reiter RE, Gu Z, Watabe T, et al. Prostate stem cell antigen: A cell surface marker overexpressed in prostate cancer. Proc Natl Acad Sci USA 1998; 95:1735–1740.
16. Schalken JA. Validation of molecular targets in prostate cancer. Br J Urol Int 2005; 96(suppl 2):23–29.
17. Fletterick RJ. Molecular modelling of the androgen receptor axis: Rational basis for androgen receptor intervention in androgen-independent prostate cancer. Br J Urol Int 2005; 96(suppl 2):2–9.
18. Kim H, Turner T, Kassis J, Souto J, Wells A. EGF receptor signaling in prostate development. Histol Histopathol 1999; 14:1175–1182.
19. Slovin SF, Kelly WK, Cohen R, et al. Epidermal growth factor receptor (EGFr) monoclonal antibody (MoAb) C225 and doxorubicin (DOC) in androgen-independent (AI) prostate cancer (PC): results of a phase Ib/IIa study [abstr 1108]. Proc Am Soc Clin Onc 1997; 16:3,11a.
20. Gross ME, Jo S, Agus DB. Update on HER-kinase-directed therapy in prostate cancer. Clin Adv Hematol Oncol 2004; 2:53–64.
21. Kaicer EK, Blat C, Harel L. IGF-1 and IGF-binding proteins: Stimulatory and inhibitory factors secreted by human prostatic adenocarcinoma cells. Growth Factors 1991; 4: 231–237.

22. Bello-DeOcampo D, Kleinman HK, Deocampo ND, Webber MM. Laminin-1 and alpha6beta1 integrin regulate acinar morphogenesis of normal and malignant human prostate epithelial cells. Prostate 2001; 46:142–153.
23. Rokhlin OW, Griebling TL, Karassina NV, Raines MA, Cohen MB. Human prostate carcinoma cell lines secrete GM-CSF and express GM-CSF-receptor on their surface. Anticancer Res 1996; 16:557–563.
24. George D. Targeting PDGF receptors in cancer—rationales and proof of concept. Adv Exp Med Biol 2003; 532:141–151.
25. Maker AV, Phan GQ, Attia P, et al. Tumor regression and autoimmunity in patients treated with cytotoxic T lymphocyte-associated antigen 4 blockade and interleukin 2: A phase I/II study. Ann Surg Oncol 2005; 12:1005–1016.
26. Blansfield JA, Beck KE, Tran K, et al. Cytotoxic T-lymphocyte-associated antigen-4 blockage can induce autoimmune hypophysitis in patients with metastatic melanoma and renal cancer. J Immunother 2005; 28:593–598.
27. Attia P, Phan GQ, Maker AV, et al. Autoimmunity correlates with tumor regression in patients with metastatic melanoma treated with anti-cytotoxic T-lymphocyte antigen-4. J Clin Oncol 2005; 23:6043–6053.
28. Wang YR, Wigington DP, Strugnell SA, Knutson JC. Growth inhibition of cancer cells by an active metabolite of a novel vitamin D prodrug. Anticancer Res 2005; 25(6B):4333–4339.
29. Wigington DP, Urben CM, Strugnell SA, Knutson JC. Combination study of 1,24(*S*)-dihydroxyvitamin D2 and chemotherapeutic agents on human breast and prostate cancer cell lines. Anticancer Res 2004; 24(5A):2905–2912.
30. Solit DB, Scher HI, Rosen N. Hsp90 as a therapeutic target in prostate cancer. Semin Oncol 2003; 30:709–716.
31. Solit DB, Zheng FF, Drobnjak M, et al. 17-Allylamino-17-demethoxygeldanamycin induces the degradation of androgen receptor and HER-2/neu and inhibits the growth of prostate cancer xenografts. Clin Cancer Res 2002; 8:986–993.
32. Papandreou CN, Daliani DD, Nix D, et al. Phase I trial of the proteasome inhibitor bortezomib in patients with advanced solid tumors with observations in androgen-independent prostate cancer. J Clin Oncol 2004; 22:2108–2121.
33. Adams J, Kauffman M. Development of the proteasome inhibitor Velcade (Bortezomib). Cancer Invest 2004; 22:304–311.
34. Lashinger LM, Zhu K, Williams SA, Shrader M, Dinney CP, McConkey DJ. Bortezomib abolishes tumor necrosis factor-related apoptosis-inducing ligand resistance via a p21-dependent mechanism in human bladder and prostate cancer cells. Cancer Res 2005; 65:4902–4908.
35. Gediya LK, Chopra P, Purushottamachar P, Maheshwari N, Njar VC. A new simple and high-yield synthesis of suberoylanilide hydroxamic acid and its inhibitory effect alone or in combination with retinoids on proliferation of human prostate cancer cells. J Med Chem 2005; 48:5047–5051.
36. Kelly WK, Richon VM, O'Connor O, et al. Phase I clinical trial of histone deacetylase inhibitor: Suberoylanilide hydroxamic acid administered intravenously. Clin Cancer Res 2003; 9(10 Pt 1):3578–88.
37. Kelly WK, Marks PA. Drug insight: Histone deacetylase inhibitors—development of the new targeted anticancer agent suberoylanilide hydroxamic acid. Nat Clin Pract Oncol 2005; 2:150–157.
38. Liu AY. Differential expression of cell surface molecules in prostate cancer cells. Cancer Res 2000; 60:3429–3434.
39. Liu AY, True LA. Characterization of prostate cell types by CD cell surface molecules. Am J Path 2002; 160(1):37–43.
40. Liu AY, Peehl D. Characterization of cultured human prostatic epithelial cells by cluster designation antigen expression. Cell Tissue Res 2001; 305:389–397.
41. Liu AY, LaTray L, van den Engh G. Changes in cell surface molecules associated with in vitro culture of prostate stromal cells. Prostate 2000; 45:303–312.
42. Lamy S, Ruiz MT, Wisniewski J, Garde S, et al. A prostate secretory protein94-derived synthetic peptide PCK3145 inhibits VEGF signaling in endothelial cells: implication in tumor angiogenesis. Int J Cancer 2006; 118:2350–2358.

43. Luo W, Tapolsky M, Earley K, et al. Tumor-suppressive activity of CD66a in prostate cancer. Cancer Gene Therapy 1999; 6:313–321.
44. Gu Z, Thomas G, Yamashiro J, et al. Prostate stem cell antigen (PSCA) expression increase with high Gleason score, advanced stage and bone metastasis in prostate cancer. Oncogene 2000; 19:1288–1296.
45. Lam JS, Yamashiro J, Shintaku IP, et al. Prostate stem cell antigen is overexpressed in prostate cancer metastases. Clin Cancer Res 2005; 11:2591–2596.
46. Zhigang Z, Wenlu S. Complete androgen ablation suppresses prostate stem cell antigen (PSCA) mRNa expression in human prostate carcinoma. Prostate 2005; 65:299–305.
47. Saffran DC, Raitano AB, Hubert RS, Witte ON, Reiter JE, Jakobovits A. Anti-PSCA mAbs inhibit tumor growth and metastasis formation and prolong the survival of mice bearing human prostate cancer xenografts. Proc Natl Acad Sci. USA 2001; 98: 2658–2663.
48. Nupponen NN, Kakkol L, Koivisto P, Visakorpi T. Genetic alterations in hormone-refractory recurrent prostate carcinomas. Am J Pathol 1998; 153:141–148.
49. Takahashi S, Oian J, Brown JA, et al. Potential markers of prostate cancer aggressiveness detected by fluorescence in situ hybridization in need biopsies. Cancer Res 1994; 54:3574–3579.
50. Dannull J, Diener PA, Prikler L, et al. Prostate stem cell antigen is a promising candidate for immunotherapy of advanced prostate cancer. Cancer Res 2000; 60:5522–5528.
51. Gu Z, Yamashiro J, Kono E, Reiter RE. Anti-Prostate stem cell antigen monoclonal antibody 1G8 induces cell death in vitro and inhibits tumor growth in vivo via a Fc-independent mechanism. Cancer Res 2005; 6:9495–9500.
52. Clynes RA, Towers TL, Presta LG, Ravetch JV. Inhibitory Fc receptors modulate in vivo cytotoxicity against tumor targets. Nature Med 2000; 6:443–446.
53. Ross S, Spencer SD, Holcomb I, et al. Prostate stem cell antigen as therapy target: tissue expression and in vivo efficacy of an immunoconjugate. Cancer Res 2002; 62:2546–2553.
54. Le Page C, Koumakpayi IH, Lessard L, Mes-Masson AM, Saad F. EGFR and Her-2 regulate the constitutive activation of NF-kappaB in PC-3 prostate cancer cells. Prostate 2005; 65:130–140.
55. Ware JL. Growth factors and their receptors as determinants in the proliferation and metastasis of human prostate cancer. Cancer Metastasis Rev 1993; 12:287–301.
56. Ravindranath N, Wion D, Brachet P, Djakiew D. Epidermal growth factor modulates the expression of vascular endothelial growth factor in human prostate. J Androl 2001; 22:432–443.
57. Peng D, Fan Z, Lu Y, DeBlasio T, Scher H, Mendelsohn J. Anti-epidermal growth factor receptor monoclonal antibody 225 up-regulates p27KIP1 and induces G1 arrest in prostatic cancer cell line DU145. Cancer Res 1996; 56:3666–3669.
58. Sherwood ER, Van Dongen JL, Wood CG, Liao S, Kozlowski JM, Lee C. Epidermal growth factor receptor activation in androgen-independent but not androgen-stimulated growth of human prostatic carcinoma cells. Br J Cancer 1998; 77:855–861.
59. Mendelsohn J. Targeting the epidermal growth factor receptor for cancer therapy. J Clin Onc 2002; 20:S1–S13.
60. Prewett MC, Hooper AT, Bassi R, Ellis LM, Waksal HW, Hicklin DJ. Enhanced antitumor activity of anti-epidermal growth factor receptor monoclonal antibody IMC-C225 in combination with irinotecan (CPT-11) against human colorectal tumor xenografts. Clin Cancer Res 2002; 8:994–1003.
61. Prewett M, Rockwell P, Rockwell RF, et al. The biologic effects of C225, a chimeric monoclonal antibody to the EGFR, on human prostate carcinoma. Tumor Immunol 1996; 19:419–427.
62. Pu YS, Hsieh MW, Wang CW, et al. Epidermal growth factor receptor inhibitor (PD168393) potentiates cytotoxic effects of paclitaxel against androgen-independent prostate cancer cells. Biochem Pharmacol. 2006; Jan 12. Epub ahead of print.
63. Veeramani S, Yuan TC, Chen SJ, et al. Cellular prostatic acid phosphatase: a protein tyrosine phosphatase involved in androgen-independent proliferation of prostate cancer. Endocr Relat Cancer 2005; 12:805–822.

64. Liu D, Aguirre-Ghiso JA, Estrada Y, Ossowski L. EGFR is a transducer of the urokinase receptor initiated signal that is required for in vivo growth of a human carcinoma. Cancer Cell 2002; 1:445–457.
65. Jo M, Thomas KS, O'Donnell DM, Gonias SL. Epidermal growth factor receptor-dependent and -independent cell-signaling pathways originating from the urokinase receptor. J Biol Chem 2003; 278:1642–1646.
66. Mamouone A, Kassis J, Kharait S, et al. DU145 human prostate carcinoma invasiveness is modulated by urokinase receptor (uPAR) downstream of epidermal growth factor receptor (EGFR) signaling. Exp Cell Res 2004; 299:91–100.
67. Formento P, Hannoun-Levi JM, Gerard F, et al. Gefitinib–trastuzumab combination on hormone-refractory prostate cancer xenograft. Eur J Cancer 2005; 41:1467–1473.
68. Formento P, Hannoun-Levi JM, Fischel JL, Magne N, Etienne-Grimaldi MC, Milano G. Dual HER 1–2 targeting of hormone-refractory prostate cancer by ZD1839 and trastuzumab. Eur J Cancer 2004; 40:2837–2844.
69. Kubler HR, van Randenborgh H, Treiber U, et al. In vitro cytotoxic effects of imatinib in combination with anticancer drugs in human prostate cancer cell lines. Prostate 2005; 1;385–394.
70. Ustach CV, Taube ME, Hurst NJ Jr., et al. A potential oncogenic activity of platelet-derived growth factor D in prostate cancer progression. Cancer Res 2004; 64:1722–1729.
71. Ko Y-J, Small EJ, Kabinavar F, et al. A multi-institutional phase II study of SU101, a platelet-derived growth factor receptor inhibitor, for patients with hormone-refractory prostate cancer. Clin Ca Res 2001; 7:800–805.
72. George D. Platelet-derived growth factor receptors: A therapeutic target in solid tumors. Semin Oncol 2001; 28(5, suppl 17):27–33.
73. Hofer MD, Fecko A, Shen R, et al. Expression of the platelet-derived growth factor receptor in prostate cancer and treatment implications with tyrosine kinase inhibitors. Neoplasia 2004; 6:503–512.
74. Roa K, Goodin S, Levitt MJ, et al. A phase II trial of imatinib mesylate in patients with prostate specific antigen progression after local therapy in prostate cancer. Prostate 2005; 62:115–122.
75. Nazarova N, Golovko O, Blauer M, Tuohimaa P. Calcitriol inhibits growth response to platelet-derived growth factor-BB in human prostate cells. J Steroid Biochem Mol Biol 2005; 94:189–196.
76. Todorova K, Zoubak S, Mincheff M, Kyurkchiev S. Biochemical nature and mapping of PSMA epitopes recognized by human antibodies induced after immunization with gene-based vaccines. Anticancer Res 2005; 25:4727–4732.
77. Mincheff M, Zoubak S, Makogonenko Y. Immune responses against PSMA after gene-based vaccination for immunotherapy-A: Results from immunizations in animals. Cancer Gene Ther 2006; 13:436–444.
78. Dunphy EJ, McNeel DG. Antigen-specific IgG elicited in subjects with prostate cancer treated with Flt 3 ligand. J Immunother 2005; 28:268–275.
79. McNeel DG, Knutson KL, Schiffman K, et al. Pilot study of an HLA-A2 peptide vaccine using Flt3 ligand as a systemic vaccine adjuvant. J Clin Immunol 2003; 23:62–67.
80. Christiansen JJ, Rajasekaran SA, Inge L, et al. *N*-glycosylation and microtubule integrity are involved in apical targeting of prostate-specific membrane antigen: implications for immunotherapy. Mol Cancer Ther 2005; 4:704–714.
81. Chambers CA, Kuhns MS, Allison JP. Cytotoxic T lymphocyte antigen-4 (CTLA-4) regulates primary and secondary peptide-specific CD4(+) T cell responses. Proc Natl Acad Sci USA 1999; 96:8603–8608.
82. Kwon ED, Foster BA, Hurwitz AA, et al. Elimination of residual metastatic prostate cancer after surgery and adjunctive cytotoxic T lymphocyte-associated antigen 4 (CTLA-4) blockade immunotherapy. Proc Natl Acad Sci USA 1999; 96:15074–15079.
83. Hurwitz AA, Sullivan TJ, Sobel RA, Allison JP. Cytotoxic T lymphocyte antigen 4 (CTLA-4) limits the expansion of encephalitogenic T cells in experimental autoimmune encephalomyelitis (EAE)-resistant BALB/c mice. Proc Natl Acad Sci USA 2002; 99: 3013–3017.

84. Leach DR, Krummel MF, Allison JP. Enhancement of antitumor immunity by CTLA-4 blockade. Science 1996; 271:1734–1736.
85. van Elsas A, Hurwitz AA, Allison JP. Combination immunotherapy of B16 melanoma using anti-CTLA-4 and GM-CSF producing vaccines induces rejection of subcutaneous and metastatic tumors accompanied by autoimmune depigmentation. J Exp Med 1999; 190:355–366.
86. van Elsas A, Sutmuller RP, Hurwitz AA. Elucidating the autoimmune and anti-tumor effector mechanisms of a treatment based on cytotoxic T lymphocyte antigen-4 (CTLA-4) blockade in combination with a B16 melanoma vaccine: Comparison of prophylaxis and therapy. J Exp Med 2001; 194:481–489.
87. Camacho LH, Ribas A, Glaspy JA, et al. Phase 1 clinical trial of anti-CTLA4 human monoclonal antibody CP-675,206 in patients (pts) with advanced solid malignancies [abstr 2505]. Proc Amer Soc Clin Onc 2004; 22:S164.
88. Jaeger M, Stroehlein MA, Schoberth A, et al. Immunotherapy with the trifunctional antibody removable leads to significant elimination of tumor cells from malignant ascites in ovarian cancer: Results of a phase I/II study [abstr 2504]. Proc Amer Soc Clin Onc 2004; 22:154s.

6 Immunologic Approaches to Prostate Cancer

Lawrence Fong and Eric J. Small
University of California, San Francisco, California, U.S.A.

INTRODUCTION

Prostate cancer has historically been considered to be a poor target for immune recognition compared with such malignancies as melanoma and renal cell carcinoma. The majority of antigens identified in the prostate, including prostate-specific antigen (PSA), prostate-specific membrane antigen (PSMA), and prostatic acid phosphatase (PAP), represent "self proteins." As a result, these proteins are thought not to be inherently immunogenic. Moreover, soluble antigens that circulate in the serum, such as PSA and PAP, can render T-cells that recognize these antigen nonfunctional or anergic (1). Nevertheless, multiple studies, which will be reviewed in this chapter, have demonstrated that immune responses can be induced to antigens expressed by prostate tissue or cancer. Moreover, a recent study has demonstrated that prostate cancer can induce spontaneous autoantibodies in patients, not unlike melanoma, and therefore may be inherently immunogenic (2).

Immunotherapy of cancer focuses on potentiating the various immune effectors to kill tumor cells. Arms of the immune system that may function in tumor recognition and clearance include (i) antibody-producing B cells, (ii) CD8 cytotoxic T-cells, (iii) CD4 helper T-cells, (iv) natural killer (NK) cells, (v) NK T-cells, and (vi) monocytes. B-cells target antigen with antibody that can mediate killing through complement, antibody-dependent cell-mediated cytotoxicity, or induction of apoptosis (e.g., anti-Her-2*neu*). T, NK, and NKT cells recognize tumor cells through cell–cell contact and mediate killing through Fas–Fas ligand interaction, or through the elaboration of cytokines (including interferons and TNFα) and lytic granules (containing granzymes and perforin). NK cells recognize target cells based upon their expression pattern of both activating and inhibitory receptors. CD4 and CD8 lymphocytes, on the other hand, recognize processed antigens presented on MHC scaffolds. CD8 cytotoxic T-cells recognize MHC class I molecules presenting 8–10 amino acid peptide fragments that are derived from endogenous proteins degraded in the cytosol. CD4 helper T-cells recognize MHC class II molecules presenting longer antigenic peptides derived from endogenous and exogenous protein.

The goal of cancer immunotherapy is target at cancer cells through recognition by antibody and/or T lymphocytes. By delivering antigens in a manner that stimulates an immune response, cancer vaccines attempt to generate cytotoxic T-cells and/or antibodies from B lymphocytes, overcoming the pre-existing immune tolerance to these antigens. The most straightforward vaccines involve admixing tumor-associated proteins with nonspecific immunostimulatory adjuvants. An alternative approach utilizes the patient's own dendritic cells (DCs) as a cellular vaccine (3). DCs are rare, bone marrow-derived antigen presenting cells that are uniquely capable of sensitizing naive T-cells to new antigens. Presumably, many of the vaccine approaches rely on targeting antigen to DC in order to generate immunity. By loading the DC themselves with tumor antigens, this approach hopes to accentuate immune responses to the targeted antigens.

DETECTING RESPONSES TO IMMUNOTHERAPY

Clinical Responses

Immunotherapies, as with other novel therapies for prostate cancer, have been initially evaluated in patients with "advanced" disease, which is arbitrarily defined as beginning at the time of serologic progression after definitive local therapy. Thus, treatments have been investigated in a wide spectrum of disease ranging from patients with asymptomatic elevations in serum PSA levels following local primary therapy, to patients with overt metastasis.

Serum PSA level is used to follow patients with advanced disease and more recently as an intermediate marker of tumor response (4). Given the long natural history of prostate cancer, defining therapeutic efficacy on the basis of survival alone generally precludes the development of therapies in a timely fashion. However, the use of PSA decline as an intermediate marker of response remains problematic because confounding factors such as the effects of ancillary treatments on PSA synthesis or secretion can affect serum levels (5,6). Nevertheless, in patients with hormone-refractory prostate cancer, treatment-related declines in PSA ≥50% lasting ≥28 days has been associated with improvement in pain end points and both progression-free and overall survival (7). PSA decline, therefore, remains a reasonable intermediate end point for evaluating novel therapies in Phase II trials in the treatment of androgen-independent prostate cancer (AIPC), with the understanding that efficacy of promising therapies so identified must ultimately be confirmed with other end points such as survival or improvements in quality of life.

The slope of PSA rise in patients with advanced disease has been described to be log-linear without treatment (8). Moreover, the PSA doubling time remains relatively constant over time as well. Thus, changes in the PSA slope or doubling time (PSADT) can potentially be used as a sensitive method for assessing responses to novel therapies (9–11). For example, PSA slopes before and following immunization with a tumor vaccine can be compared for statistical significance. It must be emphasized that a change in the PSADT has not been shown to correlate with clinical outcome. Thus the observation that a novel agent prolongs the PSADT should be interpreted solely as a sign that the agent has a biologic effect, not clinical benefit. Nevertheless, a change in the PSADT can be considered as a screen to identify agents that should be further investigated. Detection of circulating prostate cancer cells by PCR has also been explored as an intermediate end point in immunotherapy trials (12). Alternative clinical end points used in prostate cancer include time to progression as measured by radiologic studies (e.g., bone scan). Finally, the ultimate end point would obviously be altering overall survival, and in fact, randomized trials are showing early signs that immunotherapy can impact on this challenging end point (13).

Immunologic Responses

In terms of defining "immunologic efficacy," defining a "positive" immune response continues to be an evolving end point. Demonstrating that antigen-specific T-cells are induced by a particular vaccine strategy has become an important element in understanding its immunologic efficacy. Methods used to identify antigen-specific CD4 T-cells include T-cell proliferation, cytokine production by enzyme-linked immunosorbent assay (ELISA), intracellular cytokine staining, and enzyme-linked immunosorbent spot (ELISPOT). Methods for detecting antigen-specific CD8 T-cells include ELISPOT, cytotoxicity assays, and MHC/peptide tetramer staining. Induction of antigen-specific antibodies can be assessed by ELISA. Delayed-type hypersensitivity (DTH) testing has also been used as an in vivo approach to determine whether patients can mount a skin reaction to the immunogen, consistent with the induction of antigen-specific T-cells. Preliminary trials that CD4 T-cell proliferation and MHC/peptide tetramer staining can even correlate with clinical outcome (14,15). Nevertheless the different immune assays that are used must be validated in large series in order to develop a consensus for acceptable immunologic end points that correlate with clinical outcome.

PROSTATE ANTIGENS RECOGNIZED BY T-CELLS

Prostate-Specific Antigen

PSA is a 34kd glycoprotein comprised of 237 amino acids represents the most widely used serum marker for prostate cancer. Several groups have induced CD8 T-cells in vitro to several epitopes derived from PSA (16,17). Clinical trials have since used PSA as the target antigen. Several groups have used recombinant viruses expressing PSA. The most commonly used viral vector thus far is vaccinia. A Phase I study using this vector was performed with six patients who had biochemical recurrence of disease after radical prostatectomy (18). Patients were treated with LHRH agonist therapy pre-vaccination until an undetectable PSA nadir was achieved and then vaccinated with the PSA expressing vaccinia. In this setting, clinical responses are difficult to interpret, but one of the six patients had delay of PSA rise for over eight months following recovery of testosterone.

Another Phase I study using PSA expressing vaccinia was performed with 33 men with biochemical progression after local therapy, locally advanced disease, or metastatic disease (19). Patients received three monthly doses of vaccinia, and the final cohort of 10 patients also received granulocyte-macrophage colony-stimulating factor (GM-CSF) for four days around the time of vaccination. Stable disease (defined as $<80\%$ decrease or $<50\%$ increase in PSA) was achieved in 14 of 33 men for at least six months. Induction of T-cells specific for $PSA_{154-163}$ could be detected by cytokine ELIPSOT in five of the seven patients with the relevant HLA allele (HLA*0201). Interestingly, four of these five patients had stable PSA levels for 6–11+ months.

More recently a Phase I trial also using PSA expressing vaccinia was performed in 42 patients with metastatic prostate cancer (20). Patients received up to three monthly injections of vaccinia. Three of the five patients who expressed the HLA allele and who could be assessed immunologically had induction of PSA-specific T-cells following vaccination. No objective clinical responses were seen, however.

Despite these early trials, pre-existing immunity to vaccinia and immunodominance of viral-derived proteins has limited the applicability of vaccinia-based strategies. Newer generation PSA trials based upon viral vectors rely on fowlpox to avoid the former, and prime-boost strategies where different viral vectors are used for subsequent immunizations to minimize the latter.

DC has also been used to vaccinate against PSA. DC loaded with PSA expressing mRNA was used to immunize 13 patients with metastatic prostate cancer (12). All patients developed PSA-specific T-cells following vaccination. Six of the seven patients had reduction in their rate of rising PSA. PSA may, therefore, represent a potential target for immunotherapy with suggestions of clinical benefit, though this benefit may be modest.

Prostate Acid Phosphatase

The gene for human PAP (hPAP) contains a 1065 nucleotide coding region that gives rise to a 354 amino acid glycoprotein that forms 102 kDa homodimers (21). PAP is specifically expressed in prostate tissue as evaluated by Northern blotting or monoclonal antibody staining and is physiologically secreted into the semen. PAP immunization in a rodent model could induce an antigen-specific CD4 and CD8 T-cell immune response that could generate autoimmune prostatitis (22).

A Phase I/II trial in AIPC patients explored whether autologous antigen-presenting cells loaded with a recombinant fusion protein consisting of hPAP and human GM-CSF (Provenge®, Dendreon Corporation, Seattle, Washington, U.S.A.) was safe and if immunogenicity to this antigen could be induced in vivo (23). In consecutive Phase I/II trials, 31 patients received three monthly infusions of Provenge with a final boost at 24 mo if disease was no worse. Provenge administration stimulated T-cell responses against native PAP in 38% of patients. T-cells collected after treatment (but not before) secreted IFN-γ. Three patients experienced PSA declines $\geq$50% from baseline (all developed immune responses to PAP), and three had PSA declines from 25% to 49%. Development of a response to native PAP appeared to correlate with time to progression. More recently, a multi-center Phase III trial was completed in 127 patients with hormone-refractory prostate cancer (24). Patients were randomized to either receive Provenge ($n = 82$) or placebo ($n = 45$) with primary end points of time to disease progression. Patients received APC8015 or placebo intravenously thrice every 2 week Time to objective disease progression was not statistically different: 11.1 week in the vaccine group compared with 10.1 week in the control group ($p = 0.061$). However, there was a statistically significant difference in the median overall survival: 25.9 months for those randomized to vaccine versus 22.0 months for those randomized to placebo ($p = 0.020$, hazard ratio 1.625) (13). Provenge, therefore, represents the first non-chemotherapeutic agent shown to provide a survival advantage in men with AIPC, although this Phase III trial had a small sample size, and requires confirmation.

Prostate-Specific Membrane Antigen

PSMA is a 100 kDa transmembrane glycoprotein produced by prostatic epithelium that functions as a protease and folate hydrolase. PSMA is expressed in primary prostate tumors and their metastases, and its expression is upregulated after androgen deprivation. In vitro, studies have identified potentially relevant T-cell epitopes derived from PSMA (25).

A Phase I trial of PSMA vaccination in 51 patients with advanced, hormone-refractory prostate cancer has been reported (26,27). Patients were divided into five groups. Two groups received injection of one of the two HLA-A2-restricted PSMA peptides, one group received autologous DC alone, and two groups received autologous DC pulsed with one of the two PSMA peptides. A T-cell response was observed in some patients infused with DC pulsed with either peptide. Seven patients had a partial response [based on National Prostate Cancer Project (NPCP) criteria and $>50\%$ PSA decrease] and eleven demonstrated stable disease. Five of the seven clinical responses were seen in the cohort receiving DC pulsed with PSMA peptide. Subsequent follow-up demonstrated four durable partial responses with an average response duration of 232 days. The NPCP response criteria were used, which have been criticized, among other reasons, for including stable disease as a response category.

A Phase II trial was then conducted in 95 patients with either locally-recurrent ($n = 37$) or hormone-refractory, metastatic ($n = 58$) prostate cancer (28,29). Six infusions of DC pulsed with both PSMA peptides from the Phase I study were administered at 6-wk intervals. A total of three complete and 16 partial responses were reported. Again, NPCP response criteria were utilized. In addition, the extent to which patients received other treatments prior to or during the study was also not controlled. Finally, the peptides used were HLA*A2-binding, but many patients did not express this allele, including several of the clinical responders (1CR and 4PR), making understanding of the biology difficult. A Phase I/II clinical trial using recombinant PSMA protein loaded onto DC was recently completed in 31 patients with AIPC. In this trial there was evidence for a delay in disease progression compared with historical controls, and 82% of the patients had either a PSMA-specific antibody or cellular immune response.

Other vaccination approaches targeting PSMA have also been explored. Twenty-six patients with varying stages of prostate cancer were enrolled (30). Patients were immunized with either a cDNA plasmid encoding either the extracellular domain of PSMA (with or without CD86 transcript), an adenoviral vector expressing PSMA, or both in a prime- and final-boost strategies. In addition some patients received GM-CSF with immunization. DTH responses to the PMSA-expressing plasmid were seen in some of the patients, including all 10 patients immunized with the PSMA adenoviral vector. The presence of a patient population with varying disease states possible concomitant hormone therapy and the use of GM-CSF (itself a modulator of PSA levels) confounded interpretation of the clinical results, however. Nonetheless, PSA declines were seen in some patients receiving vaccination only.

In aggregate, these reports demonstrate the ability to induce T-cell responses against PSMA in vivo in prostate cancer patients.

Telomerase

Telomerase is thought to be a universal cancer antigen since tumor cells express this molecule to avoid cellular senescence. The enzymatic portion of telomerase, TERT, has been used as an antigenic target in the setting of prostate cancer (31). Clinical trials using DC loaded with TERT expressing mRNA (32) or a TERT derived peptide (33) as a vaccine platform have demonstrated the induction of TERT reactive T-cells following vaccination. Moreover, the former study demonstrated reductions in PSA doubling time in some patients.

PROSTATE ANTIGENS TARGETED BY ANTIBODIES

Passive administration of antibodies or active vaccination to induce antibodies can target cells that express target proteins on their cell surface. Unlike antibodies against CD20 in nonHodgkin's lymphoma and against Her2*neu* in breast cancer, specific antibodies that trigger cell death in prostate cancer have yet to be identified, although a preclinical study has demonstrated some activity of anti-Her2*neu* antibodies against prostate cancer xenografts (34). Unfortunately, Her2*neu* does not appear to be frequently overexpressed in prostate cancer specimens (35). With most antibody trials currently underway, antibodies are coupled to cytotoxic agents, such as radioisotopes and toxins, and used to target the complexes to sites of tumor.

Prostate-Specific Membrane Antigen

An antibody against PSMA that has been used in prostate imaging may also have therapeutic applications. Antibodies directed to the extracellular domain of PSMA and coupled to radioisotopes or toxins have been shown to have antitumor effects in both cell lines and murine models (36,37). In a Phase I study in 12 patients with AIPC, patients received a yttrium [^{90}Y]-labeled anti-PSMA antibody (CYT-356, IgG_1 murine antibody) (38). While no patient achieved a clinical response as measured by PSA or radiologic criteria, two patients did report a subjective improvement in pain. Antibody infusions were well-tolerated with myelosuppression as the dose-limiting toxicity. Another anti-PSMA antibody (J591, a humanized antibody) coupled to [^{90}Y] or lutetium [^{177}Lu] has been used in a Phase I study (39). Twenty-seven patients with AIPC received increasing doses of antibody with toxicity limited to reversible myelosuppression. Three patients had PSA declines of $\geq$50%.

TAG-72

TAG-72 represents a tumor-associated mucin found on many adenocarcinomas including prostate cancer. CC49, a murine IgG_1 antibody that recognizes the pancarcinoma antigen TAG-72, has been shown to generate disease responses in ovarian cancer (40). This antigen is expressed on prostate cancer cells (41), and is being studied in clinical trials for prostate cancer. Problems with specificity and adequate delivery of antibodies into tumor tissues must be addressed as this treatment approach is developed clinically (42).

CC49 labeled with radioactive iodine (^{131}I) was used in a preliminary clinical trial of AIPC but failed to show any objective clinical responses (43). A subsequent study has combined this treatment with administration of interferon-γ to upregulate TAG-72 expression and thus enhances the antitumor response (42). Sixteen patients with progressive AIPC were studied, and twelve patients had antibody localization to tumor. No patient achieved a radiologic response or $\geq$50% decline in PSA. Four patients achieved moderate, short-term palliative benefit from painful bone metastases. Dosimetry estimates demonstrated that, despite upregulation of antigen expression in three of four assessable cases, only modest radiation doses (10–15 Gy) were delivered to tumor sites. Thrombocytopenia was the dose-limiting toxicity and rapid development of human anti-mouse antibodies (HAMA) precluded repetitive dosing. A subsequent trial with similar design and rationale treated 14 patients with interferon-α before administration of 75 mCi/m^2 of ^{131}I-CC49 (44). Two patients had a minor radiographic response and three had PSA reductions $\geq$50%. No biopsies were undertaken to demonstrate antigen upregulation because of IFN-α, yet the authors note a significantly (approximately fourfold) higher radiation dose to tumors versus the previous trial of ^{131}I-CC49 alone. Development of a humanized antibody would eliminate HAMA development and allow for the repetitive dosing needed to achieve an adequate radiation dose to tumor sites.

Prostate-Specific Antigen

Generation of a bispecific antibody that recognizes both PSA and the CD3 on T-cells has also been explored (45). Such an antibody would direct nonspecific $CD3^+$ T-cells to PSA. These antibodies could redirect pre-activated human peripheral blood mononuclear cells to lyse PSA-expressing prostate carcinoma cells in vitro. Antitumor activity in vivo was also demonstrated in nude mice. Further human studies are required to define potential clinical benefit. Nevertheless, because PSA circulates in the serum, targeting of this antigen with antibodies presents significant challenges.

Carbohydrates

Globo H hexasaccharide (globo H) is a carbohydrate with enhanced expression on both primary and metastatic prostate cancer specimens. Preclinical murine studies have demonstrated the ability to induce high-titer antibodies against globo H via immunization with globo H conjugated to keyhole limpet hemocyanin and administered with the immunologic adjuvant QS-21. A Phase I trial of 18 prostate cancer patients with biochemical relapse after local therapy or metastatic disease was undertaken (46). Anti-globo H antibody responses, predominantly IgM, were demonstrated in almost all patients with a peak at week 9 and declining titers thereafter. Sera from nine patients showed an increase in complement-mediated lysis versus globo H expressing cell lines. Clinical benefit was limited to a decreasing slope of PSA rise in two of the five patients with only biochemically detected disease who did not receive subsequent hormone therapy. This report demonstrates the ability to generate IgM antibodies versus this carbohydrate in advanced prostate cancer patients.

TUMOR VACCINES UTILIZING PROSTATE CANCER AS A SOURCE OF ANTIGEN

Prostate tumor cells have also been used as cancer vaccines. Preclinical models have demonstrated that tumor cells, when transduced with cytokine genes (47) or costimulatory molecules (48), can be used to immunize animals and protect them from developing tumors. One approach used GM-CSF to promote uptake of tumor antigens by DC (29). Prostate cancer cells were removed at surgery, expanded, and transfected to secrete high levels of GM-CSF via ex vivo retroviral transduction with cDNA encoding GM-CSF. These cells were then irradiated and injected subcutaneously into patients. Vaccine could be prepared in 8 of 11 enrolled patients with locally advanced prostate cancer. Patients received vaccination every 21 days until the supply was depleted (three to six vaccinations). Biopsies of vaccine sites revealed infiltration of DC, macrophages, T-cells, and eosinophils, more pronounced at the higher dose level. DTH against irradiated, unmodified autologous tumor cells and recall antigens was tested in pretreatment and post-treatment to assess induction of specific antitumor immune responses. DTH response against autologous tumor cells was present in two of the eight patients before vaccination and in seven of the eight patients following vaccination. Biopsy of DTH sites revealed 80% of T-cells expressing the activation marker CD45RO as well as presence of both type-1 helper (Th1) and type-2 helper (Th2) $CD4^+$ T-cells. Three of eight patients developed serum antibodies against prostate polypeptides from prostate cancer cell lines. No clinical responses were observed. This study demonstrated the effective induction of an immune response using this vaccination strategy. A higher proportion of patients with a DTH response against autologous tumor cells after vaccination is evidence for generation of a tumor-specific cellular response, while the lack of clinical benefit highlights the need for other manipulations for effective immunotherapy.

An attempt to broaden the applicability of this approach has been investigated by transducing the allogeneic prostate cancer cell lines LNCaP and PC-3 with the GM-CSF gene (GVAX®, Cell Genesys, South San Francisco, California, U.S.A.). A preliminary report demonstrates induction of antibody responses to proteins expressed by the cell lines and suggestions of improved time to progression in patients receiving higher doses of the vaccine (49). In a Phase II study of the cell line-based vaccine, 34 patients with metastatic AIPC were treated with an initial vaccination followed by 12 booster vaccinations at two-week intervals, with patients separated into two cohorts receiving different doses. At the two year, 9 of the 24 patients at the lower dose were still alive (41%) while 7 of the 10 patients at the higher dose were alive (70%) suggesting that there may be a dose–response to this vaccine (50). Two Phase III trials in patients with AIPC are currently underway.

CYTOKINE THERAPY

Cytokines have been used as an immunotherapeutic approach for prostate cancer. While some cytokines can be cytotoxic to tumor cells, most of the cytokines studied in prostate cancer are directed at enhancing the presentation of antigens from the prostate. Treatment with GM-CSF (Leukine®, Berlex, Montville, New Jersey, U.S.A.) has been explored in a Phase II trial of patients with androgen insensitive prostate cancer. Thirty-six patients received GM-CSF with minimal side effects. Ten of 22 patients who received intermittent GM-CSF (14 out of 28 days) had evidence of a saw tooth pattern with PSA declines on GM-CSF and PSA rises while off treatment. Fourteen patients were subsequently treated with maintenance GM-CSF after a two-week induction period. Thirteen had declines in their PSA, with one patient having a greater than 99% decline and improving bone scan for more than a year (51). GM-CSF has since been studied in patients with biochemical relapses following primary therapy (11). Thirty patients received the same schedule of 14 days of GM-CSF given monthly. Significantly, three patients had a 50% reduction in PSA without any other intervention and patients for which the on-treatment PSA doubling-time could be calculated, the median PSA double time increased from 8.4 months to 15 months ($p = 0.001$). The presumed mechanism of action of GM-CSF is through in vivo stimulation of function and/or number of antigen presenting cells including DC.

IMMUNOMODULATORY TREATMENT

We now know that a myriad of immunosuppressive factors are exist within cancer patients that may serve to dampen antitumor immune responses. Some of these molecules represent natural pathways to inhibit autoimmunity, while some molecules may have been usurped by the tumor to evade immune recognition. Novel approaches are now being developed to target these pathways.

For example, CTLA-4 is an inhibitory molecule that blocks binding of B7 to CD28, thereby preventing co-stimulation and down-modulating T-cell activation (52). By preventing the action of CTLA-4, an anti-CTLA-4 antibody can augment and prolong T-cell immune responses. In animal models, anti-CTLA-4 antibody can induce tumor rejection in immunogenic tumors, and in combination with antitumor vaccination, can induce rejection of minimally immunogenic tumors, including in the TRAMP prostate cancer model (53). In a Phase I study, 14 patients with androgen insensitive prostate cancer were treated with a humanized anti-CTLA-4 antibody (MDX-010, Medarex, Inc., Bloomsbury, New Jersey, U.S.A.). There was no evidence of polyclonal T-cell activation, therapy was well tolerated, and two patients had ≥50% decline in their PSA (54). Clearly, the combination of CTLA-4 blockade with vaccination is of interest and is under investigation.

FUTURE DIRECTIONS

Clinical efficacy with the majority of the discussed emerging treatments has been tested in patients with advanced prostate cancer. These patients, however, possess a high frequency of underlying immune suppression despite not have recent chemotherapy or radiation (10). Immunotherapy may therefore be more effective in patients with earlier stage disease. Moreover, studying patients in settings of minimal residual disease will be important given the issues of immunologic tolerance.

Combining various treatment modalities will also be important in determining the best setting to perform immunotherapy. The National Cancer Institute is currently sponsoring vaccine protocols combining vaccination against PSA with radiation therapy, hormonal therapy, or docetaxel chemotherapy. Combining immunotherapeutic modalities may also lead to improved efficacy. Combining vaccine with immunomodulatory treatments (e.g., anti-CTLA-4 antibodies) also provides exciting opportunities in potentiating tumor vaccines. The combination of anti-CTLA-4 blockade together with GM-CSF is currently being tested. Androgen ablation has also been show to affect the immune system by enhance the generation of new T-cells (55,56). In an animal model of prostate cancer, androgen ablation was shown to in fact enhance antitumor responses to a tumor vaccine (57). These studies provide a rationale for combining immunotherapies with hormonal therapy.

Finally, new prostate antigens continue to be characterized, including prostate stem cell antigen (PSCA), Trp-p8, prostein, and EphA2 (58–62). With the ongoing developments in genomics and the advent of microarrays, the genetic and molecular defects involved in prostate carcinogenesis will most certainly be more thoroughly dissected in the coming years. This knowledge will lead the way for improved immunotherapies for patients with prostate cancer.

REFERENCES

1. Lohr J, Knoechel B, Nagabhushanam V, et al. T-cell tolerance and autoimmunity to systemic and tissue-restricted self-antigens. Immunol Rev 2005; 204:116–127.
2. Wang X, Yu J, Sreekumar A, et al. Autoantibody signatures in prostate cancer. N Engl J Med 2005; 353:1224–1235.

3. Fong L, Engleman EG. Dendritic cells in cancer immunotherapy. Annu Rev Immunol 2000; 18:245–273.
4. Hudson MA, Bahnson RR, Catalona WJ. Clinical use of prostate specific antigen in patients with prostate cancer. J Urol 1989; 142:1011–1017.
5. Plowman PN, Perry LA, Chard T. Androgen suppression by hydrocortisone without aminoglutethimide in orchiectomised men with prostatic cancer. Br J Urol 1987; 59:255–257.
6. Storlie JA, Buckner JC, Wiseman GA, et al. Prostate specific antigen levels and clinical response to low dose dexamethasone for hormone-refractory metastatic prostate carcinoma. Cancer 1995; 76:96–100.
7. Small EJ, McMillan A, Meyer M, et al. Serum prostate-specific antigen decline as a marker of clinical outcome in hormone-refractory prostate cancer patients: association with progression-free survival, pain end points, and survival. J Clin Oncol 2001; 19: 1304–1311.
8. Schmid HP, McNeal JE, Stamey TA. Observations on the doubling time of prostate cancer. The use of serial prostate-specific antigen in patients with untreated disease as a measure of increasing cancer volume. Cancer 1993; 71:2031–2040.
9. Slovin SF, Scher HI. Peptide and carbohydrate vaccines in relapsed prostate cancer: immunogenicity of synthetic vaccines in man–clinical trials at Memorial Sloan-Kettering Cancer Center. Semin Oncol 1999; 26:448–454.
10. Fong L, Brockstedt D, Benike C, et al. Dendritic cell-based xenoantigen vaccination for prostate cancer immunotherapy. J Immunol 2001; 167:7150–7156.
11. Rini BI, Weinberg V, Bok R, et al. Prostate-specific antigen kinetics as a measure of the biologic effect of granulocyte-macrophage colony-stimulating factor in patients with serologic progression of prostate cancer. J Clin Oncol 2003; 21:99–105.
12. Heiser A, Coleman D, Dannull J, et al. Autologous dendritic cells transfected with prostate-specific antigen RNA stimulate CTL responses against metastatic prostate tumors. J Clin Invest 2002; 109:409–417.
13. Small EJ, Schellhammer PF, Higano C, et al. Immunotherapy (APC8015) for androgen independent prostate cancer (AIPC): final survival data from a phase 3 randomized placebo-controlled trial. J Clin Onc 2006; 24:3089–3094.
14. Yamamoto JK, Kruzel ML, Louie H, et al. Inhibition of human immunodeficiency virus type 1 replication by human interferons alpha, beta and gamma. Arch Immunol Ther Exp 1993; 41:185–191.
15. Savage PA, Boniface JJ, Davis MM. A kinetic basis for T cell receptor repertoire selection during an immune response. Immunity 1999; 10:485–492.
16. Correale P, Walmsley K, Nieroda C, et al. In vitro generation of human cytotoxic T lymphocytes specific for peptides derived from prostate-specific antigen. J Natl Cancer Inst 1997; 89:293–300.
17. Xue BH, Zhang Y, Sosman JA, et al. Induction of human cytotoxic T lymphocytes specific for prostate-specific antigen. Prostate 1997; 30:73–78.
18. Sanda MG, Smith DC, Charles LG, et al. Recombinant vaccinia-PSA (PROSTVAC) can induce a prostate-specific immune response in androgen-modulated human prostate cancer. Urology 1999; 53:260–266.
19. Eder JP, Kantoff PW, Roper K, et al. A phase I trial of a recombinant vaccinia virus expressing prostate-specific antigen in advanced prostate cancer. Clin Cancer Res 2000; 6:1632–1638.
20. Gulley J, Chen AP, Dahut W, et al. Phase I study of a vaccine using recombinant vaccinia virus expressing PSA (rV-PSA) in patients with metastatic androgen-independent prostate cancer. Prostate 2002; 53:109–117.
21. Vihko P, Virkkunen P, Henttu P, et al. Molecular cloning and sequence analysis of cDNA encoding human prostatic acid phosphatase. FEBS Lett 1988; 236:275–281.
22. Fong L, Benike C, Brockstedt D, et al. Immunization with dendritic cells pulsed with xenogeneic prostatic acid phosphatase administered via different routes induces cellular immune responses in prostate cancer patients. Proc Am Assoc Cancer Res 1999; 40:85.

23. Small EJ, Fratesi P, Reese DM, et al. Immunotherapy of hormone-refractory prostate cancer with antigen-loaded dendritic cells. J Clin Oncol 2000; 18:3894–3903.
24. Small EJ, Rini B, Higano C, et al. A randomized, placebo-controlled phase III trial of APC8015 (Provenge™) in patients with androgen-independent prostate cancer (AiPCa). Proc ASCO 2003; 22:1534.
25. Lu J, Celis E. Recognition of prostate tumor cells by cytotoxic T lymphocytes specific for prostate-specific membrane antigen. Cancer Res 2002; 62:5807–5812.
26. Murphy G, Tjoa B, Ragde H, et al. Phase I clinical trial: T-cell therapy for prostate cancer using autologous dendritic cells pulsed with HLA-A0201-specific peptides from prostate-specific membrane antigen. Prostate 1996; 29:371–380.
27. Murphy GP, Tjoa BA, Simmons SJ, et al. Phase II prostate cancer vaccine trial: report of a study involving 37 patients with disease recurrence following primary treatment. Prostate 1999; 39:54–59.
28. Tjoa BA, Simmons SJ, Elgamal A, et al. Follow-up evaluation of a phase II prostate cancer vaccine trial. Prostate 1999; 40:125–129.
29. Simons JW, Mikhak B, Chang JF, et al. Induction of immunity to prostate cancer antigens: results of a clinical trial of vaccination with irradiated autologous prostate tumor cells engineered to secrete granulocyte-macrophage colony-stimulating factor using ex vivo gene transfer. Cancer Res 1999; 59:5160–5168.
30. Mincheff M, Tchakarov S, Zoubak S, et al. Naked DNA and adenoviral immunizations for immunotherapy of prostate cancer: a phase I/II clinical trial. Eur Urol 2000; 38: 208–217.
31. Nair SK, Heiser A, Boczkowski D, et al. Induction of cytotoxic T cell responses and tumor immunity against unrelated tumors using telomerase reverse transcriptase RNA transfected dendritic cells. Nat Med 2000; 6:1011–1017.
32. Su Z, Dannull J, Yang BK, et al. Telomerase mRNA-transfected dendritic cells stimulate antigen-specific $CD8^+$ and $CD4^+$ T cell responses in patients with metastatic prostate cancer. J Immunol 2005; 174:3798–3807.
33. Vonderheide RH, Domchek SM, Schultze JL, et al. Vaccination of cancer patients against telomerase induces functional antitumor CD8+ T lymphocytes. Clin Cancer Res 2004; 10:828–839.
34. Agus DB, Scher HI, Higgins B, et al. Response of prostate cancer to anti-Her-2/neu antibody in androgen-dependent and -independent human xenograft models [In Process Citation]. Cancer Res 1999; 59:4761–4764.
35. Reese DM, Small EJ, Magrane G, et al. HER2 protein expression and gene amplification in androgen-independent prostate cancer. Am J Clin Pathol 2001; 116:234–239.
36. McDevitt MR, Barendswaard E, Ma D, et al. An alpha-particle emitting antibody ([213Bi]J591) for radioimmunotherapy of prostate cancer. Cancer Res 2000; 60: 6095–6100.
37. Fracasso G, Bellisola G, Cingarlini S, et al. Anti-tumor effects of toxins targeted to the prostate specific membrane antigen. Prostate 2002; 53:9–23.
38. Deb N, Goris M, Trisler K, et al. Treatment of hormone-refractory prostate cancer with 90Y-CYT-356 monoclonal antibody. Clin Cancer Res 1996; 2:1289–1297.
39. Bander NH, Trabulsi EJ, Yao D, et al. Phase I radioimmunotherapy (RIT) trials of humanized monoclonal antibody (mAb) J591 to the extracellular domain of prostate specific membrane antigen (PSMA ext) radiolabeled with 90 yttrium (90Y) or 177 lutetium (177Lu) in advanced prostate cancer (Pca). J Urol 2003; 170:1717–1721.
40. Alvarez RD, Partridge EE, Khazaeli MB, et al. Intraperitoneal radioimmunotherapy of ovarian cancer with 177Lu-CC49: a phase I/II study. Gynecol Oncol 1997; 65:94–101.
41. Myers RB, Meredith RF, Schlom J, et al. Tumor associated glycoprotein-72 is highly expressed in prostatic adenocarcinomas. J Urol 1994; 152:243–246.
42. Slovin SF, Scher HI, Divgi CR, et al. Interferon-gamma and monoclonal antibody 131I-labeled CC49: outcomes in patients with androgen-independent prostate cancer. Clin Cancer Res 1998; 4:643–651.
43. Meredith RF, Bueschen AJ, Khazaeli MB, et al. Treatment of metastatic prostate carcinoma with radiolabeled antibody CC49. J Nucl Med 1994; 35:1017–1022.

44. Meredith RF, Khazaeli MB, Macey DJ, et al. Phase II study of interferon-enhanced 131I-labeled high affinity CC49 monoclonal antibody therapy in patients with metastatic prostate cancer. Clin Cancer Res 1999; 5:3254s–3258s.
45. Katzenwadel A, Schleer H, Gierschner D, et al. Construction and in vivo evaluation of an anti-PSA × anti-CD3 bispecific antibody for the immunotherapy of prostate cancer. Anticancer Res 2000; 20:1551–1555.
46. Slovin SF, Ragupathi G, Adluri S, et al. Carbohydrate vaccines in cancer: Immunogenicity of a fully synthetic globo H hexasaccharide conjugate in man. Proc Natl Acad Sci USA 1999; 96:5710–5715.
47. Dranoff G, Jaffee E, Lazenby A, et al. Vaccination with irradiated tumor cells engineered to secrete murine granulocyte-macrophage colony-stimulating factor stimulates potent, specific, and long-lasting anti-tumor immunity. Proc Natl Acad Sci USA 1993; 90: 3539–3543.
48. Baskar S, Glimcher L, Nabavi N, et al. Major histocompatibility complex class II+B7-1+ tumor cells are potent vaccines for stimulating tumor rejection in tumor-bearing mice. J Exp Med 1995; 181:619–629.
49. Simons J, Carducci MA, Mikhak B, et al. Phase II trials of a GM-CSF gene-transduced prostate cancer cell line vaccine (GVAX) in hormone refractory prostate cancer. Clin Cancer Res 2006; 12:3394–4401.
50. Sacks N, Small E, Higano C, et al. A phase I/II study of high dose allogeneic GM-CSF gene-transduced prostate cancer cell line vaccine in patients with metastatic hormone-refractory prostate cancer. Mol Ther 2003; 7:S447.
51. Small EJ, Reese DM, Um B, et al. Therapy of advanced prostate cancer with granulocyte macrophage colony-stimulating factor. Clin Cancer Res 1999; 5:1738–1744.
52. Egen JG, Kuhns MS, Allison JP. CTLA-4: New insights into its biological function and use in tumor immunotherapy. Nat Immunol 2002; 3:611–618.
53. Hurwitz AA, Foster BA, Kwon ED, et al. Combination immunotherapy of primary prostate cancer in a transgenic mouse model using CTLA-4 blockade. Cancer Res 2000; 60:2444–2448.
54. Davis TA, Tchekmedyian S, Korman A, Keler T, Deo Y, Small EJ. MDX-010 (human anti-CTLA4): a phase 1 trial in hormone refractory prostate carcinoma (HRPC). Proc ASCO 2002; 21:74.
55. Mercader M, Bodner BK, Moser MT, et al. T cell infiltration of the prostate induced by androgen withdrawal in patients with prostate cancer. Proc Natl Acad Sci USA 2001; 98:14565–14570.
56. Sutherland JS, Goldberg GL, Hammett MV, et al. Activation of thymic regeneration in mice and humans following androgen blockade. J Immunol 2005; 175:2741–2753.
57. Drake CG, Doody AD, Mihalyo MA, et al. Androgen ablation mitigates tolerance to a prostate/prostate cancer-restricted antigen. Cancer Cell 2005; 7:239–249.
58. Dannull J, Diener PA, Prikler L, et al. Prostate stem cell antigen is a promising candidate for immunotherapy of advanced prostate cancer. Cancer Res 2000; 60:5522–5528.
59. Kiessling A, Schmitz M, Stevanovic S, et al. Prostate stem cell antigen: Identification of immunogenic peptides and assessment of reactive $CD8^+$ T cells in prostate cancer patients. Int J Cancer 2002; 102:390–397.
60. Tsavaler L, Shapero MH, Morkowski S, et al. Trp-p8, a novel prostate-specific gene, is up-regulated in prostate cancer and other malignancies and shares high homology with transient receptor potential calcium channel proteins. Cancer Res 2001; 61:3760–3769.
61. Kiessling A, Stevanovic S, Fussel S, et al. Identification of an HLA-A*0201-restricted T-cell epitope derived from the prostate cancer-associated protein prostein. Br J Cancer 2004; 90:1034–1040.
62. Alves PM, Faure O, Graff-Dubois S, et al. EphA2 as target of anticancer immunotherapy: Identification of HLA-A*0201-restricted epitopes. Cancer Res 2003; 63:8476–8480.

7 Gene Therapy and Novel Clinical Trial Design

Henry T. Tsai and Jonathan W. Simons
Department of Hematology and Oncology, Winship Cancer Institute, Emory University School of Medicine, Atlanta, Georgia, U.S.A.

INTRODUCTION

Gene therapy, which aims to restore, modify or enhance cellular functions through the introduction of a functional gene into a target cell, has captured attention. The intuitive concepts of gene therapy together with exciting early results in animal models have led to the worldwide enthusiasm for this new direction in medicine. Over 900 gene therapy clinical trials were approved worldwide from March 1989 to July 2005 (http://www.wiley.co.uk/genetherapy/clinical/). Of these clinical trials, 66% are directed toward cancer therapy. Seventy-two of these gene therapy trials specifically involving prostate cancer (PCA) are currently registered with National Institute of Health in December 2005 (http://www.gemcris.od.nih.gov). Early results of these trials were hampered by three areas of major problems: vector efficiency, expression of the recombinant gene, and adverse immunological reaction to the vector.

In 1999, a patient with ornithine transcarbamylase deficiency died from the immunological reaction to the gene vector. However, in 2000 at Paris, Cavazzana-Calvo et al. (1) successfully corrected the immune defect in infants with life-threatening X-linked severe combined immune deficiency (SCID-X1) with gene therapy. This breakthrough was followed by equally impressive proof of concept in children with SCID because of adenosine deaminase (ADA) deficiency by Aiuti et al. (2). The success story of a total 18 children SCID-X1 and seven ADA children so far is dampened by three children who have developed T-cell lymphoproliferative disease 3 years from the gene therapy; it is a reminder that at the current stage of gene therapy, success comes with a cost. However, with advancing discoveries and improving technology, gene therapy will continue to evolve. In this chapter, we will discuss the current gene therapy strategies for prostate cancer and explore ideas behind new clinical trial designs that may facilitate and enhance a more efficient approach to finding optimal gene therapy for our patients.

Rationale for PCA Gene Therapy

PCA is the second leading cause of cancer related deaths among men in the United States. It is estimated that 232,090 men will be diagnosed in 2005 and that 30,350 deaths will occur. Currently, the treatment for organ-confined PCA includes radiation, brachytherapy, and surgery, with variations of neoadjuvant or adjuvant hormonal therapy. Nevertheless, a significant proportion of the localized PCA patients eventually relapse. These relapsed patients will eventually progress to metastatic disease, which, at current time, clinicians have limited treatment options. The major weapon for metastatic disease has been androgen ablation

TABLE 1 Prostate Cancer Gene Therapy Targets

	PCA-specific features	Significance to gene therapy
Natural history	Long pre-clinical latency	Preventive gene therapy
	Propensity for metastatic spread to lymphatics and bone	Systemic target gene therapy to the lymphatic and bone
Anatomy	Localized tumor accessible for procedures	Introduce localized gene therapy in combination with standard therapy in vivo by transurethral or transrectal route
	Accessory organ	Complete ablation of the normal organ in addition to the tumor is clinically undeleterious
Biology	Low mitotic rate	Target both nondividing and dividing cells
	Androgen dependence to independence	Define gene target for each state
Prostate-specific genes and antigens	500+ prostate-specific targets	Prostate-specific promoter/ antigen targeting

Source: From Ref. 5.

for 60 years. While this provides cytoreduction and palliation, progression to hormone-refractory disease typically occurs within 18–24 months. With the landmark TAX-327 multi-center study (3), docetaxel plus prednisone has now become the standard of care for treatment of men with hormone-refractory PCA. Chemotherapy, however, does not add much more to the overall survival of patients, with a median survival of 18.9 mo for the hormone-refractory group in the TAX-327 trial. Yet, with better understanding of the disease pathway of the PCA, we now have available approaches designed to target signal transduction, angiogenesis, apoptosis, immune response, and the metastatic cascade.

PCA is unique in that it has a myriad of molecular targets. The Prostate Expression Database is an online resource that stores gene expression information derived from the human prostate (4). It has revealed more than 55,000 expressed sequence tags from 43 cDNA libraries, with approximately 500 that are prostate-specific.

The large number of prostate-unique promoters and candidate antigens gives investigators ample targets to design prostate-specific gene therapy. By taking into account the specific properties of PCA, natural history, anatomy, biology, etc., clinicians can design multi-targeted gene therapy approach (Table 1) (5).

Cancer gene therapy may be defined as the transfer of recombinant DNA into human cells to achieve an antitumor effect. Depending upon the strategy, DNA may be introduced either into cells removed from the body, the ex vivo approach, or introduced directly into cells in their normal location, the in vivo approach (6).

GENE VECTOR

All vectors contain as a minimum the transgene of interest linked to a promoter (7). The ideal vector should be specific to the target cell and efficient in its delivery of the gene. It should also ideally be nontoxic, nonmutagenic, and nonimmunogenic.

Our current gene therapy vectors have not met all of the ideal situations. At present, we have many vectors available at our disposal, both viral and synthetic, each with its advantages and limitations (Table 2) (5). However, most vectors used for gene therapy contain promoters that are tissue-nonspecific; therefore gene expression may occur in unintended tissues and result in potential for systemic toxicity. When a gene vector is chosen, the size of the virus titer, the transgene size, amount of inflammatory/immune response, persistence of gene expression, ability to transduce nondividing cells, transduction efficiency, and target specificity must be considered. One should also keep in mind the overall goal. Are we looking to cyto-reduce the tumor or aiming for gene correction? These overall strategies will be discussed further later in the chapter.

Viral Vectors

Viral vectors are used in the vast majority of gene therapy trials; it is in general much more efficient than the synthetic vectors. Viral vectors can be broken down into RNA or DNA virus-based. RNA viruses include the retroviruses (RVs) from which the oncoviruses such as murine leukemia virus (MuLV) and mouse mammary tumor virus (MMTV), the lentiviruses derived from human immunodeficiency virus (HIV), and the spumaviruses such as human foamy virus (HFV) are members. The DNA viruses include herpes simplex virus (HSV), vaccinia virus, adenovirus (Ad), and adeno-associated viruses (AAVs). Safety concerns with the viral vectors have led to designing replication deficient viral vectors. In essence, the replication deficient viral vector delivers the gene product to the target cell, and the vector then dies without regenerating itself. Situations may also call for the viral vectors to be replication-competent or replication-attenuated, in which case viral replication can occur in permissive cells.

RNA Virus

Retrovirus

RVs of the oncovirus subfamily are single-stranded RNA viruses with a 7–10 kb genome. The RV attaches to a cell-surface receptor via an envelope (env) surface protein. RVs may be either amphotropic, able to infect all species, or ecotropic, able to infect only mouse cells, depending on the (env) protein. The amphotropic variety of MuLV attaches to cells via the RAM-1 receptor (8), a widely expressed inducible sodium phosphate symporter. Receptor-mediated endocytosis follows. Upon entering, RV virus sheds its outer env protein coat, and the virus genome undergoes reverse transcription. Subsequently, the viral nucleoprotein complex enters the cell nucleus and integrates randomly via the viral long-terminal repeat sequences into the host genome. At this stage, the provirus is stable within the host genome, and it can sustain transgene expression by transmitting to the progeny when the host replicates, a major advantage particularly for corrective gene therapy strategies (9). However, retroviral entry into the cell nucleus depends on cell division, which may be a significant problem when considering the treatment of cancers with low mitotic rates, such as prostate carcinoma.

Other potential problems are the risk of insertional mutagenesis, low transduction rate, nonspecific transduction as RAM-1 receptor is ubiquitous, and rapid inactivation of the viral vector by complements. Because of all these potential problems, RV is best used in an ex vivo setting (10).

TABLE 2 Gene Therapy Vector

Vector	Gene therapy application	Advantages	Disadvantages	Insert size (kb)	Immune responses
RNA virus RV vectors					
RVs	MMLV-based used in majority of current clinical trials; ex vivo transduction for stable gene expression	Transmitted to progeny of transduced cell; potentially long-term transgene expression	Infect actively dividing cells only; risk of insertional mutagenesis; relatively low titers; low transduction efficiency; inactivated by complement in vivo; difficult to target attachment	6–8	No
Lentiviruses	Phase II trial underway; infection of nondividing cells	Can infect nondividing cells; long-term transgene expression; not inactivated by human serum	Safety: possible recombination with endogenous HIV/other viruses; risk of insertional mutagenesis	6–8	No
HFVs	Preclinical testing, stable infection of nondividing cells	Nonpathogenic; infect nondividing cells; polycations not required for efficient transduction; not inactivated by human serum	Low titers	5–7	No
DNA virus vectors					
Vaccinia	Vaccine-based gene therapy	Large insert size replicates in vivo	Low-efficiency pre-existing immunity from prior vaccinations limits expression duration to 1 mo	25	Yes
HSV	Neural tropism	Potentially large insert size (amplicons); episomal no-risk insertional mutagenesis; infect nondividing cells; moderate efficiency	Expression transient; cytopathic; difficult to produce high titers	10–100	Yes
Ad	In vivo use	Infect nondividing cells; wide target cell range; concentrate to high titers; high transduction	Transient expression without passage to progeny; Ad infection provokes cell-	7.5	Yes

(*Continued*)

TABLE 2 Gene Therapy Vector (*Continued*)

Vector	Gene therapy application	Advantages	Disadvantages	Insert size (kb)	Immune responses
		efficiency; episomal, no risk of insertional mutagenesis; high transgene expression	mediated immune response limiting duration of expression; humoral response makes reinfection less feasible with rapid clearance of vector; local tissue inflammation		
AAV	In vivo use	Nonpathogenic; infect non-dividing cells; wide target cell range; high transduction efficiency; site-specific integration Chr 19	Limited insert size; propensity for rearrangement during integration; risk of helper Ad and wild-typed AAV contamination; insertional mutagenesis possible if *rep* gene deleted	2–4.5	No
Synthetic vectors					
Naked DNA	DNA vaccines	Low cost; simple preparation; nontoxic	Poor efficiency	Unlimited	No
Liposomes	In vivo/ex vivo use	Large insert size; safe for repeated administration; nontoxic; low cost; suited for targeting	Poor efficiency; prone to degradation/short expression	50	No
DNA–protein complex	In vivo	Large insert size; safe for repeated administration; non-toxic; low cost; suited for targeting	Poor efficiency; prone to degradation/short expression	50	No

Abbreviations: AAV, adeno-associated virus; Ad, adenovirus; HSV, herpes simplex virus; HFV, human foamy virus; MMLV, moloney murine leukemia virus; RV, retrovirus.
Source: From Ref. 5.

Lentivirus and Spumavirus

The lentiviruses are a subfamily of the RVs, which includes HIV, bovine leukemia virus, and human T-cell leukemia virus-1 (HTLV) and HTLV-2. While members of the oncoviridae subfamily such as moloney murine leurkemia virus (MMLV) and MMTV, cannot integrate into nondividing cells as discussed, the lentiviruses are able to integrate into nondividing cells, an important advantage for gene therapy in vivo. HIV does it by its viral proteins vpr and viral matrix protein p17 (11,12). Even without mitosis, p17 with the phosphorylation of a terminal tyrosine residue, permits transport of the HIV pre-integration complex into the nucleus (12,13). Lentiviral vectors can sustain transgene expression for greater than six months (14). As commonly known, HIV targets primarily $CD4^+$ cells. Experimentally, researchers have been able to substitute env sequences from other RVs for those of HIV to confer varying and broader cell specificity (15,16).

Safety concerns about the small risk of pathogenic recombination in vivo while using HIV-based vector has driven the search for nonHIV-based/ nonhuman lentiviral vectors. Loimas et al. (17) has found that lentiviral vectors carrying a fusion gene of HSV-thymidine kinase (HSV-TK) were efficient vehicles for three human PCA cell lines DU-145, LNCaP, and PC-3.

In December 2002, VIRxSYS Corporation, Gaithersburg, Maryland in conjunction with the University of Pennsylvania, received approval to conduct a first-in-class human gene therapy trial using HIV-based lentiviral vectors. The Phase I trial used VRX496, which is an HIV-derived lentiviral vector from which the disease-causing aspects of the virus have been removed. This vector is then equipped with an anti-HIV gene consisting of a long anti-sense molecule that blocks HIV replication by targeting the HIV envelope gene (18,19). This is achieved by taking autologous $CD4^+$ T cells from HIV-positive subjects and transducing the $CD4^+$ T cells with VRX496. The $CD4^+$ T cells are then reintroduced to the patients. The reintroduced $CD4^+$ T cells may delay or prevent the progression of HIV disease by repopulating a patient's immune system with HIV resistant CD4 T cells. This potentiates the immune response against HIV and protects or restores normal immune function against other infections. The Phase I trial was finished in May 2005 with finding of decrease in HIV viral load. A Phase II trial is currently underway.

The spumaviruses are another subfamily of the RVs and include the HFVs. HFV is nonpathogenic; it can also has integrate into the genome of a wide range of nondividing cells (20). These are not inactivated by human serum as are the oncoviruses and may represent a safer alternative for clinical gene therapy than HIV. HFVs cellular properties are being actively explored and refined for gene therapy. Liu et al. (21) has demonstrated therapeutic gene expression in cultured rat hippocampal neurons mediated by HFV vectors.

Retrovirus- and lentiviral-based vectors will continue to play an important role in gene therapy. While these vectors offer advantages of long-term expression, low toxicity, high capacity and low anti-vector immunity allowing repeat administration, safety issues remain as evidenced in the serious adverse events (AEs) in the X-SCID trial using MuLV-based vectors by the three children. Currently, a better understanding of the science behind the integration site preferences within the family of retroviruses, along with better vector design, and controlled integration should help to reduce the likelihood of insertional mutagenesis. The first clinical trial with a lentiviral vector in HIV patients is encouraging, and may signal the advent of the lentiviral vector era for clinical applications for PCA.

DNA Virus

Vaccinia Virus

The vaccinia virus, a member of the pox virus family, has several characteristics that are advantageous as gene therapy vector. Vaccinia has a large genome of 186 kb, allowing a large transgene insert, as large as up to 25 kb, facilitating multi-gene transfer (22). Vaccinia virus replicates and transcribes in the cytoplasm without the need to be transported to the cell nucleus, avoiding any potential insertional mutagenesis. By its ability to replicate in vivo, vaccinia increases its efficiency of host cell transduction.

Disadvantages start with a strong immune response they elicit, and patients' pre-existing anti-vaccinia immunity is common as a result of childhood smallpox vaccination. The immunological elimination of the vaccinia-transduced cells therefore restricts gene expression to about four weeks. Nevertheless, for the vaccinia applications for which vaccinia vectors are typically used, this duration of expression is sufficient to initiate an immune response. Booster vaccine administrations may be given secondarily effective if given via a heterologous vector, avoiding immunological cross-reactivity (23).

For the above reasons, vaccinia virus has been used extensively for delivery of antigen and immune-stimulatory genes for vaccine-based gene therapy (24). Most recently, Pantuck et al. (25) have conducted a Phase I trial using vaccinia virus expressing MUC-1 and IL-2 genes (VV/MUC-1/IL-2) in patients with advanced PCA. In advance PCA, tumor infiltrating lymphocytes are often found, however, with little or no immune activity, or anergic. The goal of immunotherapy is to prime the immune system to the tumor antigen and allows immune system to do the tumor destruction. Aberrant glycosylation of MUC-1 (a transmembrane glycoprotein expressed on both normal and malignant epithelium) on human tumors leads to exposure of cryptic peptide epitopes that play a role in tumor immunity. It has been identified as a potential target for immunotherapy. In combination with IL-2, an antitumor cytokine, the VV/MUC-1/IL-2 model has demonstrated promise in vitro and animal studies to reverse the anergic state and restoring the full competence of immune cells. This Phase I trial has demonstrated a possibility of future immunotherapy treatment options of patients with advanced PCA.

Herpes Simplex Virus

The herpes viruses are enveloped DNA viruses of the family Herpesviridae. The HSV-1 genome has a double stranded linear DNA of 152 kb. Other members of the herpes virus family include HSV-2, varicella zoster, cytomegalovirus, Epstein–Barr virus, human herpes virus-6 (HHV) and HHV-7. The herpes viruses replicate in the nucleus episomally. From the nucleus, the viral particles reach the cell surface via the endoplasmic reticulum. HSV-1-based vectors have been used extensively in gene therapy for neural tissue and tumors, mainly because of their inherent neural tropism.

Like vaccinia virus, HSV-1-based vectors also have large insert capacity of 35 kb, and their ability to infect dividing as well as nondividing cells. Disadvantages of the HSV-based vectors include their potential pathogenicity, poor transduction efficiency and the short duration of gene expression achieved. For the above disadvantages, research is focusing to bypass the disadvantages. Parkinson et al. (26) have been able to use a disabled infectious single cycle–HSV (DISC–HSV) system for gene delivery/expression of granulocyte-macrophage colony-stimulating factor (GM-CSF) in human PCA, with promising results with cell lines and xenograft tumor models. The disabled single cycle virus is designed to limit pathogenic properties, and the current evidence shows durable expression. Further experiments are needed before this vector functions fully as a vector for patients with PCA.

Adenovirus

Ad vectors are the most common viral vehicles used for PCA gene therapy in human clinical studies; it is because of the advantages of efficient transduction, low potential for pathogenicity, broad host range, and easy manipulation in vitro.

Ad has a linear double-stranded DNA genome of 30–40 kb. The initial binding of Ad to target cells relies on the presence of the coxsackie Ad receptor (CAR) and of the $\alpha_V\beta_3$ and $\alpha_V\beta_5$ integrins (27,28). The Ad fiber protein knob domain (28) mediates the binding of Ad and CAR. This fiber protein is reengineered to target of cell-surface molecules like prostate-specific membrane antigen (PSMA) along with prostate-specific promoter/enhancers (29–31). Once attached, Ad is internalized through coated pits into endosomes; subsequently, it is disassembled and extruded into the cytosol prior to lysosomal fusion, avoiding lysosomal degradation (32). The DNA–protein core then enters the nuclear pores into the nucleus and gene expression starts. Ad gene expression goes through two phases. The first phase has the expression of the early genes (E1–E4) that are essential to DNA replication and hiding from the host's anti-viral defenses.

If replication-competent, the Ad proceeds to replicate episomally, eschewing the problem of insertional mutagenesis. Moreover, the lack proviral integration also means that gene expression that is less sustainable as comparing with RV.

Ad vectors are generally safe with their mild clinical pathogenicity. Furthermore, Ad vectors trigger both cellular and humoral immune responses, which clear the remaining viruses and the transduced cells, limiting the duration of transgene expression. The anti-Ad immune response has the consequence of restricting further vector injection (33).

To combat the immune response and increase Ad transgene expression, researchers have utilized cytotoxic T-lymphocyte (CTL) blocking agents such as cytotoxic T-lymphocyte antigen-4Ig (34) or immunosuppressive drugs (35). In addition to their immunogenicity, another problem of Ad vectors is their limited transgene capacity of approximately 8 kb. Modified Ad vectors known as "gutless" Ad vectors, or as encapsidated Ad minichromosomes (EAMs). In EAMs, almost the entire Ad genome has been deleted except the inverted repeats necessary for replication and the encapsidation/packaging signals (36). EAMs can take up to cloning capacity of 36 kb. The large carrying capacity facilitate the transfer of genes with large regulatory regions intact, or of multiple gene cassettes. "Ad dodecahedron," which is composed of only 2 of the 11 Ad structural proteins with no Ad DNA, just enough for attachment, cell entry and avoidance of endosomal degradation (37). Comparing with the EAMs which have already limited viral DNAs, one finds the dodecahedron to be even more suited for repeat application with avoidance of immunogenicity by having no viral DNA and limited viral proteins. Trudel et al. (38) have conducted a Phase I trial with Ad carrying interleukin-2, and others are focusing on various apoptotic components as transgene targets in various cell line and tumor models. Ad will continue to be a viable vector options.

Adeno-Associated Virus

AAV, as a gene transfer system vector, has become more feasible during the last decade. AAVs are a nonenveloped DNA virus in the family of Parvoviridae. With a linear 4.7 kb genome, AAVs have a group of regulatory genes, the *rep* genes, and a group of structural genes, the *cap* genes. To propagate, AAVs must be coinfected with a helper virus such as Ad for productive lytic infection; otherwise they remain latent. It is the Ad E1/E4 gene products that are essential for AAV transcription and the AAV lytic phase (39). AAVs integrate in a site-specific manner. The preferred site of integration for wild-type AAV is chromosome 19q14.3 (40). However, the capacity for site-specific integration is *rep* gene-dependent. Hence, the deletion of *rep* will result in random integration. AAVs are limited to a small transgene size of approximately 4.5 kb, smaller than the capacity of what Ad can carry. Unlike RVs, AAVs may infect nondividing cells. Moreover, the AAVs generate little inflammatory response. The low immunogenicity, the pathogenicity and its site-specific integration make AAVs an ideal vector for repeated administrations and stable long-term transduction. Advances in the production of high-titer purified rAAV vector stocks have made the transition to human clinical trials a reality (41). One such application uses an allogeneic cell line modified with an AAV vector (GVAX) expressing GM-CSF by taking advantage of the ability to select rare events of integration of AAV vectors into cells cultured in vitro. Clinical studies of this cancer vaccine for PCA have advanced to Phase III currently, "A Phase III Randomized, Open-Label Study of CG1940 and CG8711 Versus Docetaxel and Prednisone in Patients with Metastatic Hormone-Refractory Prostate Cancer Who are Chemotherapy-Naïve" (http://www.gemcris.od.nih.gov/).

Synthetic Vectors

Plasmids

Plasmid is the simplest form of gene therapy. An appropriate promoter along with the transgene is injected directly into a desired site. The efficiency of transgene uptake/expression is very low. There is no integration of the plasmid into the host genome; the duration of the expression is limited. The one tissue that has the greatest transduction efficiency is seen in (42), for which a brief low-level expression may be sufficient for eliciting a therapeutic immune response. The use of syngeneic dendritic cells (DCs) that has been transfected ex vivo with DNA for tumor-specific antigen results in tumor regression and decreased number of metastases in the animal model.

Mincheff et al. (43) have initiated a clinical trial for immunotherapy of PCA with PSMA and CD86. No immediate or long-term side effects following immunizations have been recorded. A Phase II clinical study to evaluate the effectiveness of the therapy is currently underway. Pavlenko et al. (44) have conducted a Phase I trial with plasmid prostate-specific antigen (PSA)/IL-2/GM-CSF combination with observed immune response against PSA proteins. Given the current success with the newer plasmid vectors, plasmids will continue be active participant for PCA.

Liposome

Liposomes are the second most frequently used gene transfer method. Liposome vectors consist of a DNA plasmid enveloped by a charged liposomal coat. The charge of the liposomal coat determines the targeting capacity, intracellular stability and transgene size capacity of the vector. Anionic liposome-based vectors have specific cell-surface binding (45). Once endocytosed, anionic liposome gets targeted to endosome and prone to degradation by lysosomal nucleases. Cationic liposomes bind nonspecifically to the cell surface and endocytosed by a non-receptor–mediated process. This way, cationic liposomes are less likely to be degraded by lysosome; it can also pack a much larger transgene. A general property of liposome is its preferential uptake in the reticuloendothelial (RES) cells. A stealth liposome by adding sialic acid residues has been designed in order to evade RES uptake (46). In summary, liposomal vectors are inexpensive and easy to prepare. They also have a large insert capacity, weak inflammatory response because of lack of proteins; on the other hand, it is not efficient, and it takes thousands of liposomes per cell to transducer successfully. Hybrid vectors combining viral and synthetic approaches have been devised to overcome their respective limitations. Ad–liposome complexes have resulted in a 1000-fold increase in gene transfer efficiency relative to naked plasmid. Transgenes of up to 48 kb have successfully been transferred using this technique (47). Ikegami et al. (48) have successfully utilized cationic liposomal vector coupled with IgM monoclonal antibody against prostate-specific membrane antigen in PCA cell lines. Liposomal gene transfer is currently used in other tumors in various Phase I trials except for PCA. Further details on the other cancer models trials will help to define the properties of a successful liposome vector, with potential usage on PCA cells.

DNA–Protein Complex and Hybrid

DNA–protein complex is a structure in which the transgene is complexed with a targeting protein. By its design, it gives the possibility of high-specificity gene transfer of large inserts with minimal immune response. DNA–protein complexes, however, is susceptible to endosomal targeting and lysosomal nuclease degradation. Generally, the major limitation of the synthetic vectors is the poor gene transfer efficiency, mainly because of the poor uptake and likely lysosomal degradation once the synthetic vectors are internalized. On the other hand, for viral vectors, the major limitation is the maximum insert size. Hybrid vectors have been designed to combine the best of both worlds. DNA segments complexed with Ad Virions, with final conjugation to polylysine or DEAE dextran (49–51), with improved gene-transfer efficiency. Another complex, Ad–liposome complex, results in a 1000-fold increase in gene transfer efficiency relative to naked plasmid (52), with a capacity of up to 48 kb (47). The virion proteins in the DNA–virus complex facilitates vector attachment and uptake, and more importantly, provide an escape of the vector DNA from endosomes prior to fusion with the lysosomes, where they may be degraded (53).

STRATEGIES IN PCA GENE THERAPY

Cytoreductive Approaches

Immunotherapy

Of the various approaches to reduce the tumor burden by gene therapy, immunotherapy is the one that has been most extensively evaluated. PCA has many unique antigen targets that can be exploited for the genetic induction of autoimmune antitumor immune responses. The goal of immunotherapy is to alert the host's immune system to direct its firepower against the evasive tumor.

Tumor cells are poor antigen presenting cells (APCs). Up to 85% of the primary PCA and 100% of metastatic PCA have defects in MHC class I expression (54). To combat this problem, researchers have primed the immune system via the targeted expression of cytokines in tumor cells. The transduced cytokines lead to improved tumor cell vaccine antigen presentation, and activation of APCs, both essential for effective priming of the cellular immune response. GM-CSF has been found to be the cytokine with significant efficacy in the induction of an antitumor immune response (55). GM-CSF is the most potent cytokine signal tested for activation of antigen processing and presentation by macrophages and DCs (56,57). GM-CSF may be transduced into tumor cells ex vivo using viral vectors. The transduced tumor cells are then irradiated in order to minimize immunogenicity and malignant potential (58). The cells are then reintroduced by vaccination into the patient. Tumor cell vaccine-expressed GM-CSF may activate APCs, leading to active immune system tumor destruction response.

One Phase I trial was designed with repeated intraprostatic vaccination with autologous GM-CSF-secreting PCA cells (GVAX®) Hayward, California every 3 week in eight men who had undergone prostatectomy for locally advanced disease (59). The approach was safe, with evidence of immune response, but no definite clinical response. However, in a subsequent Phase II trial (60), with transduction of the GM-CSF into allogeneic PCA cells, there are some suggestions of clinical activity. Out of 96 men (41 with hormone-naïve and 55 with hormone-refractory disease), one man with hormone-naive disease had a partial biochemical response (a decline in serum PSA), and there was one complete response (including normalization of PSA with regression of a lesion on bone scan) in a man with metastatic hormone-refractory PCA (HRPC). A second Phase II trial of GVAX vaccine for cancer in patients with metastatic hormone-refractory PCA with 22 patients who received the highest dose, the dosing regimen comparable to that being employed in Phase III trial, indicate that the median survival has not been reached and the final median survival will be no less than 24.1 months based on the current median follow-up time for these patients (61), (http://www.cellgenesys.com/clinicaltrials-prostate-cancer.shtml). Previously reported findings from the first Phase 2 trial of GVAX vaccine for PCA indicated an overall median survival of 26.2 mo. These median survival results from both Phase 2 trials compare favorably to the recently reported median survival of 18.9 months for hormone-refractory metastatic PCA patients treated with Taxotere® Bridgewater, New Jersey plus prednisone, the current standard of care.

There are other strategies involving either GM-CSF or Interleukin (IL-2) in combination with various PCA antigens; we will not address them here. However, with cautious optimism, we can expect more positive results from immunotherapy. Nevertheless, we must keep in mind the limitations of the cytoreductive immunotherapy. One is the limited tumor burden (10^3–10^6) which the immune system can eliminate in experimental models. Thus, the most feasible setting would probably be to the low bulk or micrometastatic disease, or in combination with other debulking therapies. Additionally, we need further technical advances in the harvesting and culture of autologous or allogeneic tumor or immune cells for ex vivo gene therapy in order to reduce the expenses and current technological difficulties.

Suicide Gene Therapy

Suicide gene therapy, or enzyme/prodrug therapy, works via the conversion of an inactive prodrug into a toxic drug using an enzyme vectored only to the target tumor cells. Spatially, the active drug is limited in the transduced cells and the surrounding bystander cells without affecting overall tissue toxicity. Two systems, cytosine deaminase (CD), which catalyzes the conversion of the nontoxic5-fluorocytosine (5-FC) to the cytotoxic 5-fluorouracil (5-FU), and HSV-TK (Thymidine Kinase) which together with cellular enzymes facilitates the conversion of GCV (ganciclovir) into the toxic GCV triphosphate, have been used. It has been shown that even when only 2% of a tumor contains CD-transduced cells, significant tumor regression is observed, suggesting the presence of a significant bystander effect (62). The cytotoxic efficacy of suicide gene therapy in vivo may be supplemented by a systemic antitumor response that comes with tumor lysis and inflammation, mediated by natural killer cells (63). A Phase I clinical trial has been carried out in patients with recurrent PCA using a replication-deficient Ad vector containing the HSV-TK gene injected directly into the prostate, with subsequent intravenous ganciclovir (64). A statistically significant prolongation of the PSA doubling time, from a mean of 9.8 to 13.3 months, was seen after the first cycle of gene therapy. Grade 4 toxicity was encountered after the vector injection in only one of the 18 patients. There was an additive response in patients receiving a second gene therapy cycle, with further prolongation of the mean PSA doubling time. A combination of CD/HSV-TK is currently underway as a Phase I trial for patients with locally recurrent PCA after radiation therapy by Kim et al. at Henry Ford Health system.

Oncolytic Viruses

Viral vectors may themselves be designed to target and kill tumor cells without any transgene. This principle was demonstrated therapeutically in 1950s with injections of wild-type Ad into patients with cervical cancer. The Ad lifecycle has a lytic phase, which can result in lysis of host cell without the necessity of the host cell going into mitosis for propagation of transgene expression. This feature is particularly attractive given that PCA has low mitotic rate. Latham et al. (65) have genetically engineered an Ad capable of replicating in PSA-producing cells that capable of destroying large LNCaP tumors and abolish PSA production in nu/nu mouse xenograft models. In another study, an Ad vector with the E1A gene placed under control of a PSA minimal promoter enhancer, the CN706 vector, showed potent PSA-selective cytotoxic activity in preclinical testing (30).

In a Phase I study of 20 men with locally recurrent PCA following radiation therapy, CV706 was administered intraprostatically at increasing doses (66). Overall, the therapy was well tolerated, with no irreversible grade 3, or any grade 4 toxicities. Five patients had a $\geq$50% decrease in serum PSA at the top two highest doses. Oncolytic Ad CV787 provides greater specificity and in vitro efficacy against PSA-positive compared with PSA-negative cells (67). It is currently being tested in men with locally recurrent PCA via intraprostatic injections, and as an intravenous infusion in men with hormone-refractory metastatic disease. CV787 is also found to be synergistic with paclitaxel and docetaxel (68), while CV706 and radiation therapy are synergistic in vivo and in vitro. Clinical trials for the combinations are underway.

Cytotoxins

Targeted expression of a cytotoxin such as the diphtheria toxin A chain, or pseudomonas exotoxin A is another cytoreductive strategy. In a screen of cytotoxins using a wide range of PCA cell lines, Rodriguez et al. (69) demonstrated a cell cycle- and p53-independent cytotoxic activity of the diphtheria toxin A chain in

PCA cell lines through both apoptotic and nonapoptotic pathways. Another cytoreductive agent is the expanded polyglutamine, which is a pro-apoptotic molecule implicated in eight inherited neurodegenerative disorders (70). Its length determines its varying pro-apoptotic potential. The major concern with the use of potent cytotoxins for cytoreductive gene therapy is safety. Specificity in tumor targeting is paramount, and unwanted expression of the cytotoxin in other cells should be minimized. Currently, Dahm and Vieweg at Duke University are conducting a trial on autologous DCs with or without IL-2 diphtheria toxin Conjugate Denileukin Difitox (ONTAK®) San Diego, California in subjects with metastatic PCA.

Corrective Approaches

Corrective gene therapy aims to replace defective genes [e.g., tumor suppressor genes such as p53, BRCA1, p21, p16 and c-myc (71–76)] that are important for normal growth. In general, these approaches are pursued to reverse the malignant phenotype; however, this would mean that one has to target each individual cancer cell. Furthermore, in tumorigenesis, multiple mutations generally occur in various pathways, and it would mean that a single gene replacement targeting one pathway may not be sufficient. In spite of the aforementioned difficulties, preliminary results of one study evaluating a replication-defective Ad containing wild-type p53 are available (77). Seventeen men with locally advanced disease received at least one course of intraprostatic injections under transrectal ultrasound guidance. Out of the seventeen men, three of those who completed a second course of therapy had a 25% reduction in tumor size after the first course. We will have to see how feasible the overall data is for corrective approach. It is currently impossible to achieve the 100% gene transfer efficiency in order to reach every single cancer cell, as well as a sustained transgene expression for each cancer cell. Even if we do overcome the efficiency problem, it is very likely that the tumor may evolve via new mutations. Hence, theoretically, a complete correction gene transfer therapy is unlikely to be done; nevertheless, its role in combination with other treatment modalities may be elucidated when more data are available.

COMBINED MODALITIES

Like conventional therapy, gene therapy success may be impeded by tumor cell resistance and intratumoral cell heterogeneity. It makes sense to employ combined treatment modalities to improve the overall clinical outcome. Within gene therapy arena, multi-gene therapy approaches already under evaluation include the transduction of dual immunostimulatory molecules for immunotherapy (78), and dual suicide genes for enzyme/ prodrug strategies (79). One combined modality approach particularly attractive in PCA is the combination of radiation and gene therapy. There is strong evidence that synergy exists between these modalities. Work done by Advani et al. (80) revealed greater than expected tumor regression of U-87MG glioma cell xenografts following combined radiation and viral treatment with the HSV mutant R3616. Radiation seems to help viral replication and viral spread in the xenograft model. Therefore, radiation may potentially be used to improve the efficacy of corrective/cytoreductive gene therapy. Gene therapy may also be used for radiosensitization for the prodrugs such as of a GCV (81) or 5-FC (82). Chemotherapy in combination with gene therapy display synergism, and we have discussed earlier the synergism between the oncolytic viruses (CV787) and chemotherapy. Combinations of three modalities have also been demonstrated, radiotherapy, viral-cytopathic (E1B-deleted Ad), and radiosensitizing double-suicide gene therapy, in vitro models (83).

NOVEL CLINICAL TRIAL DESIGN

Goals of the Gene Therapy Trials

Cancer trials typically proceed through several distinct phases. The major goal in Phase I trials is to identify a working dose for subsequent studies; on the other hand, the major end point in Phase II and III trials is treatment efficacy. These goals are set and defined in a rigid system that is often not flexible enough to accommodate changing variables and patient differences. For gene therapy, it faces usual considerations of the efficacy, safety, and optimal dosing that conventional therapy development faces; however, there is also the constraint of expense. Because gene therapy is a novel treatment modality with long and uncertain research and development costs, and because it entails smaller patient base over which to realize scale economies, there is a limited amount of resources in terms of money and time to support full clinical trials of all the various potential gene therapy treatment strategies discussed above. We will examine the problems surrounding traditional clinical trial designs, and we will present a new clinical trial paradigm that will facilitate an efficient way of quickly eliminating the nonworking options and focusing on the development of the most promising gene therapy treatment option.

Problems with Traditional Clinical Trial Designs for Gene Therapy

Traditional drug development is slow for the following reasons. First of all, the clinical trials are usually too large; a certain number of patients have to be reached to complete the trial. Secondly, each stage of the clinical trial is written in stone. Once the design of the trial is set up, there is not much adjustment. Thirdly, the clinical trial often focuses on a single therapeutic strategy, without the ability to simultaneously evaluate multiple combinations. There are often different end points involved at the different stage of the clinical trial; for example, an early efficacy end point in Phase II is chosen, and a long-term end point such as survival is use in Phase III. For statistical analysis, the researchers restrict the inference only to the available information in the present trial, without incorporation and historical information from other trials. To think about it, one can see the predetermined confine of the traditional trial design. Let us say that we want to find the "best dose" of a drug X. Traditionally, one would calculate a predetermined sample size and the balanced randomization to several *chosen* doses to see which dose is the appropriate dose. This is akin to telling a student that he should study a medical textbook for X amount of time and then he will become a doctor. As we all know that there are other factors involved in training someone to become a physician. A simplistic set of doses do not do justice to the complex human physiology that may require adaptive dosing. In other words, there are other characteristics and factors involved that the traditional clinical trial design cannot incorporate or adjust to.

New Paradigm: Bayesian's Approach

An ideal clinical trial design should mimic our life choices. The trial should continue to experiment until the objective is met or that the objective does not warrant further pursuit. The new paradigm should have the following components: flexible design that can be modified based on the latest information, multiple experimental drugs running together to efficiently narrow down to the promising ones, efficiently and effectively, continuous trial flow without breaking down to distinct phases, continual adaptation of historical and current trial information, and decision analyses to guide the next step of development. Flexible designs allow the data that are accruing to guide the trial, like deciding when to stop or extend accrual, rather than a pre-determined number. For cancer treatment trials especially, it is going to be a selection of multiple experimental drugs from a list of many that would most likely offer the best chance for treatment, given that cancer evolution often involves multiple errors and mutations that a single-drug therapy is unlikely to be the answer. Therefore, the new paradigm would allow us to study many drugs in the trials. By designing the clinical trial to flow from one phase to another (Fig. 1), we do not have to stop patient accrual. Moreover, with continuous flow, one can model a relationship between early end points and late clinical end points, allowing early decision making in trials, increasing efficiency. The new paradigm would incorporate data from historical data, related trials or even other types of cancer.

The new paradigm approach is based on Bayesian philosophy. A Bayesian approach to a problem starts with the formulation of a model that is based on our previous studies. We then formulated a prior distribution over the unknown parameters of the model, which is meant to capture our beliefs about the situation before the trial. After observing some data, we apply Bayes' Rule to obtain a posterior distribution for these unknowns. Now the posterior distribution takes into account the prior and the current clinical data. From this posterior distribution we can compute predictive distributions for future observations. Bayesian methods

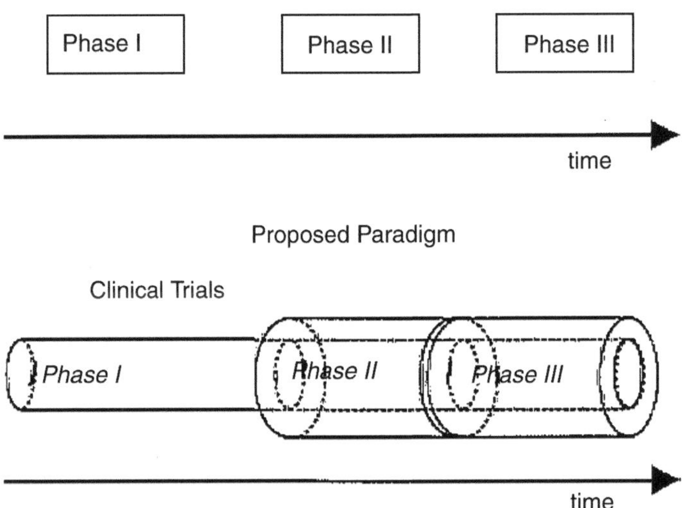

FIGURE 1 New clinical trial paradigm. *Source*: From Ref. 84.

support sequential learning. Once we collect a data point from the trial, we can update the probability distributions of the various parameters; we can then continue to collect data, and continue to update the distribution. During this process, we can stop and predict what the next observation is going to be, finding the next optimal dose for the next patient via the predictive distribution. The Bayesian paradigm utilizes historical information and results of other trials, whether they involve the same drug, similar drugs or possibly the same drug but with different patient populations.

Predictive Probability

Donald Berry, Professor and Chair of the Department of Biostatistics and Applied Mathematics at M.D. Anderson Cancer Center, has discussed examples of Bayesian method that was applied to the several clinical trials (85). We will discuss these examples to illustrate the salient points of the Bayesian methods. As mentioned earlier, predictive probability is where Bayesian allows clinicians to monitor trial and to come up with early prediction. From what is already known about the covariates of patients and current outcome, one can predict how likely it is for the trial to achieve a statistically significant answer if the trial completes. If the predictive probability is small, then the clinicians may decide that further trial may be futile or harmful or that further continuation of the trial is viable. Buzdar et al. (86) conducted a clinical trial to determine whether the addition of trastuzumab to chemotherapy in the neoadjuvant setting could increase pathologic complete response (pCR) rate in breast cancer patients with human epidermal growth factor receptor 2-positive disease.

Originally, the design has a balanced randomization of 164 patients of two arms; one with chemotherapy with trastuzumab, one arm has only chemotherapy as control. After 34 patients were enrolled and studied, the Data Safety and Monitoring Board reviewed the data. Out of 16 control patients, four (25%) achieved pCRs. Of 18 patients receiving trastuzumab, 12 (67%) achieved pCRs. Bayesian predictive probability of statistical significance was calculated. It turned out that if the trial were to continue to reach 164 patients, the probability of reaching a statistical significant result would be 95%. Hence, the trial was stopped early because of the superior result, in spite of the smaller patient sample. At the time of stopping the result, the accrual rate of patients was down to less than two patients per month. Had the trial continue to its full sample size, it would have taken many years before the positive results can be shared with research community.

Adaptive Randomization

Giles et al. (87) conducted a clinical trial that illustrates the flexibility of the Bayesian method. It was comparing troxacitabine to other chemotherapy agents for the treatment of acute myelogenous leukemia. Three treatment strategies were compared: idarubicin plus ara-C (IA), troxacitabine plus ara-C (TA), and troxacitabine plus idarubicin (TI). The maximum trial size was 75. The end point was complete response (CR). However, early CR was important in providing prognosis, and time to CR within the first 50 days was modeled in the design. The randomization process was adjusted based what was known. For instance, when a patient entered the trial, probabilities were calculated indicating that TI and TA were better than IA, and the probability that TA was better than IA, and used those current probabilities to assign the patient's therapy. If one arm performed poorly, its assignment probability would be lowered, with better performing therapies getting higher probabilities. The TI arm was dropped after 24 patients. Arm TA was dropped (and the trial ended) after 34 patients. IA group with 10 of 18 patients achieved CR in 50 days (56%), whereas TA group had 27% and TI had 0% (0 out of 5). This example illustrates that the original assumption was modified based on ongoing trial results and it was quickly established that TA and TI were not as good. Some cancer researchers argued that the finding of zero successes out of five is not definitive enough to give up on a treatment. This argument is valid except that an alternative can produce a 56% CRs. Calculating the Bayesian probability, one finds the probability of either TA or TI is better than IA is small. Furthermore, if TA or TI does have the probability of a CR rate that is greater than that of IA, it is not much greater. This case demonstrates the adaptability of Bayesian method in guiding the trial and avoiding putting more patients in the arms that is unlikely to work.

Screening Phase II Agents

The traditional approach in drug development is to focus on one drug at a time. It is usually not until Phase III does the new drug get compared to the standard therapy. By examining one drug at a time, there are going to be hundreds of other drugs that have to wait for their turn, and chances are, given the large number of experimental therapy, as seen in the gene therapy arena alone, that there is likely a better drug waiting in line than the one that is being studied. With Bayesian approach, one can screen drugs in Phase II like the way it is done in the preclinical setting. The goal is to learn about toxicity and efficacy of the candidate drugs as fast and efficiently as possible. In Bayesian approach, one can assign patients to a treatment in proportion to the probability that a response rate is >20%. We can add drugs and drop drugs based on their probability of having the 20% response rate. Those drugs that work together to achieve a high response rate can then move to Phase III. Let us say that we have a trial with 10 experimental drugs with a sample size of 200 patients. Nine of the drugs have a mix of response rates (20% and 40%). We have one strong candidate with a 60% response rate.

The standard trial design will have a 70% chance of finding the strong candidate drug because it may take up to the 7th try before one identifies the candidate drug, if one approaches the drug one at a time, for the candidate drug may not be in the first seven drugs tested. On the other hand, the Bayesian design has a 99% chance of being finding candidate drug because all drugs are being studied relatively early. The strong candidate drug will show up earlier. This design is ideal of gene therapy; given its high developmental cost, gene therapy with Bayesian design will quickly narrow down to the candidate drug without wasting time and money.

Extraim Analysis

Extraim analysis focuses on whether to continue beside a certain target sample size, as opposed in interim analysis, in which the goal is early stopping. In many clinical trials, even after one reaches the final sample size, one may not have enough to get either a positive or a negative result. Bayesian framework would allow expanding accrual, if one has a drug trial with 800 patients with a power of 80%. Let us say that around 450 patients, we have information for us calculate predictive probability on whether the probability of reaching statistical significance would be if one were to continue to full accrual, as previously illustrated in the trastuzumab trial. If the probability is not high, then it is indicated to expand the trial size to say 1400. Statistical adjustment can be make to keep the type I error down. With the continual accrual, the power increases to 95%. By performing extraim analysis, one can continue to seek for answer. If one were to use the traditional approach, one would have to stop the original trial at the predetermined number, and in order to address the ambiguity, start a second trial to find the answer—much more time consuming and expensive then simply keeping the trial going.

Assessing Drug Synergy

FDA approved a combination of pravastatin with aspirin in 2003. This was the first time that a combination drug was approved based on Bayesian method (88). A meta-analysis of data from five previous pravastatin preventive trials was used in the Bayesian analysis. Aspirin has been thought to be most effective in immediate postmyocardial infarction (MI) period. Pravastatin had been considered to have more of a long-term benefits rather than immediate effect like aspirin. However, the analysis revealed a synergy probability of more than 90% of all end points studied. By using Bayesian method, one can estimate the probability of additive benefits by examining the data from each individual drug.

Hierarchical Modeling and Safety Monitoring

Safety assessment of drugs needs to consider lots of different adverse effects and drug–drug interactions. Some adverse effects are expected. Some are incidental observations that are collected and compared with a baseline control rate. Statistically, it is challenging to tease apart whether the hundreds of observed difference between the drugs and the controls are real. Berry et al. (89) proposed a hierarchical modeling system based on Bayesian approach. A three-level hierarchical model is constructed. The most basic level is the type of AE. The second level is the body system, each of which contains a number of types of possibly related AEs. The highest level is the collection of all body systems. The model analysis allows for borrowing across body systems; with higher probability given based on the actual data within each body system. The probability that a drug has caused a type of AE is greater if its rate is elevated for several types of AEs within the same body system than if the AEs with elevated rates were in different body systems. Another way to think about the hierarchy is to break it down into the patient, the patient within the body system, and body system within the set of body systems. By calculating the probability of adverse effect based on the hierarchical structure and actual data, one can be more confident that a particular adverse effect is because of the drug, rather than by chance.

Escalation with Overdose Control Method

Lastly, we will briefly touch on a Bayesian method-based dose-finding procedure that is used here at the Winship Cancer Institute with potential applications to gene therapy. The escalation with overdose control method (EWOC) is the first dose-finding procedure, based on Bayesian approach, to address the ethical constraint of minimizing the chance of treating patients at unacceptably high doses that a typical clinical trial of MTD (maximum tolerated dose) will require. It defines an expected proportion of patients treated at doses above MTD as boundary. As demonstrated by Zacks et al. (90) that among designs with this defining property, EWOC approaches MTD as fast as possible while keeping the proportion of patients treated above MTD to a set minimum. Without addressing details, EWOC uses the basic Bayesian concept of setting up a prior distribution, a posterior distribution based on data, and constant update to come to a predictive probability that allows fine adjustment of dosing. Comparing to the common Phase I "modified Fibonacci" 3 + 3 dose escalation design, EWOC avoids the problems of having more patients treated with doses outside of the therapeutic window, and more accurately arrive at the proper dose.

FUTURE DIRECTIONS

PCA gene therapy is constantly evolving. With better technical advances in vector development, increased transgene size, minimizing adverse immunogenic reaction, improving targeting and transduction efficiency, gene therapy will play a significant role in PCA prevention and treatment, complementing other treatment modalities. However, to facilitate a more efficient gene therapy development, clinicians should design and analyze future gene therapy trials using Bayesian approaches.

By using predictive probabilities to adaptively randomize, to address whether to proceed to the next stage of drug development via extraim analysis, to borrow historical data and strength across other studies, and hierarchical modeling to monitor AEs, clinicians using Bayesian clinical trial design in PCA gene therapy will be able to come up with a more rapid progress, more accurate dosage, lower costs, and ultimately provide better treatment for our patients.

REFERENCES

1. Cavazzana-Calvo M, Hacein-Bey S, de Saint Basile G, et al. Gene therapy of human severe combined immunodeficiency (SCID)-X1 disease. Science 2000; 288(5466):669–672.
2. Aiuti A, Slavin S, Aker M, et al. Correction of ADA-SCID by stem cell gene therapy combined with nonmyeloablative conditioning. Science 2002; 296(5577):2410–2413.
3. Tannock IF, de Wit R, Berry WR, et al. Docetaxel plus prednisone or mitoxantrone plus prednisone for advanced prostate cancer [see comment]. N Engl J Med 2004; 351(15):1502–1512.
4. Nelson PS, Clegg N, Eroglu B, et al. The prostate expression database (PEDB): status and enhancements in 2000. Nucleic Acids Res 2000; 28(1):212–213.
5. Mabjeesh N, Zhong H, Simons J. Gene therapy of prostate cancer: current and future directions. Endocr Relat Cancer 2002; 9(2):115–139.
6. Anderson WF. Human gene therapy. Nature 1998; 392(suppl 6679):25–30.
7. Galanis E, Vile R, Russell SJ. Delivery systems intended for in vivo gene therapy of cancer: targeting and replication competent viral vectors. Crit Rev Oncol Hematol 2001; 38(3):177–192.
8. Kavanaugh MP, Miller DG, Zhang W, et al. Cell-surface receptors for gibbon ape leukemia virus and amphotropic murine retrovirus are inducible sodium-dependent phosphate symporters. Proc Natl Acad Sci USA 1994; 91(15):7071–7075.
9. Lin X. Construction of new retroviral producer cells from adenoviral and retroviral vectors. Gene Ther 1998; 5(9):1251–1258.
10. Cornetta K, Moen RC, Culver K, et al. Amphotropic murine leukemia retrovirus is not an acute pathogen for primates. Hum Gene Ther 1990; 1(1):15–30.
11. Bukrinsky MI, Haggerty S, Dempsey MP, et al. A nuclear localization signal within HIV-1 matrix protein that governs infection of non-dividing cells [see comment]. Nature 1993; 365(6447):666–669.
12. Gallay P, Swingler S, Aiken C, et al. HIV-1 infection of nondividing cells: C-terminal tyrosine phosphorylation of the viral matrix protein is a key regulator. Cell 1995; 80(3):379–388.

13. Gallay P, Swingler S, Song J, et al. HIV nuclear import is governed by the phosphotyrosine-mediated binding of matrix to the core domain of integrase. Cell 1995; 83(4): 569–576.
14. Miyoshi H, Takahashi M, Gage FH, et al. Stable and efficient gene transfer into the retina using an HIV-based lentiviral vector. Proc Natl Acad Sci USA 1997; 94(19):10319–10323.
15. Naldini L, Blomer U, Gallay P, et al. In vivo gene delivery and stable transduction of nondividing cells by a lentiviral vector [see comment]. Science 1996; 272(5259):263–267.
16. Nascone N, Mercola M. Organizer induction determines left-right asymmetry in Xenopus. Dev Biol 1997; 189(1):68–78.
17. Loimas S, Toppinen MR, Visakorpi T, et al. Human prostate carcinoma cells as targets for herpes simplex virus thymidine kinase-mediated suicide gene therapy. Cancer Gene Ther 2001; 8(2):137–144.
18. Lu X, Humeau L, Slepushkin V, et al. Safe two-plasmid production for the first clinical lentivirus vector that achieves >99% transduction in primary cells using a one-step protocol. J Gene Med 2004; 6(9):963–973.
19. Humeau LM, Binder GK, Lu X, et al. Efficient lentiviral vector-mediated control of HIV-1 replication in CD4 lymphocytes from diverse HIV+ infected patients grouped according to CD4 count and viral load. Mol Ther 2004; 9(6):902–913.
20. Russell DW, Miller AD. Foamy virus vectors. J Virol 1996; 70(1):217–222.
21. Liu W, He X, Cao Z, et al. Efficient therapeutic gene expression in cultured rat hippocampal neurons mediated by human foamy virus vectors: a potential for the treatment of neurological diseases. Intervirology 2005; 48(5):329–335.
22. Peplinski GR, Tsung K, Norton JA. Vaccinia virus for human gene therapy. Surg Oncol Clin N Am 1998; 7(3):575–588.
23. Irvine KR, Chamberlain RS, Shulman EP, et al. Enhancing efficacy of recombinant anticancer vaccines with prime/boost regimens that use two different vectors. J Natl Cancer Inst 1997; 89(21):1595–1601.
24. Hodge JW, Abrams S, Schlom J, et al. Induction of antitumor immunity by recombinant vaccinia viruses expressing B7-1 or B7-2 costimulatory molecules. Cancer Res 1994; 54(21):5552–5555.
25. Pantuck AJ, van Ophoven A, Gitlitz BJ, et al. Phase I trial of antigen-specific gene therapy using a recombinant vaccinia virus encoding MUC-1 and IL-2 in MUC-1-positive patients with advanced prostate cancer. J Immunother 2004; 27(3):240–253.
26. Parkinson RJ, Mian S, Bishop MC, et al. Disabled infectious single cycle herpes simplex virus (DISC-HSV) is a candidate vector system for gene delivery/expression of GM-CSF in human prostate cancer therapy. Prostate 2003; 56(1):65–73.
27. Wickham TJ, Mathias P, Cheresh DA, et al. Integrins alpha v beta 3 and alpha v beta 5 promote adenovirus internalization but not virus attachment. Cell 1993; 73(2):309–319.
28. Roelvink PW, Lizonova A, Lee JG, et al. The coxsackievirus–adenovirus receptor protein can function as a cellular attachment protein for adenovirus serotypes from subgroups A, C, D, E, and F. J Virol 1998; 72(10):7909–7915.
29. Lee CH, Liu M, Sie KL, et al. Prostate-specific antigen promoter driven gene therapy targeting DNA polymerase-alpha and topoisomerase II alpha in prostate cancer. Anticancer Res 1996; 16(4A):1805–1811.
30. Rodriguez R, Schuur ER, Lim HY, et al. Prostate attenuated replication competent adenovirus (ARCA) CN706: a selective cytotoxic for prostate-specific antigen-positive prostate cancer cells. Cancer Res 1997; 57(13):2559–2563.
31. Gotoh A, Ko SC, Shirakawa T, et al. Development of prostate-specific antigen promoter-based gene therapy for androgen-independent human prostate cancer. J Urol 1998; 160(1):220–229.
32. Silman NJ, Fooks AR. Biophysical targeting of adenovirus vectors for gene therapy. Curr Opin Mol Ther 2000; 2(5):524–531.
33. Yang Y, Su Q, Wilson JM. Role of viral antigens in destructive cellular immune responses to adenovirus vector-transduced cells in mouse lungs. J Virol 1996; 70(10):7209–7212.
34. Kay MA, Holterman AX, Meuse L, et al. Long-term hepatic adenovirus-mediated gene expression in mice following CTLA4Ig administration. Nat Genet 1995; 11(2):191–197.

35. Dai Y, Schwarz EM, Gu D, et al. Cellular and humoral immune responses to adenoviral vectors containing factor IX gene: tolerization of factor IX and vector antigens allows for long-term expression. Proc Natl Acad Sci USA 1995; 92(5):1401–1405.
36. Kumar-Singh R, Farber DB. Encapsidated adenovirus mini-chromosome-mediated delivery of genes to the retina: application to the rescue of photoreceptor degeneration. Hum Mol Genet 1998; 7(12):1893–1900.
37. Fender P, Ruigrok RW, Gout E, et al. Adenovirus dodecahedron, a new vector for human gene transfer [see comment]. Nat Biotechnol 1997; 15(1):52–56.
38. Trudel S, Trachtenberg J, Toi A, et al. A phase I trial of adenovector-mediated delivery of interleukin-2 (AdIL-2) in high-risk localized prostate cancer. Cancer Gene Ther 2003; 10(10):755–763.
39. Richardson WD, Westphal H. A cascade of adenovirus early functions is required for expression of adeno-associated virus. Cell 1981; 27(1 Pt 2):133–141.
40. Kotin RM, Siniscalco M, Samulski RJ, et al. Site-specific integration by adeno-associated virus. Proc Natl Acad Sci USA 1990; 87(6):2211–2215.
41. Monahan PE, Samulski RJ. AAV vectors: Is clinical success on the horizon? Gene Ther 2000; 7(1):24–30.
42. Wolff JA, Malone RW, Williams P, et al. Direct gene transfer into mouse muscle in vivo. Science 1990; 247(4949 Pt 1):1465–1468.
43. Mincheff M, Tchakarov S, Zoubak S, et al. Naked DNA and adenoviral immunizations for immunotherapy of prostate cancer: a phase I/II clinical trial. Eur Urol 2000; 38(2):208–217.
44. Pavlenko M, Roos AK, Lundqvist A, et al. A phase I trial of DNA vaccination with a plasmid expressing prostate-specific antigen in patients with hormone-refractory prostate cancer. Br J Cancer 2004; 91(4):688–694.
45. Lee RJ, Huang L. Folate-targeted, anionic liposome-entrapped polylysine-condensed DNA for tumor cell-specific gene transfer. J Biol Chem 1996; 271(14):8481–8487.
46. Lasic DD, Martin FJ, Gabizon A, et al. Sterically stabilized liposomes: a hypothesis on the molecular origin of the extended circulation times. Biochim Biophys Acta 1991; 1070(1):187–192.
47. Cotten M, Wagner E, Zatloukal K, et al. High-efficiency receptor-mediated delivery of small and large (48 kilobase gene constructs using the endosome-disruption activity of defective or chemically inactivated adenovirus particles. Proc Natl Acad Sci USA 1992; 89(13):6094–6098.
48. Ikegami S, Tadakuma T, Yamakami K, et al. Selective gene therapy for prostate cancer cells using liposomes conjugated with IgM type monoclonal antibody against prostate-specific membrane antigen. Hum Cell 2005; 18(1):17–23.
49. Forsayeth JR, Garcia PD. Adenovirus-mediated transfection of cultured cells. Biotechniques 1994; 17(2):354–356.
50. Wagner E, Zatloukal K, Cotten M, et al. Coupling of adenovirus to transferrin-polylysine/DNA complexes greatly enhances receptor-mediated gene delivery and expression of transfected genes. Proc Natl Acad Sci USA 1992; 89(13):6099–6103.
51. Curiel DT. High-efficiency gene transfer employing adenovirus–polylysine–DNA complexes. Nat Immun 1994; 13(2–3):141–164.
52. Raja-Walia R, Webber J, Naftilan J, et al. Enhancement of liposome-mediated gene transfer into vascular tissue by replication deficient adenovirus. Gene Ther 1995; 2(8): 521–530.
53. Cristiano RJ, Xu B, Nguyen D, et al. Viral and nonviral gene delivery vectors for cancer gene therapy. Cancer Detect Prev 1998; 22(5):445–454.
54. Blades RA, Keating PJ, McWilliam LJ, et al. Loss of HLA class I expression in prostate cancer: implications for immunotherapy. Urology 1995; 46(5):681–686; discussion 686–687.
55. Dranoff G, Jaffee E, Lazenby A, et al. Vaccination with irradiated tumor cells engineered to secrete murine granulocyte-macrophage colony-stimulating factor stimulates potent, specific, and long-lasting anti-tumor immunity. Proc Natl Acad Sci USA 1993; 90(8):3539–3543.

56. Cella M, Engering A, Pinet V, et al. Inflammatory stimuli induce accumulation of MHC class II complexes on dendritic cells [see comment]. Nature 1997; 388(6644):782–787.
57. Cella M, Sallusto F, Lanzavecchia A. Origin, maturation and antigen presenting function of dendritic cells. Curr Opin Immunol 1997; 9(1):10–16.
58. Simons JW, Mikhak B. Ex-vivo gene therapy using cytokine-transduced tumor vaccines: molecular and clinical pharmacology. Semin Oncol 1998; 25(6):661–676.
59. Simons JW, Mikhak B, Chang JF, et al. Induction of immunity to prostate cancer antigens: results of a clinical trial of vaccination with irradiated autologous prostate tumor cells engineered to secrete granulocyte-macrophage colony-stimulating factor using ex vivo gene transfer. Cancer Res 1999; 59(20):5160–5168.
60. Simons J, Small, E, Nelson, W, et al. Phase II trials of a GM-CSF gene-transduced prostate cancer cell line vaccine (GVAX®) demonstrate anti-tumor activity [abstr]. Proc Am Soc Clin Oncol 2001; 20:1073a.
61. Simons J, Higano, C, Smith, D et al. Clinical and immunologic findings in a phase 2 study of a GM-CSF-secreting prostate cancer cell line vaccine in patients with metastatic hormone-refractory prostate cancer (met HPRC). 2005 ASCO Ann Meet 2005.
62. Kim JJ, Trivedi NN, Wilson DM, et al. Molecular and immunological analysis of genetic prostate specific antigen (PSA) vaccine [erratum appears in Oncogene 1999; 18(14):2411. Note: Shoemaker H [corrected to Schoemaker H]]. Oncogene 1998; 17(24):3125–3135.
63. Hall SJ, Sanford MA, Atkinson G, et al. Induction of potent antitumor natural killer cell activity by herpes simplex virus-thymidine kinase and ganciclovir therapy in an orthotopic mouse model of prostate cancer. Cancer Res 1998; 58(15):3221–3225.
64. Herman JR, Adler HL, Aguilar-Cordova E, et al. In situ gene therapy for adenocarcinoma of the prostate: A phase I clinical trial. Hum Gene Ther 1999; 10(7):1239–1249.
65. Latham JP, Searle PF, Mautner V, et al. Prostate-specific antigen promoter/enhancer driven gene therapy for prostate cancer: construction and testing of a tissue-specific adenovirus vector. Cancer Res 2000; 60(2):334–341.
66. DeWeese TL, van der Poel H, Li S, et al. A phase I trial of CV706, a replication-competent, PSA selective oncolytic adenovirus, for the treatment of locally recurrent prostate cancer following radiation therapy. Cancer Res 2001; 61(20):7464–7472.
67. Yu DC, Chen Y, Seng M, et al. The addition of adenovirus type 5 region E3 enables calydon virus 787 to eliminate distant prostate tumor xenografts [erratum appears in Cancer Res 2000; 60(4):1150]. Cancer Res 1999; 59(17):4200–4203.
68. Yu D-C, Chen Y, Dilley J, et al. Antitumor Synergy of CV787, a Prostate Cancer-specific Adenovirus, and Paclitaxel and Docetaxel. Cancer Res 2001; 61(2):517–525.
69. Rodriguez R, Lim HY, Bartkowski LM, et al. Identification of diphtheria toxin via screening as a potent cell cycle and p53-independent cytotoxin for human prostate cancer therapeutics. Prostate 1998; 34(4):259–269.
70. Ikeda H, Yamaguchi M, Sugai S, et al. Expanded polyglutamine in the Machado-Joseph disease protein induces cell death in vitro and in vivo. Nat Genet 1996; 13(2):196–202.
71. Gotoh A, Kao C, Ko SC, et al. Cytotoxic effects of recombinant adenovirus p53 and cell cycle regulator genes (p21 WAF1/CIP1 and p16CDKN4) in human prostate cancers. J Urol 1997; 158(2):636–641.
72. Allay JA, Steiner MS, Zhang Y, et al. Adenovirus p16 gene therapy for prostate cancer. World J Urol 2000; 18(2):111–120.
73. Steiner MS, Anthony CT, Lu Y, et al. Antisense c-myc retroviral vector suppresses established human prostate cancer. Hum Gene Ther 1998; 9(5):747–755.
74. Kim M, Wright M, Deshane J, et al. A novel gene therapy strategy for elimination of prostate carcinoma cells from human bone marrow. Hum Gene Ther 1997; 8(2):157–170.
75. Ko SC, Gotoh A, Thalmann GN, et al. Molecular therapy with recombinant p53 adenovirus in an androgen-independent, metastatic human prostate cancer model. Hum Gene Ther 1996; 7(14):1683–1691.
76. Eastham JA, Hall SJ, Sehgal I, et al. In vivo gene therapy with p53 or p21 adenovirus for prostate cancer. Cancer Res 1995; 55(22):5151–5155.
77. Pisters L, Pettaway C, Hossan E, et al. Intraprostatic AD-p53 gene therapy followed by radical prostatectomy: feasibility and preliminary results. Prostate Cancer Prostatic Dis 1999; 2(4, suppl 3):pS27.

78. Albertini MR, Emler CA, Schell K, et al. Dual expression of human leukocyte antigen molecules and the B7-1 costimulatory molecule (CD80) on human melanoma cells after particle-mediated gene transfer. Cancer Gene Ther 1996; 3(3):192–201.
79. Uckert W, Kammertons T, Haack K, et al. Double suicide gene (cytosine deaminase and herpes simplex virus thymidine kinase) but not single gene transfer allows reliable elimination of tumor cells in vivo. Hum Gene Ther 1998; 9(6):855–865.
80. Advani SJ, Sibley GS, Song PY, et al. Enhancement of replication of genetically engineered herpes simplex viruses by ionizing radiation: a new paradigm for destruction of therapeutically intractable tumors. Gene Ther 1998; 5(2):160–165.
81. Nishihara E, Nagayama Y, Mawatari F, et al. Retrovirus-mediated herpes simplex virus thymidine kinase gene transduction renders human thyroid carcinoma cell lines sensitive to ganciclovir and radiation in vitro and in vivo. Endocrinology 1997; 138(11): 4577–4583.
82. Hanna NN, Mauceri HJ, Wayne JD, et al. Virally directed cytosine deaminase/5-fluorocytosine gene therapy enhances radiation response in human cancer xenografts. Cancer Res 1997; 57(19):4205–4209.
83. Freytag SO, Rogulski KR, Paielli DL, et al. A novel three-pronged approach to kill cancer cells selectively: concomitant viral, double suicide gene, and radiotherapy [see comment]. Hum Gene Ther 1998; 9(9):1323–1333.
84. Rogatko A, Babb JS, Tighiouart M, et al. New paradigm in dose-finding trials: patient-specific dosing and beyond phase I. Clin Cancer Res 2005; 11(15):5342–5346.
85. Berry DA. Introduction to Bayesian methods III: Use and interpretation of Bayesian tools in design and analysis. Clin Trial 2005; 2(4):295–300.
86. Buzdar AU, Ibrahim NK, Francis D, et al. Significantly higher pathologic complete remission rate after neoadjuvant therapy with trastuzumab, paclitaxel, and epirubicin chemotherapy: results of a randomized trial in human epidermal growth factor receptor 2-positive operable breast cancer [see comment]. J Clin Oncol 2005; 23(16):3676–3685.
87. Giles FJ, Kantarjian HM, Cortes JE, et al. Adaptive randomized study of idarubicin and cytarabine versus troxacitabine and cytarabine versus troxacitabine and idarubicin in untreated patients 50 years or older with adverse karyotype acute myeloid leukemia [see comment]. J Clin Oncol 2003; 21(9):1722–1727.
88. Couzin J. The new math of clinical trials. Science 2004; 303(5659):784–786.
89. Berry SM, Berry DA. Accounting for multiplicities in assessing drug safety: a three-level hierarchical mixture model. Biometrics 2004; 60(2):418–426.
90. Zacks S, Rogatko A, Babb J. Optimal Bayesian-feasible dose escalation for cancer phase I trials. Statist Prob Lett 1998; 38(3):215–220.

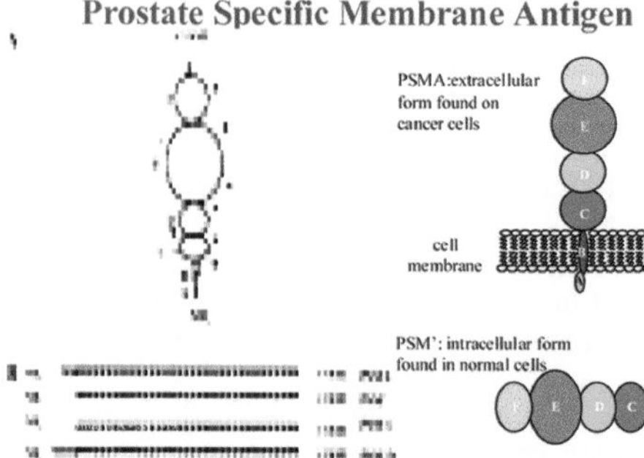

Figure 5.2 Prostate-specific membrane antigen as a globular molecule with demonstration of the extracellular, transmembrane, and intracellular domains. (*See p. 77*)

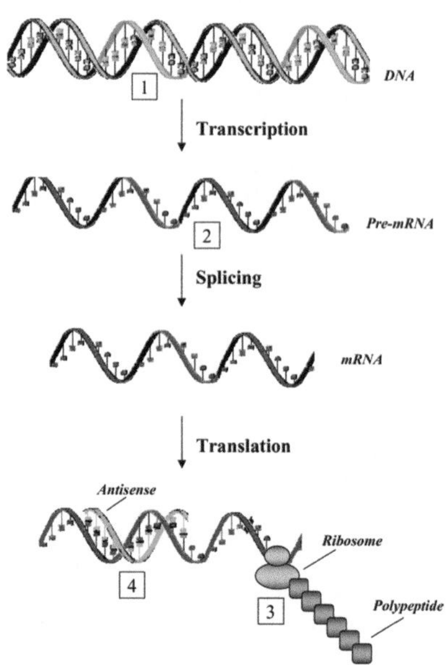

Figure 9.1 Mechanisms of antisense action on target genes. (*See p. 144*)

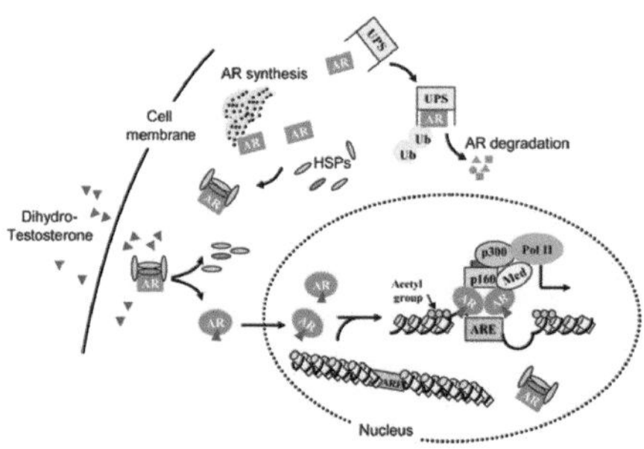

Figure 10.2 Ligand-induced AR activation. (*See p. 165*)

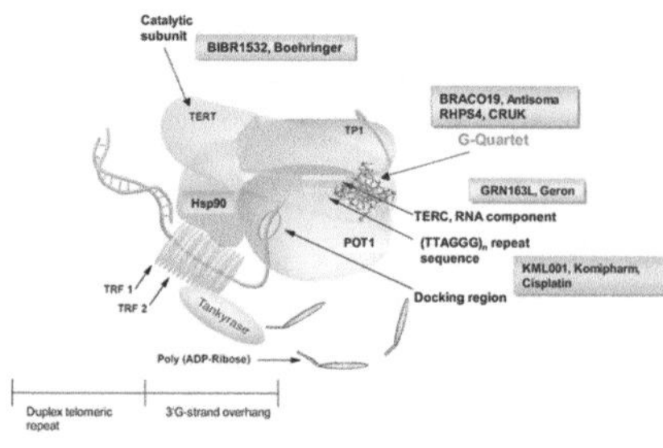

Figure 12.1 The human telomere/telomerase complex. (*See p. 196*)

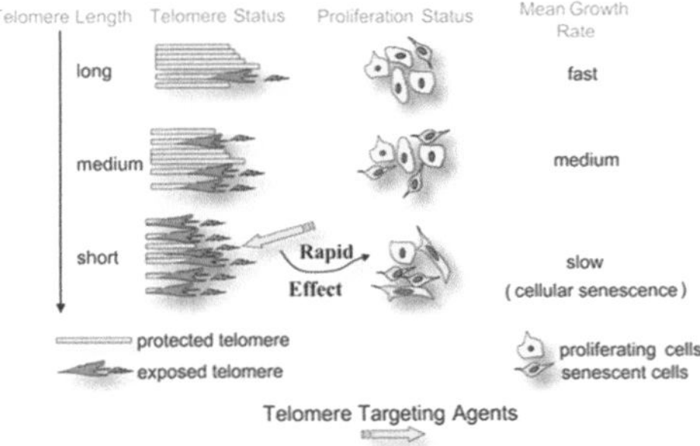

Figure 12.2 Uncapping of telomeres and cellular senescence. (*See p. 197*)

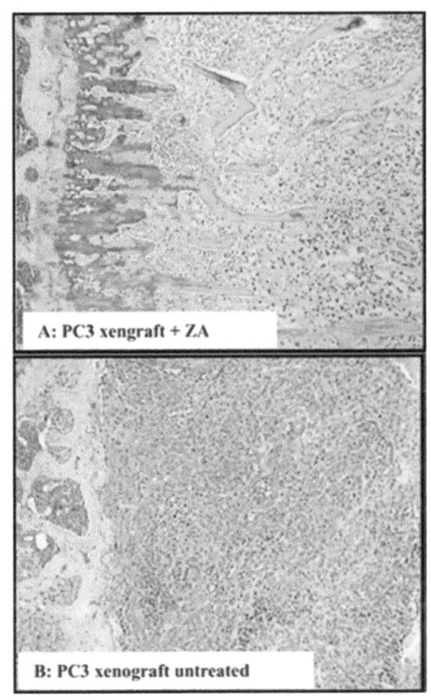

Figure 14.3 Prostate cancer xenografts ± ZA. (*See p. 227*)

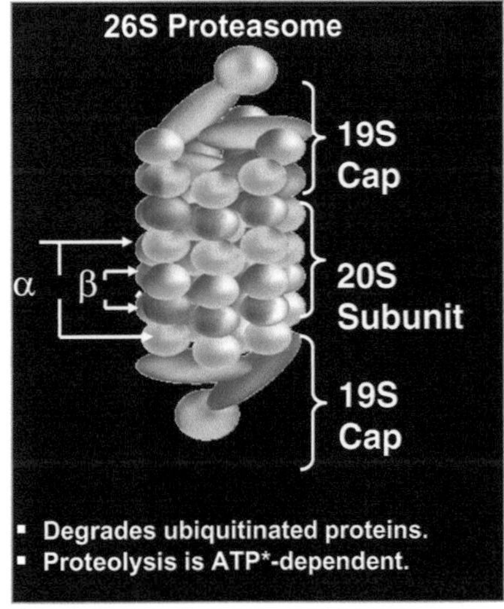

Figure 15.1 26S Proteasome. (*See p. 238*)

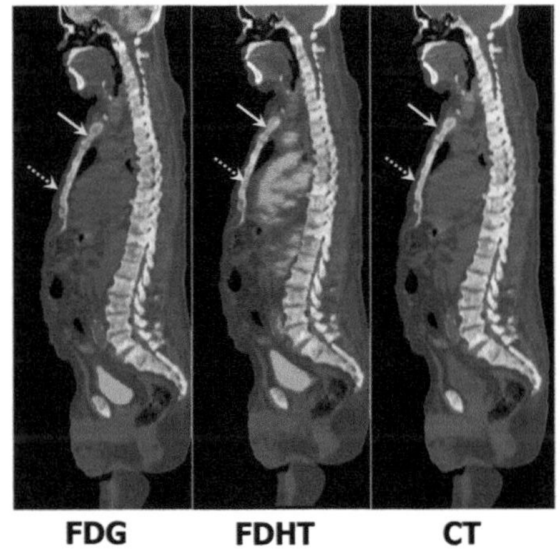

Figure 19.1 Shown is a PET CT fusion study of a patient with castrate metastatic prostate cancer. (*See p. 296*)

8 Angiogenesis Inhibitors in Prostate Cancer

William D. Figg, Michael C. Cox, Tania Alachalabi, and William L. Dahut
Medical Oncology Branch, Center for Cancer Research, National Cancer Institute, National Institutes of Health, Bethesda, Maryland, U.S.A.

INTRODUCTION

Angiogenesis is defined by Merriam Webster dictionary as "the formation and differentiation of new blood vessels." The British surgeon John Hunter was the first to describe this phenomenon, detailing vascular networks formed within a healing wound (1). Hertig (2) first used "angiogenesis" in describing the formation of blood vessels to bring oxygen and nutrients to the developing placenta. In 1971, Folkman (3,4) used this same term to describe the production of vasculature to support a tumor's growth. Without angiogenesis, tumorigenesis, tumor invasion, and metastasis would not occur (5,6). In order for a tumor to grow past 0.5 mm^3, the limit of diffusion to provide adequate oxygenation and nutrients, vascularization must occur (7). Gimbrone et al. (8) showed that blocking angiogenesis caused tumor cells to become dormant. Although this dormancy was due to mechanical isolation of the implanted tumor cells into avascular areas, improved understanding of tumor biology and drug design has brought forth compounds that target the production or receptor binding of these proangiogenic stimulators. With this chapter, we will review the tumor biology of angiogenesis and examine therapeutic uses of anti-angiogenesis in the context of treating prostate cancer.

BIOLOGIC CONTROL OF ANGIOGENESIS

A balance between angiogenesis and anti-angiogenesis is found with homeostasis (5). Naturally occurring proangiogenic agents include basic fibroblast growth factor (bFGF), vascular endothelial growth factor (VEGF), hypoxia inducible growth factor, and IL-8, as well as various cytokines, matrix molecules, and metalloproteinases, whereas anti-angiogenic agents include interferon (IFN), angiostatin, endostatin, and thrombospondin (5,9). Inhibitors of this process include thrombospondin-1, angiostatin, endostatin, platelet factor 4, and TIMPs (9–15).

Tumor growth occurs when there is an imbalance between cell proliferation and cell death (16). It has been postulated that angiogenesis requires complex, interdependent processes, similar to that of tissue invasion (17). Endothelial cell function is altered by the release of angiogenic cytokines, growth factors, and matrix remodeling. This loss of function results in a break down of the basement membrane of surrounding capillaries, followed by invasion of endothelial cells into the surrounding stroma, and finally, journey of endothelial cells towards the proangiogenic factors. As this column advances, it begins to take on the shape of a new capillary (6,18).

PROANGIOGENIC FACTORS

Basic Fibroblast Growth Factor

Basic fibroblast growth factor(bFGF) was isolated from the bovine brain in 1978 (19). bFGF is found in the basement membrane and subendothelial extracellular matrix of blood vessels. In tumor development, the action of heparin sulfate degrading enzymes activates bFGF, thus mediating the formation of new blood vessels. Overproduction of bFGF has been shown to increase angiogenesis in numerous in vitro and in vivo models (20), whereas inhibiting bFGF prevents angiogenesis (20). bFGF is a nonspecific mediator of angiogenesis produced by endothelial cells, which is found outside normal angiogenic sites (21).

It has been demonstrated that bFGF and other members of the FGF family are important for prostate organogenesis (22–24) as well as the progression for normo-organogenesis to carcinoma (24–27). Twenty-three FGFs have been identified to date (28,29) which bind to one of four identified receptors (30). Increased expression of bFGF receptors 1 and 4 have been demonstrated in prostate cancer (24,25,31). This increased expression has not been correlated with prostate cancer prognosis or microvessal density (MVD) of the tumor (32–35).

HYPOXIA INDUCIBLE FACTOR-1

Hypoxia inducible factor-1 (HIF-1) is involved in the transcribing of genes encoding for a variety of normo-physiologic functions, including erythropoietin and transferring production, endothelin-1, inducible nitric oxide synthase, heme oxygenase 1, VEGF, insulin-like growth factor-2, glucose transporters, and glycolytic enzymes (36). HIF-1 consists of an α and a β subunit. Increased HIF-1α has been shown to be up-regulated in benign prostatic hypertrophy as well as adjacent prostate cancer lesions, signaling a potential target for early prostate cancer therapy (37). This HIF-1α overexpression has not been correlated with a poorer treatment outcome in patients with prostate cancer (38).

ANGIOPOIETIN

The angiogenesis promoter angiopoietin-1 (ang-1) and its antagonist angiopoietin-2 (ang-2) act through their own receptor, tie-2, to interact with VEGF during the angiogenic process (39). These two factors appear to have increased expression in prostate cancer (39), and ang-2 expression has been correlated to increased Gleason score, time to metastasis, and patient survival (40).

PLATELET-DERIVED GROWTH FACTOR

Platelet-derived growth factor (PDGF) binds to one of the two receptors PDGFR-α or PDGFR-β (41). Platelet derived growth factor inhibits phosphorylation of platelet derived growth factor receptor by treatment with PDGFR kinase inhibitor (imatinib) and the chemotherapeutic agent pacitaxel reduce the incidence and size of human prostate cancer bone lesions on nude mice. PDGF consists of one of the four different polypeptide chains, PDGF-A, -B, -C, and -D, which dimerize into the isoforms PDGF-AA, -AB, -BB, -CC, and -DD (41). PDGF-AA, -AB, -BB, and -CC can bind to PDGFR-α, whereas binding to PDGFR-β is limited to PDGF-BB and -DD (42). Activation of the PDGFR-β tyrosine kinase after PDGF binding promotes endothelial, pericyte and smooth muscle cell, proliferation, and migration (43,44), whereas disturbing the genes that encode for PDGF-B or PDGFR-β will cause death in mice (43). PDGFR may play an important role in prostate cancer-related osteoblastic metastases, as well as assisting in apoptosis (45). PDGF and PDGFR appear to have an important role in angiogenesis related to androgen-independent prostate cancer, stimulating cell signaling and participating in cell signaling pathways (46–52).

Epidermal Growth Factor

Epidermal growth factor (EGF) is a generic classification for a number of factors that are implicated in angiogenesis associated with cancer. EGF is overexpressed in a number of cancers, including prostate carcinoma (53–55). Epidermal growth factor receptor (EGFR) has four members, all parts of the erbB receptor family: EGFR (erbB1), HER2 (erbB2), HER3 (erbB3), and HER4 (erbB4) (56). EGFR overexpression is common among many solid tumors, including prostate cancer (57,58). Signaling occurs following activation and dimerization of the EGFR, leading to autophosphorylation. HER2, known to be overexpressed in approximately 30% of all breast cancers, which has also shown overexpression in prostate cancer (59–61). Di Lorenzo et al. (62) demonstrated that the aggressiveness of prostate cancer, as documented by rate of progression and change from androgen-dependent to androgen-independent, was correlated with increased expression of EGFR and HER2.

Preclinical model systems have shown that VEGF secretion can be altered by EGF and EGFR activation (35,63–68). The androgen receptor interacts with EGFR during the crucial loss of hormonal responsiveness of advancing prostate cancer (69). Increased EGF secretion leads to up-regulation of EGFR in the local vasculature. Therefore, if EGFR is inhibited, it may be possible to elicit an anti-vascular and an antitumor effect (70).

VASCULAR ENDOTHELIAL GROWTH FACTOR

In 1988, VEGF was purified from xenografts of ovarian cancer (15). First attributed to acting as a contributing factor for ascities formation in patients with ovarian cancer, VEGF was initially called as vascular permeability factor (71). VEGF's many roles include vascular endothelial cell growth, induction of capillary tube formation, increased vascular permeability and protein extravasation, stimulation of endothelial-cell migration, and promotion of endothelial cell division and survival (72–74).

There are six related glycoprotein members of the EGF family: VEGF-A, VEGF-B, VEGF-C, VEGF-D, placental growth factor (PIGF)-1, and PIGF-2 (15,75–77). In addition, there are three known receptors, VEGFR1 (Flt-1), VEGFR2 (Flk-1/KDR), and VEGFR3 (Flt-4) (67). VEGF-A, the first known form of VEGF, has been found in four isoforms, appearing as molecules of 121, 165, 189, and 206 amino acids in length (76,77). These smaller isoforms can be secreted, whereas the larger ones are found in the stromal compartment of the extracellular matrix, and require activation by proteases (78–80). VEGF-A is important physiologically for wound healing, ovulation, menstruation, pregnancy, and blood pressure maintenance (81). VEGF-A also plays a role in the pathophysiologic conditions of arthritis, psoriasis, macular degeneration, and diabetic retinopathy, to name a few (15).

Both VEGFR1 and VEGFR2 are high-affinity receptors, with each playing a role in physiologic and pathophysiologic angiogenesis (82,83). VEGFR1 has the highest affinity for VEGF, with a weaker affinity shown by VEGFR2, and almost no binding capacity for VEGFR3 (84). It has been hypothesized that VEGFR1 gene encodes two different polypeptides, one the receptor form of VEGFR1 which is a full-length membrane protein, and the other being a soluble VEGF-binding protein, also known as soluble VEGFR-1 (84). VEGFR3 is responsible for lymphangiogenesis. VEGF2 is a ubiquitous receptor found on endothelial cells, whereas VEGFR1 and VEGFR3 are found only on endothelial cells in distinct vascular beds (75). It has been postulated that soluble VEGFR-1 may work as a negative regulator of VEGF activity (85,86), whereas the VEGFR2 receptor has been shown to be most important in elucidating angiogenic activity (85–87). Developmental and physiologic angiogenesis is dependent on activation of VEGFR1 (88), whereas VEGF-A activation of VEGFR2 leads to microvascular permeability, endothelial cell proliferation, invasion, migration, and survival (87,89,90).

It has been suggested that VEGF acts as a paracrine factor, with expression occurring in tumor, stroma, and endothelial cells. Increased expression of VEGF is a negative risk factor for survival in many solid tumors, including prostate cancer (32,33,91–95). Increased expression of VEGF in prostate cancer may be indicative of the progression from androgen-dependent to -independent disease (92). To assess the impact of VEGF expression in prostate cancer, a study examining 67 prostatectomy specimens, in addition to 20 cases of benign prostatic hyperplasia was undertaken. Sixty-seven percent (45 of 67) of the prostatectomy samples were positive for cytoplasmic VEGF staining. Seventy-one percent of these samples showed positivity for VEGF in the stroma, particularly around tumor cells. With multivariate analysis, increased VEGF was related to increased serum prostate-specific antigen (PSA) levels ($p = 0.01$) and a higher Gleason score ($p = 0.04$). High stromal VEGF expression resulted in poorer survival ($p = 0.037$) as well. Another paper examined tissues from 25 patients following transurethral prostatectomy (94). They noted an increase in VEGFR-3 expression in the prostate. In addition, expression of VEGFR-3 correlated with increased PSA, Gleason score, and the risk for metastatic disease to the lymph nodes, preoperatively.

PROSTATE CANCER AND THE DEPENDENCE ON ANGIOGENESIS

Microvessel density, MVD (the number of vessels per microscope viewing field) is a standard in quantifying angiogenesis in a tissue specimen. Higher MVD counts have been correlated with advanced pathologic stage (96,97), increased PSA levels (98,99), higher tumor grade (98), increased metastatic potential (97,100,101), and survival of patients with prostate cancer (98,102–104).

Prostate cancer cells secrete multiple angiogenic factors. Interleukin-8 (IL-8) expression was determined at the invasive edge of prostate tumor samples from 41 patients (105). Increased expression of IL-8 was correlated with Gleason score and pathologic stage ($p = 0.002$) and could be used to determine organ-confined from nonorgan-confined tumors. However, bFGF expression in the same tumors did not correlate with Gleason score or pathologic stage (105). Another group looked at circulating bFGF and vascular endothelial growth factor (VEGF) in patients with PSA-stable versus PSA-progressive hormone-sensitive prostate cancer (106). Although there was no difference in circulating VEGF levels

(801.5 vs. 655.5 pg/mL) the authors suggested that anti-VEGF therapy must be a potential target (106), due to the overall high levels of VEGF in patients with prostate cancer. In addition, only 4 of the 41 patients had measurable urine levels of bFGF with no patients exhibiting circulating levels of bFGF.

Patients enrolled on the Cancer and Leukemia Group B (CALGB) 9480 suramin trial were used to elicit prognostic markers for those patients with androgen-independent prostate cancer. One hundred patients of the 390 patients enrolled on this prospective, Phase III trial had urine collected for VEGF and bFGF concentration analysis (32) on day 1 and day 29 of the first cycle of therapy. Patients with higher baseline urine VEGF had a greater risk of death and shorter survival. For those patients with a urine VEGF >28 pg/mL, their overall survival was 10 versus 17 month for those with a urine VEGF <28 pg/mL ($p = 0.024$) (32). bFGF levels were not prognostic for survival.

The change from an androgen-dependent to an androgen-independent tumor, in context with angiogenesis has also been studied (62,107). Di Lorenzo et al. (62) reviewed four studies which looked at the EGFR family, and its expressional changes during the progression from androgen-dependent to androgen-independent disease. Three of the four studies demonstrated a statistically significant increase in ErbB-2 (Her-2/*neu*) expression. The authors also report a significantly increased expression of EGFR following hormonal manipulation therapy. This group postulates an interaction between the androgen receptor and members of the EGFR family, suggesting a possible cross-talk signaling between the androgen-receptor and ErbB-2 (62). In addition, in vivo data utilizing an LnCAP cell line in a murine model. They demonstrated that as an LnCAP cell progresses from androgen-dependent to androgen-independent, the MVD within that cell increases (107).

ANTI-ANGIOGENIC THERAPY FOR PROSTATE CANCER

As angiogenesis is better understood, and various molecular targets are identified, the excitement for new and improved drug therapies grows. While many of the first agents preformed well in in vivo and in vitro studies, but not so well in human trials, newer agents are proving to impact the care of men with prostate cancer.

TNP-470

TNP-470 is an analog of fumagillin, an antibiotic derived from *Aspergillus fumigatus* Fresenius. In vitro and in vivo studies have shown this agent's ability in inhibit bFGF and downstream angiogenesis (108). It has also shown significant activity against a wide variety of tumor cells explanted in mice. Methionine aminopeptidase-z has recently identified as the potential target for TNP-470, A Phase I study of TNP-470 in patients with androgen-independent prostate cancer has been published recently (109). The dose-limiting toxicity was neuropsychiatric symptoms (including anesthesia, gait disturbance and agitation) all of which resolved following discontinuation of therapy, and a maximum tolerated dose was established as 70.88 mg/m^2. With 33 men treated, there was no clear sign of activity for this agent in AIPC. TNP-470 has been demonstrated to up-regulate PSA secretion by 1.4-fold, and androgen-receptor transcription by 1.2-fold (110), making PSA a problematic end point with this agent.

CARBOXYTRIAMIDAZOLE (CAI)

Carboxytriamidazole acts by disrupting calcium-dependent signal transduction by inhibiting nonvoltage gated calcium channels. In vivo and in vitro experiments have shown anti-invasive, anti-metastatic, and anti-angiogenic activity (111,112). No clinical activity was shown in a Phase II trial of this agent, despite maintenance of targeted drug concentrations (113).

SU5416

SU5416 has been shown to block the ATP binding site in the kinase domain of VEGFR-2, thereby inhibiting VEGF-induced phosphorylation of VEGFR-2, and inhibiting endothelial cell proliferation in vitro (114,115). Thirty-six patients were treated on a Phase II study of SU5416 in men with AIPC (116). The study randomized patients to dexamethasone alone or dexamethasone plus SU5416. Crossover to the combination arm was allowed. No additional activity with the combination over single-agent dexamethasone was shown.

SU101

SU101 has been developed as a tyrosine kinase inhibitor with activity on PDGFR-a and PDGFR-b (117). A Phase II study enrolling 35 patients has been published (49). Three patients exhibited a decrease in PSA of at least 50%.

2-METHOXYESTRADIOL (PANZAM, 2ME$_2$)

2-Methoxyestradiol is an orally available metabolite of 17β-estradiol. While a metabolite of estrogen, there is little to no effect on estrogen receptors and has exhibited preclinical anticancer properties in tumors without estrogen receptors (118). 2-ME$_2$ may be able to exert antitumor properties by destabilizing microtubules, which in turn may be more destructive to endothelial cells as opposed to tumor cells (119). HIF-1α signaling may be inhibited as well. In vivo and in vitro work has shown the inhibition of angiogenesis and proliferation of prostate cancer cells (120–124).

A Phase II trial of 2-ME$_2$, in which patients were randomized to 400 or 1200 mg daily was undertaken (125). Treatment was well tolerated, with grade 2–3 liver function test increases seen in the high-dose group. None of the 33 patients had a PSA response, nor a radiographic response. Eight patients had a PSA decline of $>20\%$. The median time to PSA progression in the 1200 mg/day group was 109 days, compared with 67 days in the 400 mg/day group. Patients in the high-dose group had a slowing of PSA velocity over the first two cycles of therapy, but was not continued following two cycles.

IMATINIB

Imatinib targets the bcr-abl gene product, a result of the nine 22 translocation present in chronic myelogenous leukemia, which has had profound activity in this disease (126,127). Additional activity of imatinib inhibiting PDGFR and c-kit has been established. In addition, VEGF has been shown to be down-regulated in K562 cell (a chronic myelogenous leukemia cell line) by imatinib in a dose–response relationship (128). A Phase I trial of imatinib combined a dose of 600 mg qd of imatinib with escalating weekly docetaxel (45). Most of these patients were pretreated with chemotherapy, and a portion had a significant PSA decline during treatment (128). Imatinib 600 mg qd with the maximally tolerated docetaxel dose of 30 mg/ m^2/wk, 4 week out of every 6, is currently in a Phase II trial in patients with AIPC.

BEVACIZUMAB (rhuMab.VEGF)

On February 26, 2004, bevacizumab (Avastin®, Genentech, Inc., South San Francisco, California) became the first anti-angiogenic agent to receive full approval by the U.S. Food and Drug Administration (FDA). Bevacizumab is a humanized variant of a murine monoclonal antibody against VEGF (129). Bevacizumab neutralizes VEGF and therefore inhibits growth of neoplastic tumors requiring VEGF for progression.

Fifteen patients with hormone-refractory prostate cancer were treated with 10 mg/kg of bevacizumab every 2 week, for six cycles (130). Seven patients had progressive disease at day 70 and seven patients had stable disease. There were no complete or partial responders. One patient had a PSA decrease of $>25\%$, and three patients had a PSA response of $<25\%$ decrease. No patients had a $>50\%$ decrease of PSA. The authors concluded that bevacizumab alone in metastatic disease did not produce meaningful responses (130). Picus (131) reported a Phase II trial in which bevacizumab was administered concurrently with docetaxel and estramustine. Forty-two percent of patients had a partial response in soft tissue disease and 79% of patients had a $>50\%$ PSA response. Toxicities included febrile neutropenia, fatigue, uncomplicated neutropenia, deep veing thombosis, including one fatal mesenteric vein thrombosis, a fatal stroke, and a perforated sigmoid colon.

On the basis of these results, the Cancer and Leukemia Group B (CALGB) has initiated trial 90401, which examines the combination of docetaxel, prednisone with or without bevacizumab. The primary end point in this trial is overall survival. Prednisone is used as opposed to estramustine, to improve the overall toxicity profile.

THALIDOMIDE

First developed by CIBA Pharmaceutical Company in 1954 (132), thalidomide was originally used as a sedative-hypnotic and an anti-emesis agent for pregnant women. A single dose of thalidomide by the mother, during the gestation of a baby led to limb and congenital abnormalities found in slightly more than 10,000 babies worldwide (133). These teratogenic side effects resulted in the drug being pulled from the European and Canadian markets (133). In 1998, the U.S. Food and Drug Administration approved thalidomide for erythema nodosum leprosum (134).

D'Amato et al. (132) postulated that the teratogenic properties associated with thalidomide were due, in part, to the drug's ability to disrupt vasculogenesis and that a comparable response could be elicited when using thalidomide to inhibit angiogenesis of tumor cells. Bauer et al. (135) went on to determine that thalidomide must undergo metabolism to an active compound, in order for its anti-angiogenic properties to occur. Ando et al. (136) reported that cytochrome P450 2C19 is responsible for this metabolism. Thalidomide's exact mechanism of action remains unclear. It is known that modulation of inflammatory cytokines [i.e., tissue necrosis factor-α (TNF-α), γ interferon, and possibly nuclear factor $\kappa\beta$

(NF-κβ)] are involved. Thalidomide has been shown to inhibit TNF-α production by increasing the breakdown of its mRNA (137,138). TNF-α, NF-κβ, and a host of other factors have been implicated in tumor angiogenesis, and by inhibiting this angiogenesis, thalidomide may exert its antitumor properties (139).

Thalidomide's clinical impact has been seen in varying disease states, including those of an autoimmune in nature, to viral to oncologic. Of the diseases thalidomide is used in, leprosy, multiple myeloma, and prostate cancer have the most compelling data (139).

SINGLE-AGENT THALIDOMIDE

Investigators at the National Cancer Institute have reported the use of thalidomide alone, in patients with androgen-independent prostate cancer (140). In this randomized, Phase II trial, men with AIPC were randomized to either a low-dose arm (200 mg/day) or a high-dose arm (200 mg/day, escalating to 1200 mg/day). Sixty-three patients were enrolled (50 on the low-dose and 13 on the high-dose arms). Nine of 50 patients (18%) on the low-dose arm achieved a ≥50% decrease in PSA, which was maintained at least 28 days. Four patients maintained this decrease in PSA for at least 150 days. There was no correlation between microvessel counts and PSA decline or radiographic changes, as well as no correlation between response and VEGF or bFGF expression. The most reported toxicities were those of constipation, dizziness, edema, fatigue, mood changes, and peripheral neuropathy.

Drake et al. (141) reported a similar Phase II study of low-dose thalidomide in patients with AIPC. Twenty men were treated with 100 mg of thalidomide daily, for up to 6 month. Three men showed a ≥50% drop in PSA, with an overall median drop in PSA of 48%. Thalidomide was well tolerated, with only three men being removed from study due to toxicity. The authors found a correlation in decreased bFGF (statistically significant, $p = 0.04$) levels concurrent with a fall in PSA.

THALIDOMIDE IN COMBINATION WITH ANTICANCER AGENTS

Two recent reports are the first reports to note an increased survival for patients undergoing treatment with docetaxel for AIPC (142,143). While the Intergroup (142) and TAX327 (143) trials were open and accruing patients, researchers at the NCI were evaluating docetaxel in combination with thalidomide (144). This randomized Phase II trial studied 75 chemotherapy-naïve patients treated with either docetaxel (30 mg/m^2/dose weekly 3 out of 4 week) or docetaxel (given as the same regimen) and thalidomide (200 mg/day, continuous). Patients were randomized in a 1:2 fashion, with 25 patients receiving docetaxel alone, and 50 patients receiving the combination. Nine of 24 patients (37%) on the docetaxel arm had a PSA decrease ≥50% versus 25 of 47 (53%) on the combination arm ($p = 0.32$). The 18 month survival was 68% for the two groups, with a median progression free survival of 3.7 versus 5.9 month, respectively. Overall survival was 14.7 versus 28.9 month, which was not statistically significant. As before, there were no significant changes in bFGF or VEGF levels during treatment. This may suggest that such markers are not sensitive enough to predict response or may not be appropriate for this agent.

While the combination was fairly well tolerated, an increased risk of venous thromboembolism (VTE) did present itself early in the study (145). None of the patients enrolled on the docetaxel alone arm developed VTE, whereas 9 of 47 (19%) on the docetaxel/thalidomide arm developed VTE ($p = 0.025$). Patients randomized to the combination arm received enoxaparin prophylaxis for VTE, and those patients enrolled after the protocol change was made remained on study without VTE (144).

SUMMARY AND FUTURE DIRECTIONS

Angiogenesis remains an important area in solid tumor and prostate cancer research. Laboratory and clinical studies have shown that progression of prostate cancer relies on neovascularization. Early trials have shown that there is a role for anti-angiogenic therapy in this disease. While the exact role of anti-angiogenic agents in the management of prostate cancer is not fully understood, multiple clinical trials are underway combining newer agents with traditional chemotherapy options. By inhibiting angiogenesis, the progression from androgen dependence to androgen independence may be avoided. Further studies need to be conducted to understand the exact role of these agents in everyday management of prostate cancer, but the data presented to date hold great excitement in future directions.

REFERENCES

1. Hunter J. Plamer JF, ed. Lectures on the Principles of Surgery: The Works of John Hunter, F.R.S. Vol. 1. London: Longman, 1835.
2. Hertig A. Contrib Embryol 1935; 25:37.
3. Folkman J, Merler E, Abernathy C. Tumour angiogenesis: therapeutic implications. N Engl J Med 1971; 285:1182–1186.
4. Folkman J, et al. Isolation of a tumor factor responsible for angiogenesis. J Exp Med 1971; 133(2):275–288.
5. Hanahan D, Folkman J. Patterns and emerging mechanisms of the angiogeneic switch during tumorigenesis. Cell 1996; 86:353–364.
6. Fidler IJ. Critical determinants of metastasis. Semin Cancer Biol 2002; 12(2):89–96.
7. Folkman J. Angiogenesis in cancer, vascular, rheumatoid and other disease. Nat Med 1995; 1(1):27–31.
8. Gimbrone MA Jr., Leapman SB, Ramzi SC, et al. Tumor dormancy in vivo by prevention of neovascularization. J Exp Med 1972; 136(2):261–276.
9. Folkman J, Klagsbrun M. Angiogenic factors. Science 1987; 235(4787):442–447.
10. Dvorak HF. Tumors: wounds that do not heal. Similarities between tumor stroma generation and wound healing. N Engl J Med 1986; 315(26):1650–1659.
11. Ingber DE, Folkman J. Mechanochemical switching between growth and differentiation during fibroblast growth factor-stimulated angiogenesis in vitro: role of extracellular matrix. J Cell Biol 1989; 109(1):317–330.
12. O'Reilly MS. Angiostatin: an endogenous inhibitor of angiogenesis and of tumor growth. Exs 1997; 79:273–294.
13. Joseph-Silverstein J, Silverstein RL. Cell adhesion molecules: an overview. Cancer Invest 1998; 16(3):176–182.
14. Yancopoulos GD, Davis S, Gale NW, et al. Vascular-specific growth factors and blood vessel formation. Nature 2000; 407(6801):242–248.
15. Ferrara N, Gerber HP, LeCouter J. The biology of VEGF and its receptors. Nat Med 2003; 9(6):669–676.
16. Holmgren L, O'Reilly MS, Folkman J. Dormancy of micrometastases: balanced proliferation and apoptosis in the presence of angiogenesis suppression. Nat Med 1995; 1(2):149–153.
17. Kohn EC, Liotta LA. Molecular insights into cancer invasion: strategies for prevention and intervention. Cancer Res 1995; 55(9):1856–1862.

18. Auerbach W, Auerbach R. Angiogenesis inhibition: a review. Pharmacol Ther 1994; 63(3):265–311.
19. Gospodarowicz D, Bialecki H, Greenburg G. Purification of the fibroblast growth factor activity from bovine brain. J Biol Chem 1978; 253(10):3736–3743.
20. Wellstein A, Czubayko F. Inhibition of fibroblast growth factors. Breast Cancer Res Treat 1996; 38(1):109–119.
21. Rak, J, Kerbel RS. Basic fibroblast growth factor and the complexity of tumour angiogenesis. Expert Opin Investig Drugs 1998; 7(5):797–801.
22. Cunha GR, Donjacour A. Stromal–epithelial interactions in normal and abnormal prostatic development. Prog Clin Biol Res 1987; 239:251–272.
23. Cunha GR, Donjacour AA, Ceoke PS, et al. The endocrinology and developmental biology of the prostate. Endocr Rev 1987; 8(3):338–362.
24. Giri D, Ropiquet F, Ittmann M. Alterations in expression of basic fibroblast growth factor (FGF) 2 and its receptor FGFR-1 in human prostate cancer. Clin Cancer Res 1999; 5(5):1063–1071.
25. Leung HY, et al. Over-expression of fibroblast growth factor-8 in human prostate cancer. Oncogene 1996; 12(8):1833–1835.
26. Dorkin TJ, Robinson MC, Marsh C, et al. FGF8 over-expression in prostate cancer is associated with decreased patient survival and persists in androgen independent disease. Oncogene 1999; 18(17):2755–2761.
27. Dorkin TJ, Robinson MC, Marsh C, et al. aFGF immunoreactivity in prostate cancer and its co-localization with bFGF and FGF8. J Pathol 1999; 189(4):564–569.
28. Ornitz DM, Itoh N. Fibroblast growth factors. Genome Biol 2001; 2(3):REVIEWS3005.
29. Yamashita T, Yoshioka M, Itoh N. Identification of a novel fibroblast growth factor, FGF-23, preferentially expressed in the ventrolateral thalamic nucleus of the brain. Biochem Biophys Res Commun 2000; 277(2):494–498.
30. Johnson DE, Williams LT. Structural and functional diversity in the FGF receptor multigene family. Adv Cancer Res 1993; 60:1–41.
31. Gowardhan B, Douglas da, Mathers me, et al. Evaluation of the fibroblast growth factor system as a potential target for therapy in human prostate cancer. Br J Cancer 2005; 92(2):320–327.
32. Bok RA, Halabi S, Fei DT, et al. Vascular endothelial growth factor and basic fibroblast growth factor urine levels as predictors of outcome in hormone-refractory prostate cancer patients: a cancer and leukemia group B study. Cancer Res 2001; 61(6): 2533–2536.
33. George DJ, Halabi S, Shepard TF, et al. Prognostic significance of plasma vascular endothelial growth factor levels in patients with hormone-refractory prostate cancer treated on Cancer and Leukemia Group B 9480. Clin Cancer Res 2001; 7(7):1932–1936.
34. Strohmeyer D, Strauss F, Rossing C, et al. Expression of bFGF, VEGF and c-met and their correlation with microvessel density and progression in prostate carcinoma. Anticancer Res 2004; 24(3a):1797–1804.
35. Trojan L, Thomas D, Knoll T, et al. Expression of pro-angiogenic growth factors VEGF, EGF and bFGF and their topographical relation to neovascularisation in prostate cancer. Urol Res 2004; 32(2):97–103.
36. Semenza GL. Angiogenesis in ischemic and neoplastic disorders. Annu Rev Med 2003; 54:17–28.
37. Zhong H, Semenza GL, Simmons JW, et al. Up-regulation of hypoxia-inducible factor 1alpha is an early event in prostate carcinogenesis. Cancer Detect Prev 2004; 28(2):88–93.
38. Du Z, et al. Expression of hypoxia-inducible factor 1alpha in human normal, benign, and malignant prostate tissue. Chin Med J (Engl) 2003; 116(12):1936–1939.
39. Wurmbach JH, Hammener P, Sevinc S, et al. The expression of angiopoeitins and their receptor Tie-2 in human prostate carcinoma. Anticancer Res 2000; 20(6D):5217–5220.
40. Lind AJ, Wikström P, Granfurs T, et al. Angiopoietin 2 expression is related to histological grade, vascular density, metastases, and outcome in prostate cancer. Prostate 2005; 62(4):394–399.
41. Fredriksson L, Li H, Eriksson U. The PDGF family: four gene products form five dimeric isoforms. Cytokine Growth Factor Rev 2004; 15(4):197–204.

42. Betsholtz C, Karlsson L, Lindahl P. Developmental roles of platelet-derived growth factors. Bioessays 2001; 23(6):494–507.
43. Roberts WG, Whalen PM, Soderstrom E, et al. Antiangiogenic and antitumor activity of a selective PDGFR tyrosine kinase inhibitor, CP-673,451. Cancer Res 2005; 65(3): 957–966.
44. Bergers G, Song S, Meyer-Morse N, et al. Benefits of targeting both pericytes and endothelial cells in the tumor vasculature with kinase inhibitors. J Clin Invest 2003; 111(9):1287–1295.
45. Mathew P, Fidler IJ, Logothelics CJ, et al. Platelet-derived growth factor receptor inhibitor imatinib mesylate and docetaxel: a modular phase I trial in androgen-independent prostate cancer. J Clin Oncol 2004; 22(16):3323–3329.
46. Hofer MD, Fecko A, Shen R, et al. Expression of the platelet-derived growth factor receptor in prostate cancer and treatment implications with tyrosine kinase inhibitors. Neoplasia 2004; 6(5):503–512.
47. Chott A, Sun Z, Morganstern D, et al. Tyrosine kinases expressed in vivo by human prostate cancer bone marrow metastases and loss of the type 1 insulin-like growth factor receptor. Am J Pathol 1999; 155(4):1271–1279.
48. Baselga J, Rischin D, Ranson M, et al. Phase I safety, pharmacokinetic, and pharmacodynamic trial of ZD1839, a selective oral epidermal growth factor receptor tyrosine kinase inhibitor, in patients with five selected solid tumor types. J Clin Oncol 2002; 20(21):4292–4302.
49. Ko YJ, Small EJ, Kablanaver F, et al. A multi-institutional phase ii study of SU101, a platelet-derived growth factor receptor inhibitor, for patients with hormone-refractory prostate cancer. Clin Cancer Res 2001; 7(4):800–805.
50. Wang D, Huang HJS, Kazlauskas A, et al. Induction of vascular endothelial growth factor expression in endothelial cells by platelet-derived growth factor through the activation of phosphatidylinositol 3-kinase. Cancer Res 1999; 59(7):1464–1472.
51. Sundberg C, Ljungstrom M, Lindmark G, et al. Microvascular pericytes express platelet-derived growth factor-beta receptors in human healing wounds and colorectal adenocarcinoma. Am J Pathol 1993; 143(5):1377–1388.
52. Plate KH, Breier G, Farrell Cl, et al. Platelet-derived growth factor receptor-beta is induced during tumor development and upregulated during tumor progression in endothelial cells in human gliomas. Lab Invest 1992; 67(4):529–534.
53. Barton J, Blackledge G, Wakeling A. Growth factors and their receptors: new targets for prostate cancer therapy. Urology 2001; 58(2 suppl 1):114–122.
54. McKeehan WL, Adams PS, Rosser MP. Direct mitogenic effects of insulin, epidermal growth factor, glucocorticoid, cholera toxin, unknown pituitary factors and possibly prolactin, but not androgen, on normal rat prostate epithelial cells in serum-free, primary cell culture. Cancer Res 1984; 44(5):1998–2010.
55. Boonstra J, et al. The epidermal growth factor. Cell Biol Int 1995; 19(5):413–430.
56. Von Pawel J. Gefitinib (Iressa, ZD1839): a novel targeted approach for the treatment of solid tumors. Bull Cancer 2004; 91(5):E70–E76.
57. Tillotson JK, Rose DP. Density-dependent regulation of epidermal growth factor receptor expression in DU 145 human prostate cancer cells. Prostate 1991; 19(1):53–61.
58. Di Lorenzo G, Tontora G, D'Armiento FP, et al. Expression of epidermal growth factor receptor correlates with disease relapse and progression to androgen-independence in human prostate cancer. Clin Cancer Res 2002; 8(11):3438–3444.
59. Signoretti S, Monitroni R, Manda J, et al. Her-2-neu expression and progression toward androgen independence in human prostate cancer. J Natl Cancer Inst 2000; 92(23):1918–1925.
60. Morris MJ, Reuter VE, Kelly Wk, et al. HER-2 profiling and targeting in prostate carcinoma. Cancer 2002; 94(4):980–986.
61. Osman I, Scher HI, Drobnjak M, et al. HER-2/neu (p185neu) protein expression in the natural or treated history of prostate cancer. Clin Cancer Res 2001; 7(9):2643–2647.
62. Di Lorenzo G, Bianco R, Tortora G, et al. Involvement of growth factor receptors of the epidermal growth factor receptor family in prostate cancer development and progression to androgen independence. Clin Prostate Cancer 2003; 2(1):50–57.

63. Kim SJ, Uehara H, Karashima T, et al. Blockade of epidermal growth factor receptor signaling in tumor cells and tumor-associated endothelial cells for therapy of androgen-independent human prostate cancer growing in the bone of nude mice. Clin Cancer Res 2003; 9(3):1200–1210.
64. Goldman CK, Kim J, Wang WL, et al. Epidermal growth factor stimulates vascular endothelial growth factor production by human malignant glioma cells: a model of glioblastoma multiforme pathophysiology. Mol Biol Cell 1993; 4(1):121–133.
65. Danielsen T, Rofstad EK. VEGF, bFGF and EGF in the angiogenesis of human melanoma xenografts. Int J Cancer 1998; 76(6):836–841.
66. Yamamoto S, Yasui W, Kitadai Y, et al. Expression of vascular endothelial growth factor in human gastric carcinomas. Pathol Int 1998; 48(7):499–506.
67. Chevalier S, Defoy I, Lacoste J, et al. Vascular endothelial growth factor and signaling in the prostate: more than angiogenesis. Mol Cell Endocrinol 2002; 189(1–2):169–179.
68. Ravindranath N, et al. Epidermal growth factor modulates the expression of vascular endothelial growth factor in the human prostate. J Androl 2001; 22(3):432–443.
69. Festuccia C, Gravina GL, Angelucci A, et al. Additive antitumor effects of the epidermal growth factor receptor tyrosine kinase inhibitor, gefitinib (Iressa), and the nonsteroidal antiandrogen, bicalutamide (Casodex), in prostate cancer cells in vitro. Int J Cancer 2005; 115(4):630–640.
70. Mathur RS, Mathur SP, Young RC. Up-regulation of epidermal growth factor-receptors (EGF-R) by nicotine in cervical cancer cell lines: this effect may be mediated by EGF. Am J Reprod Immunol 2000; 44(2):114–120.
71. Senger DR, Galli SJ, Dvorak AM, et al. Tumor cells secrete a vascular permeability factor that promotes accumulation of ascites fluid. Science 1983; 219(4587):983–985.
72. Ferrara N, Houck K, Jakeman L, et al. Molecular and biological properties of the vascular endothelial growth factor family of proteins. Endocr Rev 1992; 13(1):18–32.
73. Connolly DT, Heuvelman DM, Nekon R, et al. Tumor vascular permeability factor stimulates endothelial cell growth and angiogenesis. J Clin Invest 1989; 84(5):1470–1478.
74. Hicklin DJ, Ellis LM. Role of the vascular endothelial growth factor pathway in tumor growth and angiogenesis. J Clin Oncol 2005; 23(5):1011–1027.
75. Thomas KA. Vascular endothelial growth factor, a potent and selective angiogenic agent. J Biol Chem 1996; 271(2):603–606.
76. Houck KA, Ferrera N, Winer J, et al. The vascular endothelial growth factor family: identification of a fourth molecular species and characterization of alternative splicing of RNA. Mol Endocrinol 1991; 5(12):1806–1814.
77. Tischer E, Mitchell R, Hartman T, et al. The human gene for vascular endothelial growth factor: multiple protein forms are encoded through alternative exon splicing. J Biol Chem 1991; 266(18):11947–11954.
78. McColl BK, Baldwin ME, Roufail S, et al. Plasmin activates the lymphangiogenic growth factors VEGF-C and VEGF-D. J Exp Med 2003; 198(6):863–868.
79. Park JE, Keller GA, Ferrara N. The vascular endothelial growth factor (VEGF) isoforms: differential deposition into the subepithelial extracellular matrix and bioactivity of extracellular matrix-bound VEGF. Mol Biol Cell 1993; 4(12):1317–1326.
80. Bergers G, Brekken R, McMahon G, et al. Matrix metalloproteinase-9 triggers the angiogenic switch during carcinogenesis. Nat Cell Biol 2000; 2(10):737–744.
81. Brown LF, Yeo KT, Berse B, Yeo TK et al. Expression of vascular permeability factor (vascular endothelial growth factor) by epidermal keratinocytes during wound healing. J Exp Med 1992; 176(5):1375–1379.
82. Veikkola T, Karkkamen M, Claesson-Welsh L, et al. Regulation of angiogenesis via vascular endothelial growth factor receptors. Cancer Res 2000; 60(2):203–212.
83. Veikkola T, Alitalo K. VEGFs, receptors and angiogenesis. Semin Cancer Biol 1999; 9(3):211–220.
84. Shibuya M. Structure and dual function of vascular endothelial growth factor receptor-1 (Flt-1). Int J Biochem Cell Biol 2001; 33(4):409–420.
85. Elkin M, Orgel A, Kleinman HK. An angiogenic switch in breast cancer involves estrogen and soluble vascular endothelial growth factor receptor 1. J Natl Cancer Inst 2004; 96(11):875–878.

86. Carmeliet P, Moons L, Lutton A, et al. Synergism between vascular endothelial growth factor and placental growth factor contributes to angiogenesis and plasma extravasation in pathological conditions. Nat Med 2001; 7(5):575–583.
87. Zeng H, Dvorak HF, Mukhopadhyay D. Vascular permeability factor (VPF)/vascular endothelial growth factor (VEGF) peceptor-1 down-modulates VPF/VEGF receptor-2-mediated endothelial cell proliferation, but not migration, through phosphatidylinositol 3-kinase-dependent pathways. J Biol Chem 2001; 276(29):26969–26979.
88. Fong GH, Rossunt J, Gertsenstein M, et al. Role of the Flt-1 receptor tyrosine kinase in regulating the assembly of vascular endothelium. Nature 1995; 376(6535):66–70.
89. Dvorak HF. Vascular permeability factor/vascular endothelial growth factor: a critical cytokine in tumor angiogenesis and a potential target for diagnosis and therapy. J Clin Oncol 2002; 20(21):4368–4380.
90. Millauer B, Wizigman-Voos S, Schnurch H, et al. High affinity VEGF binding and developmental expression suggest Flk-1 as a major regulator of vasculogenesis and angiogenesis. Cell 1993; 72(6):835–846.
91. Kohli M, Fink LM, Spencer HJ, et al. Advanced prostate cancer activates coagulation: a controlled study of activation markers of coagulation in ambulatory patients with localized and advanced prostate cancer. Blood Coagul Fibrinol 2002; 13:1–5.
92. Nicholson B, Schaefer G, Theodorescu D. Angiogenesis in prostate cancer: biology and therapeutic opportunities. Cancer Metastasis Rev 2001; 20(3–4):297–319.
93. West AF, O'Donnell M, Chartton RG, et al. Correlation of vascular endothelial growth factor expression with fibroblast growth factor-8 expression and clinico-pathologic parameters in human prostate cancer. Br J Cancer 2001; 85(4):576–583.
94. Li R, Younes M, Wheeler TM, et al. Expression of vascular endothelial growth factor receptor-3 (VEGFR-3) in human prostate. Prostate 2004; 58(2):193–199.
95. Borre M, Nerstrom B, Overgaard J. Association between immunohistochemical expression of vascular endothelial growth factor (VEGF), VEGF-expressing neuroendocrine-differentiated tumor cells, and outcome in prostate cancer patients subjected to watchful waiting. Clin Cancer Res 2000; 6(5):1882–1890.
96. Brawer MK, Deering RE, Brown M, et al. Predictors of pathologic stage in prostatic carcinoma: the role of neovascularity. Cancer 1994; 73(3):678–687.
97. Bettencourt MC, Bauer JJ, Sesterhom IA, et al. CD34 immunohistochemical assessment of angiogenesis as a prognostic marker for prostate cancer recurrence after radical prostatectomy. J Urol 1998; 160(2):459–465.
98. Hall MC, Troncoso P, Pollock A, et al. Significance of tumor angiogenesis in clinically localized prostate carcinoma treated with external beam radiotherapy. Urology 1994; 44(6):869–875.
99. Di Lorenzo G, De Placido S, Autorino R, et al. Expression of biomarkers modulating prostate cancer progression: implications in the treatment of the disease. Prostate Cancer Prostatic Dis 2005; 8(1):54–59.
100. Silberman MA, Partin AW, Veltri RW, et al. Tumor angiogenesis correlates with progression after radical prostatectomy but not with pathologic stage in Gleason sum 5 to 7 adenocarcinoma of the prostate. Cancer 1997; 79(4):772–779.
101. Weidner N, Carroll PR, Flax AJ, et al. Tumor angiogenesis correlates with metastasis in invasive prostate carcinoma. Am J Pathol 1993; 143(2):401–409.
102. Offersen BV, Borre M, Overgaard J. Immunohistochemical determination of tumor angiogenesis measured by the maximal microvessel density in human prostate cancer. Apmis 1998; 106(4):463–469.
103. Borre M, Offerson BV, Nerstorm B, et al. Microvessel density predicts survival in prostate cancer patients subjected to watchful waiting. Br J Cancer 1998; 78(7): 940–944.
104. Lissbrant IF, Stuttin P, Damber JE, et al. Vascular density is a predictor of cancer-specific survival in prostatic carcinoma. Prostate 1997; 33(1):38–45.
105. Uehara H, Troncoso P, Johnston D, et al. Expression of interleukin-8 gene in radical prostatectomy specimens is associated with advanced pathologic stage. Prostate 2005; 64(1):40–49.

106. Kohli M, Kaushal V, Spencer HJ, et al. Prospective study of circulating angiogenic markers in prostate-specific antigen (PSA)-stable and PSA-progressive hormone-sensitive advanced prostate cancer. Urology 2003; 61(4):765–769.
107. Gustavsson H, Welen K, Damber JE. Transition of an androgen-dependent human prostate cancer cell line into an androgen-independent subline is associated with increased angiogenesis. Prostate 2005; 62(4):364–373.
108. Ingber D, Fujita T, Kishimoto S, et al. Synthetic analogues of fumagillin that inhibit angiogenesis and suppress tumour growth. Nature 1990; 348(6301):555–557.
109. Logothetis CJ, Wu kk, Finn LD, et al. Phase I trial of the angiogenesis inhibitor TNP-470 for progressive androgen-independent prostate cancer. Clin Cancer Res 2001; 7(5):1198–1203.
110. Horti J, Dixon SC, Logothetis CS, et al. Increased transcriptional activity of prostate-specific antigen in the presence of TNP-470, an angiogenesis inhibitor. Br J Cancer 1999; 79(9–10):1588–1593.
111. Kohn EC, Sandeen MA, Liotta LA. In vivo efficacy of a novel inhibitor of selected signal transduction pathways including calcium, arachidonate, and inositol phosphates. Cancer Res 1992; 52(11):3208–3212.
112. Kohn EC, Liotta LA. L651582: a novel antiproliferative and antimetastasis agent. J Natl Cancer Inst 1990; 82(1):54–60.
113. Bauer KS, Figg WD, Hamilton JM, et al. A pharmacokinetically guided Phase II study of carboxyamido-triazole in androgen-independent prostate cancer. Clin Cancer Res 1999; 5(9):2324–2329.
114. Fong TA, Shawver LK, Sun L, et al. SU5416 is a potent and selective inhibitor of the vascular endothelial growth factor receptor (Flk-1/KDR) that inhibits tyrosine kinase catalysis, tumor vascularization, and growth of multiple tumor types. Cancer Res 1999; 59(1):99–106.
115. Mendel DB, Laird AD, Smolich BD, et al. Development of SU5416, a selective small molecule inhibitor of VEGF receptor tyrosine kinase activity, as an anti-angiogenesis agent. Anticancer Drug Des 2000; 15(1):29–41.
116. Stadler WM, Cao D, Vogelzang NJ, et al. A randomized Phase II trial of the antiangiogenic agent SU5416 in hormone-refractory prostate cancer. Clin Cancer Res 2004; 10(10):3365–3370.
117. Shawver LK, Schwartz DP, Mann T, et al. Inhibition of platelet-derived growth factor-mediated signal transduction and tumor growth by N-[4-(trifluoromethyl)-phenyl]5-methylisoxazole-4-carboxamide. Clin Cancer Res 1997; 3(7):1167–1177.
118. Reiser F, Way D, Berna SM, et al. Inhibition of normal and experimental angiotumor endothelial cell proliferation and cell cycle progression by 2-methoxyestradiol. Proc Soc Exp Biol Med 1998; 219(3):211–216.
119. Mabjeesh NJ, et al. 2ME2 inhibits tumor growth and angiogenesis by disrupting microtubules and dysregulating HIF. Cancer Cell 2003; 3(4):363–375.
120. Davoodpour P, Landstrom M. 2-Methoxyestradiol-induced apoptosis in prostate cancer cells requires Smad7. J Biol Chem 2005; 280(15):14773–14779.
121. Davoodpour P, Bergstrom M, Landstrom M. Effects of 2-methoxyestradiol on proliferation, apoptosis and PET-tracer uptake in human prostate cancer cell aggregates. Nucl Med Biol 2004; 31(7):867–874.
122. Bu S, Blaukat A, Fu X, et al. Mechanisms for 2-methoxyestradiol-induced apoptosis of prostate cancer cells. FEBS Lett 2002; 531(2):141–151.
123. Kumar AP, Garcia GE, Slaga TJ. 2-Methoxyestradiol blocks cell-cycle progression at G(2)/M phase and inhibits growth of human prostate cancer cells. Mol Carcinog 2001; 31(3):111–124.
124. Qadan LR, Perez-Stable CM, et al. 2-Methoxyestradiol induces G2/M arrest and apoptosis in prostate cancer. Biochem Biophys Res Commun 2001; 285(5):1259–1266.
125. Sweeney C, Anderson C, Liu G, Yiannartso SC, et al. A phase II multicenter, randomized, double-blind, safety trial assessing the pharmacokinetics, pharmacodynamics, and efficacy of oral 2-methoxyestradiol capsules in hormone-refractory prostate cancer. Clin Cancer Res 2005; 11(18):6625–6633.

126. Druker BJ, Tamura S, Bachdunger E, et al. Effects of a selective inhibitor of the Abl tyrosine kinase on the growth of Bcr-Abl positive cells. Nat Med 1996; 2(5):561–566.
127. Druker BJ, Talpaz M, Resta DJ, et al. Efficacy and safety of a specific inhibitor of the BCR-ABL tyrosine kinase in chronic myeloid leukemia. N Engl J Med 2001; 344(14):1031–1037.
128. Ebos JM, Tran J, Master Z, et al. Imatinib mesylate (STI-571) reduces Bcr-Abl-mediated vascular endothelial growth factor secretion in chronic myelogenous leukemia. Mol Cancer Res 2002; 1(2):89–95.
129. Hurwitz H, Fehrenbacher L, Novority W, et al. Bevacizumab plus irinotecan, flourouracil, and leucovorin for metastatic colorectal cancer. N Engl J Med 2004; 350(23):2335–2342.
130. Reese D, et al. A phase II trial of humanized monoclonal anti-vascular endothelial growth factor antibody (rhuMAb VEGF) in hormone refractory prostate cancer (HRPC). Proc Am Soc Clin Oncol 1999; 35 [Abstr #1355].
131. Picus J. Docetaxel/bevacizumab (Avastin) in prostate cancer. Cancer Invest 2004.
132. D'Amato R, Loughnan MS, Flynn E, et al. Thalidomide is an inhibitor of angiogenesis. Proc Natl Acad Sci USA 1994; 91:4082–4085.
133. Lenz W. A short history of thalidomide embryopathy. Terat 1988; 38(3):203–215.
134. Teo SK, Resztak KE, Scheffler MA, et al. Thalidomide in the treatment of leprosy. Microbes Infect 2002; 4(11):1193–202.
135. Bauer KS, Dixon SC, Figg WD. Inhibition of angiogenesis by thalidomide requires metabolic activation, which is species-dependent. Biochem Pharmacol 1998; 55(11):1827–1834.
136. Ando Y, Fuse E, Figg WD. Thalidomide metabolism by the CYP2C subfamily. Clin Cancer Res 2002; 8(6):1964–1973.
137. Moreira AL, Sampaio EP, Zmudzinas A, et al. Thalidomide exerts its inhibitory action on tumor necrosis factor alpha by enhancing mRNA degradation. J Exp Med 1993; 177(6):1675–1680.
138. Sampaio EP, Samo EN, Galilly R, et al. Thalidomide selectively inhibits tumor necrosis factor alpha production by stimulated human monocytes. J Exp Med 1991; 173(3):699–703.
139. Franks ME, Macpherson GR, Figg WD. Thalidomide. Lancet 2004; 363(9423):1802–1811.
140. Figg W, Dahut W, Duray P, et al. A randomized phase II trial of thalidomide, an angiogenesis inhibitor, in patients with androgen-independent prostate cancer. Clin Cancer Res 2001; 7:1888–1893.
141. Drake MJ, Robson W, Mehta P, et al. An open-label phase II study of low-dose thalidomide in androgen-independent prostate cancer. Br J Cancer 2003; 88(6):822–827.
142. Petrylak DP, Tangen CM, Hussain MHA, et al. Docetaxel and estramustine compared with mitoxantrone and prednisone for advanced refractory prostate cancer. N Engl J Med 2004; 351(15):1513–1520.
143. Tannock IF, de wit R, Berry WR, et al. Docetaxel plus prednisone or mitoxantrone plus prednisone for advanced prostate cancer. N Engl J Med 2004; 351(15):1502–1512.
144. Dahut W, Gulley JL, Arlen PM, et al. Randomized phase II trial of docetaxel plus thalidomide in androgen-independent prostate cancer. J Clin Oncol 2004; 22(13):2532–2539.
145. Horne MK III, Figg WD, Arlen P, et al. Increased frequency of venous thromboembolism with the combination of docetaxel and thalidomide in patients with metastatic androgen-independent prostate cancer. Pharmacotherapy 2003; 23(3):315–318.

9 What Antisense Oligonucleotides Have Promise in Prostate Cancer

Kim N. Chi
BC Cancer Agency, Vancouver, British Columbia, Canada

Martin E. Gleave
Vancouver Hospital D-9, Vancouver, British Columbia, Canada

INTRODUCTION

Prostate cancer is the most common cancer diagnosed and the second most common cause of cancer death in men in North America (1). Many patients with localized disease have an excellent long-term survival and high cure rates with standard approaches (2). However, patients with high risk, locally advanced metastatic disease have a poor prognosis, and although hormonal therapy in the form of medical or surgical castration can induce significant long-term remissions, development of androgen-independent (AI) disease is inevitable. AI disease, also termed hormone-refractory prostate cancer (HRPC), is clinically detected by a rise in prostate-specific antigen (PSA) and/or worsening of symptoms while on hormone therapy. The current standard of care for HRPC is palliative in its intent and includes analgesia, radiation, and chemotherapy such as docetaxel (3,4). Thus, new and active agents are desperately needed for those patients at high risk of death from prostate cancer.

Over the last two decades, with the increase in understanding of the biological basis for prostate cancer progression that has been fueled in part from the development of high throughput genomic, transcriptomic, and proteomic technologies (5), a plethora of potential therapeutic targets has been identified. Many of these targets are not easily amenable to inhibition by small molecules or antibodies, and thus strategies to inhibit them at a gene expression level are an attractive concept. Antisense oligonucleotides (ASOs) are single-stranded, chemically modified DNA-like molecules designed to specifically inhibit a target gene's expression, which holds clinical promise as a therapeutic intervention. Although previously reported Phase III clinical trials with ASOs have failed to demonstrate a benefit, recent advances in the antisense field suggest that the limitations of the first generation ASOs that were used in these studies can be overcome. This chapter will review the current concepts behind ASO and their targets in preclinical and clinical testing for prostate cancer.

ANTISENSE OLIGONUCLEOTIDES

Mechanism of Action

The concept of using ASOs to inhibit expression of a specific gene arose in the 1960s with in vitro proof of concept performed in 1978 (6,7) when it was demonstrated that viral replication could be blocked using an oligonucleotide complementary to the Rous sarcoma virus. ASOs are single strands of 17–22 nucleotides designed to be complementary to a selected genes mRNA and thereby specifically inhibit expression of that gene. The specificity of the antisense approach is based on the calculation that a particular sequence of 17 bases in DNA occurs only once within the human genome. Thus, expression of specific proteins can be reduced by blocking translation, and subsequent cascades of protein–protein signaling control of cellular proliferation, differentiation, homeostasis, and apoptosis can be altered.

Several mechanisms of how ASO inhibits translation have been proposed (Fig. 1). The most accepted and important mechanism is that the mRNA–ASO duplexes formed by Watson–Crick binding results in degradation of the target mRNA by RNase H-mediated cleavage (8). Other proposed mechanisms of action of ASO include prevention of mRNA transport, alternate splicing or translational arrest, and formation of a triple-helix by binding of the ASO to the target duplex DNA in the nucleus resulting in inhibition of transcription. Additionally, certain ASOs, especially those with a CpG repeat or G quartets in their sequences, have also been found to have broad immunostimulatory activity and other non-sequence-specific (i.e., "off-target" effects) (9).

Design and Synthesis of ASOs

The first step in identifying useful ASO sequences for target inhibition is to identify those sites on the target mRNA that are both unique to that particular gene and

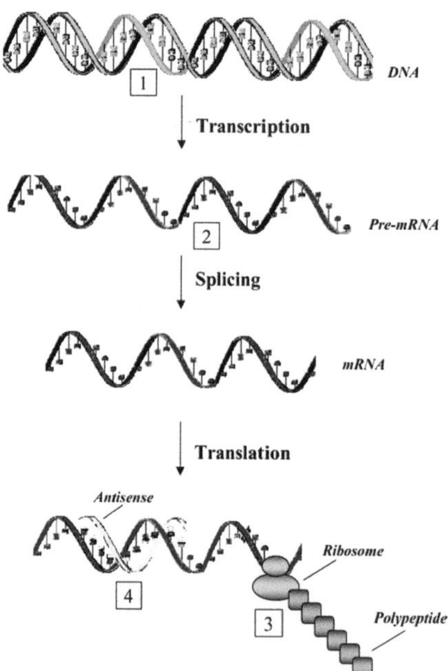

FIGURE 1 (*See color insert*) Mechanisms of antisense action on target genes. Several mechanisms of antisense action have been determined including (1) inhibition of transcription, (2) inhibition of splicing, (3) inhibition of ribosomal read through, and perhaps most important (4) activation of RNase H-mediated cleavage of target mRNA.

accessible to hybridization. The AUG start site is often accessible for oligonucleotide hybridization and ASOs targeting this codon have been used successfully for various target genes, although other sites can prove even more effective (10). To facilitate the process of selecting target sites for antisense action, a variety of in vitro techniques have been employed, many of these are combinatorial approaches based on annealing reactions with arrays of antisense species (11) and/or monitoring accessibility of target structures by RNase H mapping (12). In addition, computational attempts to predict the secondary structure and folding pattern of mRNAs have been described and target screening using computer programs, such as "mfold" or "RNAstructure," could prove to be a valid strategy to select effective antisense sequences (13). Although this approach ignores other parameters affecting antisense efficacy, such as the 3D structure of RNA in vivo or accessibility of the target site for RNase H, it may significantly reduce the number of ASOs needed for screening. By comparing sequences of the most effective versus less effective or ineffective ASO reported in the literature, the tetranucleotide motif TCCC was identified in 20 of the 42 most effective antisense sequences (12). Thus, in addition to the techniques described above, the prediction of target sites based on this motif may further assist in the design of antisense therapeutics.

Next, an ASO must be synthesized in a form that distributes effectively and resists degradation in vivo, and yet is easy to administer and is well tolerated in patients. The affinity of ASO to the target mRNA is a measure of stability of the nucleic acid hybrid, and higher affinity translates into higher gene-repressing activity (14,15). Unmodified phosphodiester oligonucleotides have no clinical utility because they distribute poorly in vivo and are rapidly degraded by endogenous nucleases, resulting in extremely short in vivo half-lives. Several useful chemical modifications of ASO backbones have yielded compounds that display good tissue distribution and enhanced resistance to nuclease digestion while retaining potent hybridization and RNase H activation.

Phosphorothioate ASO employ a substitution of a nonbridging phosphoryl oxygen of DNA with sulfur, which increases resistance to nuclease digestion and prolongs half-life. Phosphorothioate ASO becomes associated with high capacity, low affinity to serum-binding proteins after parental administration, and currently the most used form of ASO in clinical trials to date. Serum half-life with a phosphorothioate ASO, however, is still relatively short, approximately two hours in serum (16), and in mouse models, minimal amounts of full-length ASO can be found in tissues after 24 hours (17). Because of this, for clinical trials, continuous or frequent intravenous infusions have been used to administer conventional phosphorothioate ASO (16,18,19). As a class, phosphorothioate ASOs have been well tolerated in the clinic, and for the most part, toxicity has been nonsequence-specific and attributable to the phosphorothioate backbone and the polyanionic nature of these compounds. General toxicities with the first generation phosphorothioate ASO have included hypotension, tachycardia, and hemodynamic changes at high doses and blood levels of drug, thrombocytopenia and leukopenia, effects on coagulation, reduction in serum complement activity, increases in transaminases, splenomegaly, renal dysfunction, and cytokine release syndromes including fever of unknown origin (16,18–20).

Considerable effort has been made to generate ASO molecules that have improved stability and efficacy of ASO by modifications of the phosphodiester-linkage, the heterocycle, or the sugar. Some "next generation" phosphorothioate ASOs have been shown to form duplexes with RNA with a significantly higher affinity, which results in improved antisense potency (17). In addition, next generation ASOs display improved resistance against nuclease-mediated metabolism, resulting in significantly improved tissue half-life in vivo, producing a longer duration of action which potentially allows for a more patient-friendly intermittent dosing schedule (17). Finally, next generation ASOs have been reported to display a more attractive safety profile and reduced nonspecific effects relative to unmodified phosphorothioate ASO (21) which may allow higher dosing.

Like antibody-based therapeutics, which evolved to become a clinically useful therapeutic class through years of optimization, ASOs are evolving through improved chemical modifications to prolong in vivo half-life, improve tissue distribution, increase potency, and reduce toxicity. Additional critically important factors, such as improved understanding of the relative importance of the therapeutic target, optimization of dose and scheduling, enrichment of trials with tumors that are most sensitive to inhibition of the relevant target, and rational use in combination regimens, will also increase the likelihood of success.

ASOs IN PROSTATE CANCER

ASOs targeting multiple different genes have been reported to specifically inhibit expression of these genes and delay progression in several types of tumors. In our lab, one method of identifying potential therapeutic targets for prostate cancer starts with use of comparative hybridization of high-density cDNA arrays to rapidly and efficiently characterize changes in gene expression after androgen withdrawal in the Shionogi and LNCaP xenograft models that mimic the human condition of castration-induced regression followed by AI progression (22). Computer-assisted subtractive analysis of arrays highlights the increases or decreases in gene expression at various time points during AI progression. Northern or western analysis is then used to confirm the array data which can then be validated in human tissue microarrays of untreated and posthormone-therapy-treated cancers. In general, androgen withdrawal results in a programmatic drift in gene expression with upregulation of multiple genes in the Shionogi (23,24), CRW22 (22), LAPC9 (26), or LNCaP (27) tumor models. In this way and others, several genes have been implicated in prostate cancer development and progression and can be broadly grouped into those regulating apoptosis (24,27,28), growth factor signaling (25,29), and androgen receptor (AR) trans activation. The AR is grouped here as a target as adaptations in the androgen pathway have been proposed that render cells AI through the AR such as mutations that induce promiscuity, AR amplification, ligand-independent activation, co-activator amplification, and corepressor downregulation (30). Several of these putative genes have been inhibited with specifically designed ASO (Table 1) and are highlighted below.

B-Cell Leukemia-Lymphoma Gene-2

The Bcl-2 gene (B-Cell leukemia-lymphoma gene 2) is the prototype of a class of oncogenes that contributes to neoplastic progression by enhancing tumor cell survival through inhibition of apoptosis (31). Initially identified in follicular lymphoma due to the characteristic t14,18 translocation, Bcl-2 is a mitochondrial membrane protein that functions to heterodimerize with Bax and other proapoptotic regulators, thereby preventing cytochrome c release and subsequent activation of the apoptotic cascade. The selective and competitive dimerization

TABLE 1 Examples of Antisense Therapeutics in Development

Target	Compound	Company/ investigator	Phase of development
Bcl-2	G3139 (Oblimersen)	Genta	I–III
PKC-α	ISIS 3521	Isis	II–III
Clusterin	OGX-011	OncoGeneX	I–II
Methyltransferase	MG98	Methylgene	II
Raf-1	ISIS 5132	Isis	I–II
Ribonucleotide reductase	GTI-2040	Lorus	I–II
Ribonucleotide reductase	GTI-2501	Lorus	I–II
XIAP	AEG35156	Aegera	I
Mdm-2	GEM240	Hybridon	Preclinical
Survivin	LY2181308	Lily	Preclinical
IGFBP-2 and IGFBP-5	OGX-225	OncoGeneX	Preclinical
HSP27	OGX-427	OncoGeneX	Preclinical
Androgen receptor	as750/15	Eder et al.	Preclinical

between pairs of these Bcl-2 family antagonists and agonists determines how a cell responds to an apoptotic signal (32). Several lines of evidence have implicated overexpression of *bcl-2* with treatment resistance (33,34). In prostate cancer, Bcl-2 has been found to be expressed in clinical samples of androgen-dependent and independent disease (35,36), and experimental and clinical studies report that increased expression of Bcl-2 confers, or is associated with, the development of androgen independence and treatment resistance (37–40). Thus, Bcl-2 is an attractive target to improve the efficacy of treatment of patients with prostate cancer by enhancing chemotherapy-induced apoptosis. G3139 (oblimersen sodium, Genta, Inc.) is an 18mer phosphorothioate ASO complementary to the first six codons of the initiating sequence of the human Bcl-2 mRNA. In preclinical prostate cancer models, G3139 and other Bcl-2 ASO have shown significant activity in inhibiting expression of Bcl-2, delaying time to the development of androgen independence, and enhancing the effects of chemotherapy by increased apoptosis (23,27,41). A Phase I trial performed at MSKCC included several patients with prostate cancer (16) with G3139 given as a prolonged continuous IV infusion. Treatment was generally well tolerated with observed side effects including fatigue, anorexia, and hypophosphatemia. Dose-limiting toxicity was reversible transaminase elevation. Maximum tolerated dose was 6.9 mg/kg/day over 14–21 days; however, steady-state serum levels associated with biological activity were achieved at lower dose levels.

As Bcl-2 is also expressed in normal cells, there were initial safety concerns about combination of G3139 and chemotherapy. A Phase I trial of G3139 in combination with mitoxantrone for patients with HRPC was performed (18) which demonstrated that standard doses of chemotherapy could be combined with G3139 without apparent increased toxicity. A Phase I trial also determined that standard doses of docetaxel could be delivered without apparent increased toxicity when combined with 7 mg/kg/day of G3139 delivered as a continuous intravenous infusion over five to seven days (42). A Phase II trial of this combination in patients with HRPC (43) reported similar toxicity of the combination to what would be expected with docetaxel as a single agent, and a 50% decrease in PSA posttreatment occurred in 56% of patients. A randomized Phase II trial of docetaxel with or without G319 is being carried out by the EORTC with PSA "response" as the primary end point. A randomized Phase III trial in patients with HRPC comparing docetaxel with docetaxel plus G3139 with overall survival as the primary end point was scheduled to begin in 2005, but with negative results from recent Phase III trials of G3139 (44,45) and other issues, this has been put on hold. Issues persist about the optimal biological dosing of this first-generation phosphorothioate ASO and whether treatment at the doses and schedules tested is enough to suppress target sufficiently (43).

Bcl-xL is another anti-apoptotic bcl-2 family member. In tumors where Bcl-2 and Bcl-xL are co-expressed, it is difficult to predict which of the two proteins is more critical for survival and some tumor cells have been reported to switch expression from Bcl-2 to Bcl-xL (46,47). Bcl-xL ASOs have been reported to induce apoptosis in various tumor cells and sensitize tumor cells to chemotherapy (41,48–50). Bcl-xL ASO marginally enhanced chemosensitivity and delayed AI progression of prostate cancer xenografts, whereas combined Bcl-xL plus Bcl-2 ASOs acted synergistically to further enhance chemotherapy beyond that of either agent alone (51). Simultaneous downregulation of both Bcl-2 and Bcl-xL protein expression by a single bispecific ASO has been accomplished by taking advantage of the similarity of specific regions of Bcl-2 and Bcl-xL mRNA. Inhibition of both Bcl-2 and Bcl-xL expression with a novel bispecific ASO with complete sequence identity to Bcl-2 and Bcl-3 mismatches to Bcl-xL inhibits expression of both Bcl-2 and Bcl-xL mRNA in tumor cells and is a potent inducer of apoptosis in several tumor cell types including PC-3 (52,53). Future clinical development plans for this particular ASO are unknown. These findings illustrate that combinatorial regimens that inhibit two or more specific gene targets can produce additive effects and provide the basis for identifying additional anti-apoptotic genes that may serve as targets. Recently, small molecule inhibitors against anti-apoptotic Bcl-2 family members through their BH3 domains have been developed (54) and several are in early phase clinical trials. This further raises the possibility of a combination strategy, in which a small molecule inhibitor is combined with antisense gene suppression of Bcl-2 family members.

Protein Kinase C-Alpha and RAF-1

ISIS 3521 and 5132 (Isis Pharmaceuticals, Carlsbad, California) are first-generation phosphorothioate ASO directed against the mRNA of protein kinase C-alpha (PKC-alpha) and Raf-1, respectively. Raf-1 is a central component of signal transduction pathways stimulated by various growth factors that play a role in AI progression, PKC, and other protein kinases (55,56). PKC belongs to a class of serine—threonine kinases that fine tune numerous intracellular responses arising from G-protein-coupled receptors, receptors with tyrosine kinase activity, and nonreceptor tyrosine kinases (57). Increased PKC expression has been implicated in both oncogenesis and tumor progression (58,59).

In Phase I clinical studies of Isis 3521 (60,61), responses were noted in two patients with low-grade lymphoma and in one patient with ovarian cancer. Dose-limiting toxicities were grade 3 fatigue at the highest dose tested, and the recommended Phase II dose was set at 2.0 mg/kg/day. Toxicity at this dose appeared mild, with one of six patients experiencing grade 3 thrombocytopenia, and one grade 1 leukopenia. A Phase I trial of Isis 5321 (62) escalated doses to 5.0 mg/kg/day, however maximum tolerated dose was not reached. The recommended Phase II dose was set at 2 mg/kg/day based on preclinical models demonstrating activity at equivalent dosing. Both these agents underwent testing in an NCI Canada—Clinical Trials Group randomized Phase II study where patients with HRPC were randomized to one or the other of the compounds (19). Scheduling for both of the ASO was 2 mg/kg/day for 21 days by continuous infusion followed by a seven days of rest period. Overall treatment was well tolerated, with fatigue, lethargy, and mild thrombocytopenia as the main treatment-related adverse events. However, no PSA or objective responses were observed, although there were some patients with stable disease. Lack of apparent clinical activity may be due to several factors. Inhibition of these targets could result in a cytostatic effect, which the study was not designed to detect. Second, patients were not assessed for expression of the target, and therefore the targets themselves may not have been relevant in the patient population studied. Third, inhibiting a single molecular target may be insufficient to exert a clinically detectable effect and that a combination strategy may be more effective as preclinical models suggested supra-additive activity when these agents were combined with chemotherapy. Finally, optimal biological dosing and target inhibition were not determined and thus the target itself may not have affected using the dose and schedule employed.

Clusterin

The clusterin gene on chromosome 8 encodes a chaperone protein which has been implicated in a variety of physiological processes. Also known as testosterone-repressed prostate message-2 (TRPM-2), or sulfated glycoprotein-2, clusterin is associated with numerous tumors, including prostate (63), neuroblastoma (64), breast (65), lymphoma (66), urothelial (67), and renal cell carcinoma (68), and with various pathological conditions including Alzheimer's (69) and nephrotoxic injury (70). Clusterin levels increase dramatically during castration-induced apoptosis in rat prostate epithelial cells (71), in androgen-dependent Shionogi tumors (24), and in human prostate cancer CRW22 (22) and PC82 (72) xenografts. In human prostate cancer, clusterin levels are low or absent in most untreated hormone-naive tissues, but increase significantly within weeks after neoadjuvant hormone therapy (73). Because clusterin binds to a wide variety of biological ligands (74,75) and is regulated by transcription factor HSF1 (heat shock factor 1) (76), an emerging view suggests that clusterin functions similar to heat shock protein (HSP) to chaperone and stabilizes conformations of proteins at time of cell stress. Indeed, clusterin is substantially more potent than other HSPs at inhibiting stress-induced protein precipitation (77). Significant differences exist, however, in amino acid sequence analysis which suggests that clusterin is a unique protein without any closely related family members yet identified. In prostate cancer, experimental and clinical studies implicate clusterin with AI progression and have a protective role against apoptotic cell death from androgen withdrawal, chemotherapy, and radiation (24,78–80). Recently, clusterin was reported to interact with and inhibit conformationally altered and activated Bax, thereby inhibiting cytochrome c release and apoptosis (81).

OGX-011 (OncoGeneX Technologies Inc., Vancouver, Canada) is an ASO complementary to the clusterin mRNA. OGX-011 incorporates a phosphorothioate backbone with next generation chemistry in the form of 2′-*O*-methoxytheyl modifications to the four bases on either end of the 21mer molecule. Such "gapmer" modifications maintain the improved tissue pharmacokinetic profile of the second-generation chemistry but preserves high affinity for target mRNA and recruitment of RNase H necessary for activity. In primates, tissue half-life of OGX-011 was in the order of seven days, and intermittent schedules of OGX-011 were therapeutically equivalent to continuous dosing of unmodified phosphorothioate clusterin antisense (17). In prostate and other preclinical cancer models, OGX-011 improves the efficacy of chemotherapy, radiation, and androgen withdrawal by inhibiting expression of clusterin and enhancing the apoptotic response (17,24,79,80). Furthermore, because of the second-generation chemistry and enhanced tissue half-life of OGX-011, more relaxed dosing schedules are possible while maintaining biological efficacy of target inhibition.

Three Phase I trials have evaluated OGX-011 given weekly by a 2 h intravenous infusion as a single agent or in combination with chemotherapy (82,83). The single agent study had a unique design in that patients with high risk localized prostate cancer were treated with the OGX-011 prior to radical prostatectomy, thus allowing for dose-dependent correlations for *clusterin* expression and OGX-011 tissue concentrations in target tissue. Surrogate tissues for markers of biological effect (*clusterin* expression in peripheral blood mononuclear cells and serum clusterin) were also assessed. OGX-011 was given by IV infusion over 2 h at a starting dose of 40 mg on days 1, 3, 5, 8, 15, 22, and 29. Androgen deprivation therapy was started on day 1 and prostatectomy was performed days 30 to 36. Twenty-five patients were enrolled to six cohorts with doses of OGX-011 up to 640 mg delivered. Toxicity was mild or moderate only, and adverse events included fevers, rigors, fatigue, and transient liver function elevations. Plasma pharmacokinetic analysis showed linear increases in OGX-011 with a half-life of 2 h and mean peak concentrations of 80 μM at 640 mg dose. More importantly, prostate tissue concentrations of OGX-011 increased with dose, and tissue concentrations associated with preclinical effect could be achieved and observed even seven days after dosing. Dose-dependent decreases in prostate cancer cell *clusterin* expression were observed. At 640 mg dosing, *clusterin* mRNA levels were decreased by approximately 92% compared with lower dose levels and historical controls as assessed by a quantitative real-time polymerase chain reaction assay of microdissected cancer cells. By immunohistochemistry, mean percentage of cancer cells staining negative for *clusterin* at 640 mg dosing was 54% compared with 2–15% for lower dose levels and historical controls. Clusterin levels were also suppressed significantly in regional lymph tissues. This Phase I trial demonstrates that OGX-011 is well tolerated and potently inhibits *clusterin* expression in prostate cancers, and the Phase II dose for OGX-011 is 640 mg based on pharmacokinetic and pharmacodynamic parameters. Of note, this dose is significantly higher than those selected for G3139 and the Isis compounds reviewed above, especially when tissue exposure is considered given the prolonged tissue half-life of OGX-011, highlighting a potential explanation for a lack of demonstrated efficacy with the first-generation ASO agents discussed earlier.

Phase I combination studies of OGX-011 with docetaxel or gemcitabine + cisplatin have also been recently completed (83). These have shown that OGX-011 can be combined at its biologically effective dose (i.e., 640 mg) with standard doses of the chemotherapy agents. A randomized Phase II study of docetaxel with or without OGX-011 in patients with metastatic HRPC began in mid-2005 and accrual is estimated to complete by mid-2006.

The IAP Gene Family

The inhibitors of apoptosis (IAP) gene family encodes proteins that protect cells from undergoing apoptosis through, at least in part, inhibition of caspases which are the key effector proteins of apoptotic cell death (84–87). In addition, IAPs have roles in seemingly caspase-unrelated functions including cell division and signaling (88–90). IAPs have been found to be expressed in multiple malignancies including human prostate cancer and cell lines (91) with limited expression in normal tissues. Second-generation ASOs have been designed against two IAP family members: *survivin* (LY2181308, Eli Lilly and Co. in collaboration with Isis Pharmaceuticals, Carlsbad, California) and *X-linked IAP* (*XIAP*) (AEG35156, Aegera Therapeutics Inc., Montreal, Canada).

Survivin

Survivin plays an important role in both cell division and apoptosis inhibition (86,92,92). Survivin is highly expressed in a wide variety of human cancer types, including lung, colon, pancreas, breast, and prostate (93,94). However, survivin is generally not expressed in normal tissue, with expression limited to a few cell types including angiogenic endothelium, thymus, testis, activated T cells, and intestinal epithelium crypts. Survivin expression levels correlate with lower apoptotic index in tumor cells and poor prognosis in cancer patients, and serial analysis of gene expression studies have indicated that survivin is one of the top (ranked fourth) "transcriptomes" uniformly expressed in cancer cells but not in normal tissues (95). Furthermore, overexpression of survivin in tumor cells inhibits chemotherapy-induced (e.g., taxol and etoposide), Bax-induced, and Fas-induced apoptosis, and expression of dominant-negative mutants of survivin induces apoptosis in tumor cell lines (96). Taken together, these observations make survivin an attractive target for novel cancer therapy.

A second-generation 2′MOE ASO has been identified (LY2181308/ISIS 23722) that potently and specifically downregulates survivin expression in a broad range of human cancer cells including lung, colon, pancreas, breast, and prostate (97,98). Survivin inhibition in tumor cells by LY2181308 results in caspase-3 dependent apoptosis, cell cycle arrest in the G2/M phase, theformation of multinucleated cells, and in the sensitization of tumor cells to chemotherapy-induced apoptosis (97–99). Moreover, LY2181308 produces potent antitumor activity against a broad range of tumor types in human tumor xenograft models (100). Antitumor activity displayed by LY2181308 in these models is oligonucleotide sequence-specific and is associated with reduced survivin levels in tumor and the production of multinucleated tumor cells. On the basis of these impressive preclinical results, LY2181308 has been selected for clinical development and Phase I studies have been initiated.

X-Linked IAP

XIAP overexpression inhibits apoptosis arising from chemotherapy, radiation, and growth factor deprivation. By inhibiting caspase-3 and -9 activity, XIAP suppresses apoptosis triggered by intrinsic, mitochondrial-related, as well as extrinsic, death receptor-related, insults (85,88). As described with bcl-2 and clusterin ASOs above, the XIAP knockdown using ASOs in cancer cells under stress and primed for apoptosis (e.g., when challenged by chemotherapeutic agents) enhances pro-apoptotic signals and tips the apoptotic rheostat towards death. XIAP is highly expressed in many tumor cell lines and in prostate, glioblastoma, acute myeloid leukemia (AML), pancreatic, gastric, and colorectal tumors (89). In AML, this overexpression has been associated with poor clinical outcome (89). AEG35156/GEM640 (Aegera Therapeutics Inc., Montreal, Canada) is a 19mer ASO targeted to human XIAP mRNA that incorporates 2′-*O*-methyl (2′OMe) chemistry with a phosphorothioate backbone. Numerous in vitro and in vivo preclinical proof-of-concept studies have demonstrated that inhibition of XIAP protein expression by AEG35156/GEM640 enhances the antitumor activity of chemotherapy in several xenograft models (101,102).

A Phase I dose-escalation tolerability study of AEG35156/GEM640 as a single agent is currently underway in the U.K. evaluating seven- and three-day continuous intravenous infusion schedules in patients with advanced tumors (103). Phase I trials evaluating shorter intravenous infusion schedules in combination with docetaxel or re-induction chemotherapy for acute myelogenous leukemia are also planned or ongoing.

Heat Shock Protein 27

Many components of survival and apoptotic pathways are regulated by molecular chaperones, such as HSPs. HSPs are a family of highly conserved proteins whose expression is induced by signals such as hyperthermia, oxidative stress, activation of the Fas death receptor, and cytotoxic drugs (104–106). HSPs have attracted attention as new therapeutic targets for cancer, especially since the discovery and characterization of geldanamycin as an inhibitor of Hsp90 (107,108) and the targeting of the Clusterin gene as discussed above, whose product has small HSP-like function.

Hsp27 is an ATP-independent molecular chaperone highly induced during stress responses and can form oligomers to increase affinity for client proteins, to either act as chaperones or to assist in repair of misfolded proteins, by either preventing their aggregation or assisting in proteasome-mediated degradation. The cytoprotective effects of Hsp27 result from its chaperone function [e.g., chaperone of signal transducers and activators of transcription 3 (STAT3)], direct interference of caspase activation, modulation of oxidative stress, and regulation of the cytoskeleton (109–111). Higher levels of Hsp27 are commonly detected in many cancers, including breast (112), ovarian (113), glial tumors (114), prostate (115), and others (116), and are associated with metastasis, poor prognosis, and resistance to chemotherapy or radiation (117,118). Moreover, Hsp27 expression is induced by hormone or chemotherapy and inhibits treatment-induced apoptosis via multiple mechanisms (117–122).

As an important regulator of cell survival and treatment stress at many different points along the apoptotic pathway, Hsp27 is now recognized as an important therapeutic target. Recently, Hsp27 ASO and siRNA targeting the human translation initiation site were reported to potently inhibit Hsp27 expression in human prostate PC3 cells with increased caspase-3 cleavage and apoptosis and 87% suppression of cell growth (117). Hsp27 ASO and siRNA also enhanced paclitaxel chemosensitivity in vitro, whereas in vivo systemic administration of Hsp27 ASO in athymic mice decreased PC-3 tumor progression and enhanced paclitaxel chemosensitivity. Overexpression of Hsp27 in human prostate LNCaP cells caused these normally androgen-dependent cells to become AI and more resistant to cytotoxic chemotherapy. Inhibition of Hsp27 expression through administration of Hsp27 ASO postcastration delayed AI progression in LNCaP xenografts, in part through enhanced modulation of STAT-3 mediated transcriptional activity (111). These findings suggest that increased levels of Hsp27 after androgen withdrawal provide a cytoprotective role during development of androgen independence and that ASO-induced silencing can enhance apoptosis and delay tumor progression. A second-generation MOE gapmer ASO targeting Hsp27 (OGX-427, OncoGenex Technologies, Inc., Vancouver, Canada) is planned to enter clinical trials in prostate and other solid cancers and in multiple myeloma in 2006.

Insulin Growth Factor Binding Proteins

Insulin-like growth factor (IGF)-I plays an important role in the pathophysiology of prostatic disease. The biological response of cells to IGFs, a potent mitogen for prostate cells, is regulated by various factors in the microenvironment, including the IGF-binding proteins (IGFBPs) (123). After castration, the expression levels of certain IGFBPs change rapidly in the rat ventral prostate (124) and Shionogi tumors (25). Differences in expression of various IGFBPs in benign and malignant prostatic epithelial cells have also been reported, with increases in IGFBP-2 and IGFBP-5 and decreases in IGFBP-3 in malignant versus benign cells (125). Increased IGFBP-5 levels after castration have been shown to be an adaptive cell survival response that helps potentiate the anti-apoptotic and mitogenic effects of IGF-I, thereby accelerating AI progression (126,127). Furthermore, IGFBP-5 is present in high concentrations in bone, the most frequent site of metastases from prostate cancer. Systemic administration of IGFBP-5 ASO in mice bearing Shionogi tumors after castration attenuated castration-induced increases in IGFBP-5 and significantly delayed time to AI progression. IGFBP-2 levels also increase in LNCaP and human prostate tumors after castration and during AI progression and, like IGFBP-5, appear to accelerate time to AI progression by enhancing IGF-1 responsiveness (128). IGFBP-2 levels are increased in HRPC (22). Forced overexpression of IGFBP-2 in LNCaP tumors produced an AI phenotype with a growth advantage compared to parental cells only in the absence of androgens. Moreover, IGFBP-2 ASO decreased IGFBP-2 levels and reduced LNCaP cell growth rates in vitro and in vivo. Increased IGFBP-5 and -2 levels after androgen ablation may represent adaptive responses to potentiate IGF-I-mediated survival and mitogenesis. Use of ASOs to target IGFBP-modulation of IGF signaling is undergoing further study, and a bispecific antisense that can simultaneously target both IGFBP-2 and -5 mRNA is under development for clinical applications (OGX-225, OncoGenex Technologies, Inc., Vancouver, Canada).

Ribonucleotide Reductase

Ribonucleotide reductase (RR) is an enzyme important for cell division and tumor growth that is required for the reductive conversion of ribonucleotides to deoxyribonucleotides, which is a crucial step in the synthesis and repair of DNA (129,130). Mammalian RR has a dimeric structure composed of two dissimilar subunits, R1 and R2, encoded on different chromosomes, each inactive on its own (131). Each subunit consists of a nucleotide-binding site (M1) and a metal-binding site (M2). The M1-affecting RR inhibitors are nucleoside analogs (e.g., gemcitabine). The M2 contains nonheme iron and a tyrosine-free radical, which are required for the enzymatic reduction of ribonucleotides. Inhibitors of M2 act by destroying the free radical. Hydroxyurea is a clinically approved RR inhibitor acting at the iron/free radical site; however, the inhibition is reversible due to the ease in regenerating the tyrosine free radical by mammalian cells (132). The R1 subunit protein levels are constant during the cell cycle; however, the expression of the R2 subunit increases in late G1/early S phase of the cell cycle when DNA replication occurs. The R2 subunit is overexpressed in tumor tissues studied and this overexpression appears to enhance the transformation and malignant potential of some oncogenes.

GTI-2501 and GTI-2040 (Lorus Therapeutics Inc., Toronto, Canada) are phosphorothioate antisense molecules that target and inhibit expression of the R1 and R2 subunit of RR, respectively (133). A Phase I trial of GTI-2040 has been reported, and dose-limiting toxicity of hepatic enzyme elevation was observed (134). The recommended Phase II dose was based on toxicity and was determined to be 185 mg/m^2/day given as a 21-day continuous intravenous infusion. Phase I trials of GTI-2501 and GTI-2040 in combination with docetaxel have been completed and Phase II trials of these regimens are underway in patients with chemo-naïve HRPC. The Phase II trial of GTI-2040 and docetaxel has been reported in abstract form (135), with seven patients out of 16 being described as having a PSA response, but it was unclear whether additional accrual was to take place at the second stage of this two-stage designed trial.

Androgen Receptor

Several mechanisms responsible for the progression of prostate cancer to androgen independence have been proposed, which involve the AR. These include mutations resulting in a promiscuous receptor that permits activation by other ligands, AR amplification, and ligand-independent activation. Nonsteroidal anti-androgens have been used to target the AR, but have had modest results in hormone-refractory disease, and can induce paradoxical worsening of the disease through activation of a promiscuous receptor (136). AR expression has been inhibited using ASO targeting the CAG repeats encoding the polyglutamine region in vitro with the LNCaP cell line with significant effects being observed on cell growth inhibition and an increase in apoptosis (137,138). Similar effects were seen in LNCaP-abl cells, a subline established after long-term androgen ablation of the parental cell line. Other ASO (Novartis AG, Basal, Switzerland) have also been identified with inhibitory activity on AR expression and subsequent AR-mediated effects (139). Further study of this approach is warranted.

SUMMARY

Antisense inhibition of relevant genes involved in prostate cancer progression continues to be a promising area for therapeutic development. ASO technology has quickly moved from in vitro and in vivo models to testing in the clinic. Controversy still exists on the mechanism of antitumor activity and the challenges of maximizing tissue exposure, cellular uptake, and demonstration of clinical biological and antitumor activity. Next generation ASO chemistry holds potential advantages for patient-friendly dosing and routes of administration, enhanced activity, and improved toxicity profile. Similar to the difficulties in developing any of the targeted therapies, there are several issues that need to be addressed in the early phase clinical trials of ASO, and the failure of the first generation ASO therapeutics in randomized trials only emphasizes this more. These issues include determination of a biologically effective dose, ensuring that the target is relevant in the patient population being studied, study designs that can detect meaningful cytostatic activity if appropriate, and rational use of combination strategies. Addressing these issues early on will allow optimal use of these agents clinically and best ensure success in Phase III trials.

REFERENCES

1. Jemal A, Murray T, Samuels A, et al. Cancer statistics, 2003. CA Cancer J Clin 2003; 53(1):5–26.
2. D'Amico AV, Whittington R, Malkowicz SB, et al. Biochemical outcome after radical prostatectomy, external beam radiation therapy, or interstitial radiation therapy for clinically localized prostate cancer. JAMA 1998; 280(11):969–974.
3. Tannock IF, Osoba D, Stockler MR, et al. Chemotherapy with mitoxantrone plus prednisone or prednisone alone for symptomatic hormone-resistant prostate cancer: a Canadian randomized trial with palliative end points. J Clin Oncol 1996; 14(6):1756–1764.
4. Kantoff PW, Halabi S, Conaway M, et al. Hydrocortisone with or without mitoxantrone in men with hormone-refractory prostate cancer: results of the cancer and leukemia group B 9182 study. J Clin Oncol 1999; 17(8):2506–2513.
5. Luo J, Duggan DJ, Chen Y, et al. Human prostate cancer and benign prostatic hyperplasia: molecular dissection by gene expression profiling. Cancer Res 2001; 61(12):4683–4688.
6. Paterson BM, Roberts BE, Kuff EL. Structural gene identification and mapping by DNA-mRNA hybrid-arrested cell-free translation. Proc Natl Acad Sci USA 1977; 74:4370–4374.
7. Zamecnik PC, Stephenson MC. Inhibition of Rous sarcoma virus replication and cell transformation by a specific oligodeoxynucleotide. Proc Natl Acad Sci USA 1978; 75:280–284.
8. Crooke ST. Molecular mechanisms of antisense drugs: RNase H. Antisense Nucleic Acid Drug Dev 1998; 8(2):133–134.
9. Carpentier AF, Chen L, Maltonti F, et al. Oligodeoxynucleotides containing CpG motifs can induce rejection of a neuroblastoma in mice. Cancer Res 1999; 59(21):5429–5432.
10. Ho SP, Bao Y, Lesher T, et al. Mapping of RNA accessible sites for antisense experiments with oligonucleotide libraries. Nat Biotechnol 1998; 16(1):59–63.
11. Matveeva O, Felden B, Audlin S, et al. A rapid in vitro method for obtaining RNA accessibility patterns for complementary DNA probes: correlation with an intracellular pattern and known RNA structures. Nucleic Acids Res 1997; 25(24):5010–5016.
12. Stull RA, Taylor LA, Szoka FC Jr. Predicting antisense oligonucleotide inhibitory efficacy: a computational approach using histograms and thermodynamic indices. Nucl Acids Res 1992; 20(13):3501–3508.
13. Butler M, McKay RA, Popoff IJ, et al. Specific inhibition of PTEN expression reverses hyperglycemia in diabetic mice. Diabetes 2002; 51(4):1028–1034.
14. Monia BP, Lesnik EA, Gonzalez C, et al. Evaluation of 2′-modified oligonucleotides containing 2′-deoxy gaps as antisense inhibitors of gene expression. J Biol Chem 1993; 268(19):14514–14522.
15. Shen L, Siwkowski A, Wancewicz EV, et al. Evaluation of C-5 propynyl pyrimidine-containing oligonucleotides in vitro and in vivo. Antisense Nucl Acid Drug Dev 2003; 13(3):129–142.
16. Morris MJ, Tong WP, Cordon-Cardo C, et al. Phase I trial of BCL-2 antisense oligonucleotide (G3139) administered by continuous intravenous infusion in patients with advanced cancer. Clin Cancer Res 2002; 8(3):679–683.
17. Zellweger T, Miyake H, Cooper S, et al. Antitumor activity of antisense clusterin oligonucleotides is improved in vitro and in vivo by incorporation of 2′-*O*-(2-methoxy)ethyl chemistry. J Pharmacol Exp Ther 2001; 298(3):934–940.

18. Chi KN, Gleave ME, Klasa R, et al. A phase I dose-finding study of combined treatment with an antisense Bcl-2 oligonucleotide (Genasense) and mitoxantrone in patients with metastatic hormone-refractory prostate cancer. Clin Cancer Res 2001; 7(12):3920–3927.
19. Tolcher AW, Reyno L, Venner PM, et al. A randomized phase II and pharmacokinetic study of the antisense oligonucleotides ISIS 3521 and ISIS 5132 in patients with hormone-refractory prostate cancer. Clin Cancer Res 2002; 8(8):2530–2535.
20. Waters JS, Webb A, Cunningham D, et al. Phase I clinical and pharmacokinetic study of bcl-2 antisense oligonucleotide therapy in patients with non-Hodgkin's lymphoma. J Clin Oncol 2000; 18(9):1812–1823.
21. Henry S, Stecker K, Brooks D, et al. Chemically modified oligonucleotides exhibit decreased immune stimulation in mice. J Pharmacol Exp Ther 2000; 292(2):468–479.
22. Bubendorf L, Kolmer M, Kononen J, et al. Hormone therapy failure in human prostate cancer: analysis by complementary DNA and tissue microarrays. J Natl Cancer Inst 1999; 91(20):1758–1764.
23. Miyake H, Tolcher A, Gleave ME. Antisense Bcl-2 oligodeoxynucleotides inhibit progression to androgen-independence after castration in the Shionogi tumor model. Cancer Res 1999; 59(16):4030–4034.
24. Miyake H, Nelson C, Rennie PS, et al. Testosterone-repressed prostate message-2 is an antiapoptotic gene involved in progression to androgen independence in prostate cancer. Cancer Res 2000; 60(1):170–176.
25. Nickerson T, Miyake H, Gleave ME, et al. Castration-induced apoptosis of androgen-dependent Shionogi carcinoma is associated with increased expression of genes encoding insulin-like growth factor-binding proteins. Cancer Res 1999; 59(14):3392–3395.
26. Craft N, Shostak Y, Carey M, et al. A mechanism for hormone-independent prostate cancer through modulation of androgen receptor signaling by the HER-2/neu tyrosine kinase. Nat Med 1999; 5(3):280–285.
27. Gleave M, Tolcher A, Miyake H, et al. Progression to androgen independence is delayed by adjuvant treatment with antisense Bcl-2 oligodeoxynucleotides after castration in the LNCaP prostate tumor model. Clin Cancer Res 1999; 5(10):2891–2898.
28. Grossfeld GD, Olumi AF, Connolly JA, et al. Locally recurrent prostate tumors following either radiation therapy or radical prostatectomy have changes in Ki-67 labeling index, p53 and bcl-2 immunoreactivity. J Urol 1998; 159(5):1437–1443.
29. Culig Z, Hobisch A, Cronauer MV, et al. Regulation of prostatic growth and function by peptide growth factors. Prostate 1996; 28(6):392–405.
30. Feldman BJ, Feldman D. The development of androgen-independent prostate cancer. Nat Rev Cancer 2001; 1(1):34–45.
31. Tsujimoto Y, Croce CM. Analysis of the structure, transcripts, and protein products of bcl-2, the gene involved in human follicular lymphoma. Proc Natl Acad Sci USA 1986; 83(14):5214–5218.
32. Reed JC. Bcl-2 and the regulation of programmed cell death. J Cell Biol 1994; 124 (1–2):1–6.
33. Miyashita T, Reed JC. Bcl-2 oncoprotein blocks chemotherapy-induced apoptosis in a human leukemia cell line. Blood 1993; 81(1):151–157.
34. Kyprianou N, King ED, Bradbury D, et al. bcl-2 over-expression delays radiation-induced apoptosis without affecting the clonogenic survival of human prostate cancer cells. Intl J Cancer 1997; 70(3):341–348.
35. Mcdonnell TJ, Navone NM, Troncoso P, et al. Expression of bcl-2 oncoprotein and p53 protein accumulation in bone marrow metastases of androgen independent prostate cancer. J Urol 1997; 157(2):569–574.
36. Colombel M, Symmans F, Gil S, et al. Detection of the apoptosis-suppressing oncoprotein bc1-2 in hormone-refractory human prostate cancers. Am J Pathol 1993; 143(2): 390–400.
37. Mcdonnell TJ, Troncoso P, Brisbay SM, et al. Expression of the protooncogene bcl-2 in the prostate and its association with emergence of androgen-independent prostate cancer. Cancer Res 1992; 52(24);6940–6944.

38. Raffo AJ, Perlman H, Chen MW, et al. Overexpression of bcl-2 protects prostate cancer cells from apoptosis in vitro and confers resistance to androgen depletion in vivo. Cancer Res 1995; 55(19):4438–4445.
39. Bubendorf L, Sauter G, Moch H, et al. Prognostic significance of Bcl-2 in clinically localized prostate cancer. Am J Pathol 1996; 148(5);1557–1565.
40. Scherr DS, Vaughan ED Jr, Wei J, et al. BCL-2 and p53 expression in clinically localized prostate cancer predicts response to external beam radiotherapy. J Urol 1999; 162(1):12–16.
41. Leung S, Miyake H, Zellweger T, et al. Synergistic chemosensitization and inhibition of progression to androgen independence by antisense Bcl-2 oligodeoxynucleotide and paclitaxel in the LNCaP prostate tumor model. Intl J Cancer 2001; 91(6):846–850.
42. Tolcher AW, Kuhn J, Schwartz G, et al. A Phase I pharmacokinetic and biological correlative study of oblimersen sodium (genasense, G3139), an antisense oligonucleotide to the bcl-2 mRNA, and of docetaxel in patients with hormone-refractory prostate cancer. Clin Cancer Res 2004; 10(15):5048–5057.
43. Tolcher AW, Chi K, Kuhn J, et al. A phase II pharmacokinetic, and biological correlative study of oblimersen sodium and docetaxel in patients with hormone refractory prostate cancer. Clin Cancer Res 2005; 11(10):3854–3861.
44. Millward MJ, Bedikian AY, Conry RM, et al. Randomized multinational phase 3 trial of dacarbazine (DTIC) with or without Bcl-2 antisense (oblimersen sodium) in patients (pts) with advanced malignant melanoma (MM): analysis of long-term survival. J Clin Oncol ASCO Annu Meeting Proc 2004; 22(14S):7505.
45. Rai KR, Moore JO. Phase 3 randomized trial of fludarabine/cyclophosphamide chemotherapy with or without oblimersen sodium (Bcl-2 antisense; genasense; G3139) for patients with relapsed or refractory chronic lymphocytic leukemia (CLL). Blood 2004; 104:100a.
46. Han Z, Chatterjee D, Early J, et al. Isolation and characterization of an apoptosis-resistant variant of human leukemia HL-60 cells that has switched expression from Bcl-2 to Bcl-xL. Cancer Res 1996; 56(7):1621–1628.
47. Arriola EL, Rodriguez-Lopez AM, Hickman JA, et al. Bcl-2 overexpression results in reciprocal downregulation of Bcl-X(L) and sensitizes human testicular germ cell tumours to chemotherapy-induced apoptosis. Oncogene 1999; 18(7):1457–1464.
48. Leech SH, Olie RA, Gautschi O, et al. Induction of apoptosis in lung-cancer cells following bcl-xL anti-sense treatment. Intl J Cancer 2000; 86(4):570–576.
49. Simoes-Wust AP, Olie RA, Gautschi O, et al. Bcl-xl antisense treatment induces apoptosis in breast carcinoma cells. Intl J Cancer 2000; 87(4):582–590.
50. Lebedeva I, Rando R, Ojwang J, et al. Bcl-xL in prostate cancer cells: effects of overexpression and down-regulation on chemosensitivity. Cancer Res 2000; 60(21):6052–6060.
51. Miyake H, Monia BP, Gleave ME. Inhibition of progression to androgen-independence by combined adjuvant treatment with antisense BCL-XL and antisense Bcl-2 oligonucleotides plus taxol after castration in the Shionogi tumor model. Intl J Cancer 2000; 86(6):855–862.
52. Gautschi O, Tschopp S, Olie RA, et al. Activity of a novel bcl-2/bcl-xL-bispecific antisense oligonucleotide against tumors of diverse histologic origins. J Natl Cancer Inst 2001; 93(6):463–471.
53. Yamanaka K, Rocchi P, Miyake H, et al. A novel antisense oligonucleotide inhibiting several antiapoptotic Bcl-2 family members induces apoptosis and enhances chemosensitivity in androgen-independent human prostate cancer PC3 cells. Mol Cancer Ther 2005; 4(11):1689–1698.
54. Oltersdorf T, Elmore SW, Shoemaker AR, et al. An inhibitor of Bcl-2 family proteins induces regression of solid tumours. Nature 2005; 435(7042):677–681.
55. Fu H, Xia K, Pallas DC, et al. Interaction of the protein kinase Raf-1 with 14-3-3 proteins. Science 1994; 266(5182):126–129.
56. Kolch W, Heidecker G, Kochs G, et al. Protein kinase C alpha activates RAF-1 by direct phosphorylation. Nature 1993; 364(6434):249–252.
57. Newton AC. Regulation of protein kinase C. Curr Opin Cell Biol 1997; 9(2):161–167.

58. Liu B, Maher RJ, Hannun YA, et al. 12(S)-HETE enhancement of prostate tumor cell invasion: selective role of PKC alpha. J Natl Cancer Inst 1994; 86(15):1145–1151.
59. O'Brian CA. Protein kinase C-alpha: a novel target for the therapy of androgen-independent prostate cancer? Oncol Rep 1998; 5(2):305–309.
60. Nemunaitis J, Holmlund JT, Kraynak M, et al. Phase I evaluation of ISIS 3521, an antisense oligodeoxynucleotide to protein kinase C-alpha, in patients with advanced cancer. J Clin Oncol 1999; 17(11):3586–3595.
61. Yuen AR, Halsey J, Fisher GA, et al. Phase I study of an antisense oligonucleotide to protein kinase C-alpha (ISIS 3521/CGP 64128A) in patients with cancer. Clin Cancer Res 1999; 5(11):3357–3363.
62. Cunningham CC, Holmlund JT, Schiller JH, et al. A phase I trial of c-Raf kinase antisense oligonucleotide ISIS 5132 administered as a continuous intravenous infusion in patients with advanced cancer. Clin Cancer Res 2000; 6(5):1626–1631.
63. Steinberg J, Oyasu R, Lang S, et al. Intracellular levels of SGP-2 (Clusterin) correlate with tumor grade in prostate cancer. Clin Cancer Res 1997; 3(10):1707–1711.
64. Cervellera M, Raschella G, Santilli G, et al. Direct transactivation of the anti-apoptotic gene apolipoprotein J (clusterin) by B-MYB. J Biol Chem 2000; 275(28):21055–21060.
65. Redondo M, Villar E, Torres-Munoz J, et al. Overexpression of clusterin in human breast carcinoma. Am J Pathol 2000; 157(2):393–399.
66. Wellmann A, Thieblemont C, Pittaluga S, et al. Detection of differentially expressed genes in lymphomas using cDNA arrays: identification of clusterin as a new diagnostic marker for anaplastic large-cell lymphomas. Blood 2000; 96(2):398–404.
67. Miyake H, Gleave M, Kamidono S, et al. Overexpression of clusterin in transitional cell carcinoma of the bladder is related to disease progression and recurrence. Urology 2002; 59(1):150–154.
68. Parczyk K, Pilarsky C, Rachel U, et al. Gp80 (clusterin; TRPM-2) mRNA level is enhanced in human renal clear cell carcinomas. J Cancer Res Clin Oncol 1994; 120(3):186–188.
69. Calero M, Rostagno A, Matsubara E, et al. Apolipoprotein J (clusterin) and Alzheimer's disease. Microsc Res Tech 2000; 50(4):305–315.
70. Rosenberg ME, Silkensen J. Clusterin and the kidney. Exp Nephrol 1995; 3(1):9–14.
71. Montpetit ML, Lawless KR, Tenniswood M. Androgen-repressed messages in the rat ventral prostate. Prostate 1986; 8(1):25–36.
72. Kyprianou N, English HF, Isaacs JT. Programmed cell death during regression of PC-82 human prostate cancer following androgen ablation. Cancer Res 1990; 50(12):3748–3753.
73. July LV, Akbari M, Zellweger T, et al. Clusterin expression is significantly enhanced in prostate cancer cells following androgen withdrawal therapy. Prostate 2002; 50(3): 179–188.
74. Koch-Brandt C, Morgans C. Clusterin: a role in cell survival in the face of apoptosis? Prog Mol Subcell Biol 1996; 16:130–149.
75. Wilson MR, Easterbrook-Smith SB. Clusterin is a secreted mammalian chaperone. Trends Biochem Sci 2000; 25(3):95–98.
76. Michel D, Chatelain G, North S, et al. Stress-induced transcription of the clusterin/apoJ gene. Biochem J 1997; 328(1):45–50.
77. Humphreys DT, Carver JA, Easterbrook-Smith SB, et al. Clusterin has chaperone-like activity similar to that of small heat shock proteins. J Biol Chem 1999; 274(11): 6875–6881.
78. Sensibar JA, Sutkowski DA, Raffo A, et al. Prevention of cell death induced by tumor necrosis factor alpha in LNCaP cells by overexpression of sulfated glycoprotein-2 (clusterin). Cancer Res 1995; 55(11):2431–2437.
79. Zellweger T, Chi K, Miyake H, et al. Enhanced radiation sensitivity in prostate cancer by inhibition of the cell survival protein clusterin. Clin Cancer Res 2002; 8(10): 3276–3284.
80. Miyake H, Chi KN, Gleave ME. Antisense TRPM-2 oligodeoxynucleotides chemosensitize human androgen-independent PC-3 prostate cancer cells both in vitro and in vivo. Clin Cancer Res 2000; 6(5):1655–1663.

81. Zhang CR, Kim JK, Edwards CA, et al. Clusterin inhibits apoptosis by interacting with activated Bax. Nat Cell Biol 2005; 7(9):909–915.
82. Chi KN, Eisenhauer E, Fazil L, et al. A phase 1 pharmacokinetic and pharmacodynamic study of OGX-011, a 2′-methoxyethyl antisense oligonucleotide to clusterin in patients with localized prostate cancer. J Natl Cancer Inst 2005; 97(17):1287–1296.
83. Chi KN, Eisenhauer E, Siu L, et al. A phase 1 study of a second generation antisense oligonucleotide to clusterin (OGX-011) in combination with docetaxel: NCIC CTG IND.154. J Clin Oncol ASCO Annu Meeting Proc 2005; 23(16S):3085.
84. Deveraux QL, Roy N, Stennicke HR, et al. IAPs block apoptotic events induced by caspase-8 and cytochrome c by direct inhibition of distinct caspases. EMBO J 1998; 17(8):2215–2223.
85. Roy N, Deveraux QL, Takahashi R, et al. The c-IAP-1 and c-IAP-2 proteins are direct inhibitors of specific caspases. EMBO J 1997; 16(23):6914–6925.
86. Deveraux QL, Takahashi R, Salvesen GS, et al. X-linked IAP is a direct inhibitor of cell-death proteases. Nature 1997; 388(6639):300–304.
87. Tamm I, Wang Y, Sausville E, et al. IAP-family protein survivin inhibits caspase activity and apoptosis induced by Fas (CD95), Bax, caspases, and anticancer drugs. Cancer Res 1998; 58(23):5315–5320.
88. Levkau B, Garton KJ, Ferri N, et al. xIAP induces cell-cycle arrest and activates nuclear factor-kappaB: new survival pathways disabled by caspase-mediated cleavage during apoptosis of human endothelial cells. Circ Res 2001; 88(3):282–290.
89. Silke J, Hawkins CJ, Ekert PG, et al. The anti-apoptotic activity of XIAP is retained upon mutation of both the caspase 3- and caspase 9-interacting sites. J Cell Biol 2002; 157(1):115–124.
90. Salvesen GS, Duckett CS. IAP proteins: blocking the road to death's door. Nat Rev Mol Cell Biol 2002; 3(6):401–410.
91. Krajewska M, Krajewski S, Banares S, et al. Elevated expression of inhibitor of apoptosis proteins in prostate cancer. Clin Cancer Res 2003; 9(13):4914–4925.
92. Li F, Ambrosini G, Chu EY, et al. Control of apoptosis and mitotic spindle checkpoint by survivin. Nature 1998; 396(6711):580–584.
93. Ambrosini G, Adida C, Altieri DC. A novel anti-apoptosis gene, survivin, expressed in cancer and lymphoma. Nat Med 1997; 3(8):917–921.
94. Lu CD, Altieri DC, Tanigawa N. Expression of a novel antiapoptosis gene, surviving, correlated with tumor cell apoptosis and p53 accumulation in gastric carcinomas. Cancer Res 1998; 58(9):1808–1812.
95. Lal A, Lash AE, Altschul SF, et al. A public database for gene expression in human cancers. Cancer Res 1999; 59(21):5403–5407.
96. Altieri DC. Survivin, versatile modulation of cell division and apoptosis in cancer. Oncogene 2003; 22(53):8581–8589.
97. Li F, Ackermann EJ, Bennett CF, et al. Pleiotropic cell-division defects and apoptosis induced by interference with survivin function. Nat Cell Biol 1999; 1(8):461–466.
98. Chen J, Wu W, Tahir SK, et al. Down-regulation of survivin by antisense oligonucleotides increases apoptosis, inhibits cytokinesis and anchorage-independent growth. Neoplasia 2000; 2(3):235–241.
99. Ansell SM, Arendt BK, Grote DM, et al. Inhibition of survivin expression suppresses the growth of aggressive non-Hodgkin's lymphoma. Leukemia 2004; 18(3):616–623.
100. Patel BK, Carrasco RA, Stamm NB, et al. Antisense inhibition of survivin expression as a cancer therapeutic. Proceedings of the AACR-NCI-EORTC International Conference on Molecular Targets and Cancer Therapeutics 2003, Abstract B62, 2003.
101. Hu Y, Cherton-Horvat G, Dragowska V, et al. Antisense oligonucleotides targeting XIAP induce apoptosis and enhance chemotherapeutic activity against human lung cancer cells in vitro and in vivo. Clin Cancer Res 2003; 9(7):2826–2836.
102. Sasaki H, Sheng Y, Kotsuji F, et al. Down-regulation of X-linked inhibitor of apoptosis protein induces apoptosis in chemoresistant human ovarian cancer cells. Cancer Res 2000; 60(20):5659–5666.
103. Ranson M, Robson L, Durkin J, et al. A phase I trial of AEG35156 (XIAP antisense) administered as a 7-day continuous intravenous infusion in patients with advanced

tumors. Proceedings of the AACR-NCI-EORTC International Conference on Molecular Targets and Cancer Therapeutics 2005. Abstract C72, 2005.
104. Garrido C, Schmitt E, Cande C, et al. HSP27 and HSP70: potentially oncogenic apoptosis inhibitors. Cell Cyc 2003; 2(6):579–584.
105. Concannon CG, Gorman AM, Samali A. On the role of Hsp27 in regulating apoptosis. Apoptosis 2003; 8(1):61–70.
106. Ciocca DR, Oesterreich S, Chamness GC, et al. Biological and clinical implications of heat shock protein 27,000 (Hsp27): a review. J Natl Cancer Inst 1993; 85(19):1558–1570.
107. Neckers L, Schulte TW, Mimnaugh E. Geldanamycin as a potential anti-cancer agent: its molecular target and biochemical activity. Invest New Drugs 1999; 17(4):361–373.
108. Ramanathan RK, Trump DL, Eiseman JL. A phase I pharmacokinetic (PK) and pharmacodynamic (PD) trial of weekly 17-allylamino-17 demethoxygeldanamycin (17AAG, NSC-704057) in patients with advanced tumors. J Clin Oncol 2004; 22(14S):3031.
109. Liang P, MacRae TH. Molecular chaperones and the cytoskeleton. J Cell Sci 1997; 110(pt 13):1431–1440.
110. Parcellier A, Gurbuxani S, Schmitt E, et al. Heat shock proteins, cellular chaperones that modulate mitochondrial cell death pathways. Biophys Res Commun 2003; 304(3):505–512.
111. Rocchi P, Beraldi E, Ettinger S, et al. Hsp27 after androgen ablation facilitates androgen-independent progression in prostate cancer via signal transducers and activators of transcription 3-mediated suppression of apoptosis. Cancer Res 2005; 65(23): 11083–11093.
112. Conroy SE, Latchman DS. Do heat shock proteins have a role in breast cancer? Br J Cancer 1996; 74(5):717–721.
113. Arts HJ, Hollema H, Lemstra W, et al. Heat-shock-protein-27 (hsp27) expression in ovarian carcinoma: relation in response to chemotherapy and prognosis. Intl J Cancer 1999; 84(3):234–238.
114. Zhang R, Tremblay TL, McDermid A, et al. Identification of differentially expressed proteins in human glioblastoma cell lines and tumors. Glia 2003; 42(2):194–208.
115. Cornford PA, Dodson AR, Parsons KF, et al. Heat shock protein expression independently predicts clinical outcome in prostate cancer. Cancer Res 2000; 60(24):7099–105.
116. Bruey JM, Paul C, Fromentin A, et al. Differential regulation of HSP27 oligomerization in tumor cells grown in vitro and in vivo. Oncogene 2000; 19(42):4855–4863.
117. Rocchi P, So A, Kojima S, et al. Heat shock protein 27 increases after androgen ablation and plays a cytoprotective role in hormone-refractory prostate cancer. Cancer Res 2004; 64(18):6595–6602.
118. Garrido C, Ottavi P, Fromentin A, et al. HSP27 as a mediator of confluence-dependent resistance to cell death induced by anticancer drugs. Cancer Res 1997; 57(13):2661–2667.
119. Vargas-Roig LM, Gago FE, Tello O, et al. Heat shock protein expression and drug resistance in breast cancer patients treated with induction chemotherapy. Int J Cancer 1998; 79(5):468–475.
120. Garrido C, Bruey JM, Fromentin A, et al. HSP27 inhibits cytochrome c-dependent activation of procaspase-9. FASEB J 1999; 13(14):2061–2070.
121. Paul C, Manero F, Gonin S, et al. Hsp27 as a negative regulator of cytochrome C release. Mol Cell Biol 2002; 22(3):816–834.
122. Concannon CG, Orrenius S, Samali A. Hsp27 inhibits cytochrome c-mediated caspase activation by sequestering both pro-caspase-3 and cytochrome c. Gene Exp 2001; 9(4–5): 195–201.
123. Jones JI, Clemmons DR. Insulin-like growth factors and their binding proteins: biological actions. Endocrine Rev 1995; 16(1):3–34.
124. Nickerson T, Pollak M, Huynh H. Castration-induced apoptosis in the rat ventral prostate is associated with increased expression of genes encoding insulin-like growth factor binding proteins 2, 3, 4 and 5. Endocrinology 1998; 139(2):807–810.
125. Figueroa JA, De Raad S, Tadlock L, et al. Differential expression of insulin-like growth factor binding proteins in high versus low Gleason score prostate cancer. J Urol 1998; 159(4):1379–1383.

126. Miyake H, Nelson C, Rennie PS, et al. Overexpression of insulin-like growth factor binding protein-5 helps accelerate progression to androgen-independence in the human prostate LNCaP tumor model through activation of phosphatidylinositol 3′-kinase pathway. Endocrinology 2000; 141(6):2257–2265.
127. Miyake H, Pollak M, Gleave ME. Castration-induced up-regulation of insulin-like growth factor binding protein-5 potentiates insulin-like growth factor-I activity and accelerates progression to androgen independence in prostate cancer models. Cancer Res 2000; 60(11):3058–3064.
128. Kiyama S, Morrison K, Zellweger T, et al. Castration-induced increases in insulin-like growth factor-binding protein 2 promotes proliferation of androgen-independent human prostate LNCaP tumors. Cancer Res 2003; 63(13):3575–3584.
129. Elford HL, Freese M, Passamani E, et al. Ribonucleotide reductase and cell proliferation. I. Variations of ribonucleotide reductase activity with tumor growth rate in a series of rat hepatomas. J Biol Chem 1970; 245(20):5228–5233.
130. Fan H, Villegas C, Huang A, et al. The mammalian ribonucleotide reductase R2 component cooperates with a variety of oncogenes in mechanisms of cellular transformation. Cancer Res 1998; 58(8):1650–1653.
131. Bjorklund S, Skog S, Tribukait B, et al. S-phase-specific expression of mammalian ribonucleotide reductase R1 and R2 subunit mRNAs. Biochemistry 1990; 29(23):5452–5458.
132. Wright JA, Chan AK, Choy BK, et al. Regulation and drug resistance mechanisms of mammalian ribonucleotide reductase, and the significance to DNA synthesis. Biochem Cell Biol 1990; 68(12):1364–1371.
133. Lee Y, Vassilakos A, Feng N, et al. GTI-2040, an antisense agent targeting the small subunit component (R2) of human ribonucleotide reductase, shows potent antitumor activity against a variety of tumors. Cancer Res 2003; 63(11):2802–2811.
134. Desai AA, Schilsky RL, Young A, et al. A phase I study of antisense oligonucleotide GTI-2040 given by continuous intravenous infusion in patients with advanced solid tumors. Ann Oncol 2005; 16(6):958–965.
135. Sridhar SS, Canil CM, Hotte SJ, et al. A Phase 2 study of GTI-2040 plus docetaxel and prednisone as 1st line treatment in hormone-refractory prostate cancer (HRPC). AACR-NCI-EORTC International Conference Proceedings Molecular Targets and Cancer Therapeutics 2005, Abstract A36, 2005.
136. Scher HI, Kelly WK. Flutamide withdrawal syndrome: its impact on clinical trials in hormone-refractory prostate cancer. J Clin Oncol 1993; 11(8):1566–1572.
137. Eder IE, Culig Z, Ramoner R, et al. Inhibition of LNCaP prostate cancer cells by means of androgen receptor antisense oligonucleotides. Cancer Gene Ther 2000; 7(7): 997–1007.
138. Eder IE, Hoffmann J, Rogatsch H, et al. Inhibition of LNCaP prostate tumor growth in vivo by an antisense oligonucleotide directed against the human androgen receptor. Cancer Gene Ther 2002; 9(2):117–125.
139. Hamy F, Brondani V, Spoerri R, et al. Specific block of androgen receptor activity by antisense oligonucleotides. Prostate Cancer Prostatic Dis 2003; 6(1):27–33.

10 Novel Approaches to Androgen Receptor Blockade

Ingo K. Mellinghoff

Department of Pharmacology, University of California, Los Angeles, California, U.S.A.

INTRODUCTION

Prostate cancer remains the most common nonskin cancer and the second leading cause of cancer deaths in North American men. Patients with disease localized to the prostate gland can be cured by surgery and/or radiation therapy. Patients with metastatic disease currently cannot be cured and receive androgen deprivation therapy in palliative intent. This therapy encompasses castration, antiandrogen therapy, and combinations thereof (1,2). Androgen deprivation therapy causes a substantial regression of tumor burden in most patients, but ultimately fails due to the outgrowth of "hormone-refractory" cancer cells. Understanding the molecular mechanisms of tumor progression during androgen deprivation therapy is prerequisite to develop therapies against this lethal form of prostate cancer.

As advanced prostate cancer is clearly a disease of great genetic diversity (3), several lines of evidence suggest that the androgen receptor (AR) axis remains critical for tumors that progress during androgen deprivation therapy. First, most of these cancers continue to express the AR protein and androgen-related genes such as prostate-specific antigen (PSA), indicating that AR remains transcriptionally active. Second, many patients with clinically "androgen-independent" disease are still responding to second-line manipulations of the AR axis, including agents that antagonize adrenal hormone production. Third, intratumoral androgen concentrations during standard androgen ablation therapy appear to be well within the range known to activate AR transcriptional activity in vitro (4). Finally, genetic experiments recently documented the causative role of AR for hormone-refractory prostate cancer growth (5). In summary, these observations suggest that current androgen deprivation therapy selects for prostate cancer cells that are capable of sustaining AR transcriptional activity at subphysiological androgen levels.

The need for more potent inhibitors of the AR signaling axis has encouraged detailed studies into the molecular mechanisms of AR function. Crystallographic studies (6–11), chromatin immunoprecipitation experiments (12–18), and fluorescence resonance energy transfer (19) have considerably refined the view of the AR during the last few years. This chapter reviews the current knowledge of AR function, its role in hormone-refractory prostate cancer, and therapeutic opportunities arising from these new insights and comparisons to the estrogen receptor (ER).

THE STRUCTURAL BASIS OF AR FUNCTION

The AR was cloned less than a decade ago (20–22) and is a member of the nuclear hormone receptor "superfamily" of transcription factors (23). This superfamily is further divided into the steroid and nonsteroid hormone receptor families. Unique to the steroid receptor family (AR, progesterone receptor, glucocorticoid receptor, mineralcorticoid receptor, and ER) is their ability to bind as ligand-induced homodimers to palindromic DNA sequences called hormone response elements.

The structure of the AR protein (Fig. 1) is highly modular and comprises of an amino-terminal domain, a central DNA-binding domain (DBD), and a carboxy-terminal ligand-binding domain (LBD). The amino-terminus contains a transcription activation function (AF1) (24) and homopolymeric stretches of amino acids (glutamine, proline, and glycine) seen in other transcription factors (25). The DBD has two zinc-finger motifs that are highly conserved within the steroid receptor family. The first zinc finger contains the recognition helix which makes base-specific contacts within the major groove. The second zinc finger stabilizes the binding of the receptor to the DNA by discriminating half-site spacing and contacting the sugar-phosphate backbone of adjacent sequences (27,28). Further sequence elements contained within the DBD and adjacent hinge region contribute to AR dimerization (29) and ligand-induced nuclear translocation (30). The carboxy-terminus of AR contains the LBD, a hydrophophic heptad repeat region critical for efficient AR homodimerization (27,31,32), and a second transcription activation function (AF2). AF2 is highly conserved within the nuclear hormone receptor family and is crucial for the recruitment of transcriptional coactivators through their short leucine-rich LxxLL motifs (L—leucine, x—any amino acid) (33–35).

Our understanding of AR functional domains has historically been shaped through comparisons with other steroid hormone receptors, mutagenesis studies, and the phenotypic characterization of spontaneously occurring germline mutations in the AR gene located on the X-chromosome (36,37). More detailed insights into the structural basis of ligand selectivity were recently gained through the determination of X-ray crystal structures for the AR LBD in complex with the synthetic agonist metribolone (R1881) (6), the natural ligand dihydrotestosterone (7), and peptides containing recognition motifs of AR coregulator proteins (COR) (8,9). Overall, the AR LBD has a similar three-dimensional structure as other nuclear hormone receptors and the numbering of the α-helices was retained to facilitate structural comparisons (helix 2 is missing in AR). The 11 α-helices of

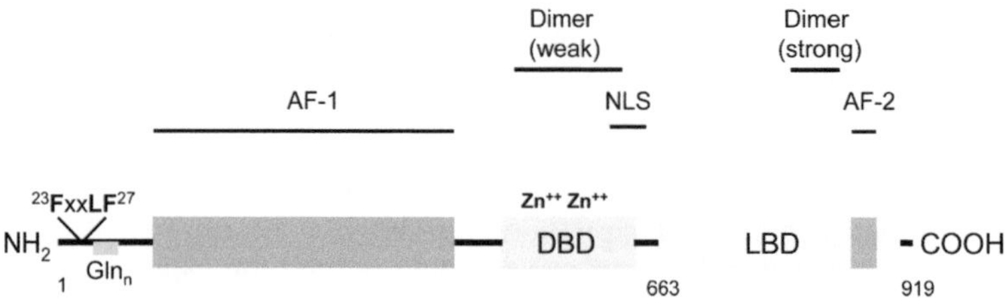

FIGURE 1 Structure of the AR protein. AR, like other nuclear receptors, is a modular protein with three major domains. The amino terminus contains a trans activation domain (AF-1). The central DBD has two highly conserved zinc-finger motifs (Zn). The carboxy-terminal LBD contains a second trans activation domain (AF-2) which is critical for interactions with transcriptional coregulator proteins and with the N-terminal FxxLF motif (F—phenylalanine, L-leucine x—any amino acid). Other functionally relevant sequence elements include an amino-terminal homopolymeric stretch of Gln_n, an NLS, and dimerization motifs (Dimer) located within the DBD and LBD. Please see text for details. *Abbreviations*: AR, androgen receptor; DBD, DNA-binding domain; Gln_n, glutamines; LBD, ligand-binding domain; NH_2, amino terminus; NLS, nuclear localization motif; AF, activation function. *Source*: From Ref. 26.

the AR LBD are arranged in an antiparallel sandwich motif. Helix 12 (H12) contains residues that are crucial for AF-2 function and serves as a movable lid over the binding pocket. The conformational change associated with agonist binding creates a shallow groove atop the LBD (H12 forms one side of this groove) which allows coactivators to dock via their LxxLL motifs. In the case of AR, LxxLL-containing peptides appear to make fewer and less optimized hydrophobic contacts with the AF2 pocket than FxxLF (F—phenylalanine, x—any amino acid) containing peptides. This preference of AF2 for aromatic-rich motifs distinguishes AR from other nuclear receptors and provides an explanation for the previously observed ligand-induced intramolecular association of the LBD with the AR N-terminal domain which contains such motifs (38–40). Current studies aim to elucidate how this N/C interaction affects AR-regulated gene transcription programs and the recruitment of AR coactivators (41) to AF-2 and/or other AR surfaces (42).

ACTIVATION OF AR SIGNALING

In the absence of ligand, the majority of AR molecules reside in the cytoplasm in a transcriptionally inactive multiprotein complex (43–45). Agonist binding triggers a series of AR conformational changes, including an intramolecular interaction between the LBD and amino-terminus, release of AR-associated proteins, and AR self-association in the nucleus (Fig. 2) (19,46). Heat shock proteins (HSPs), such as HSP 90, appear to participate in this conformational maturation of AR by maintaining it in a high-affinity ligand-binding conformation (47). Most steroid

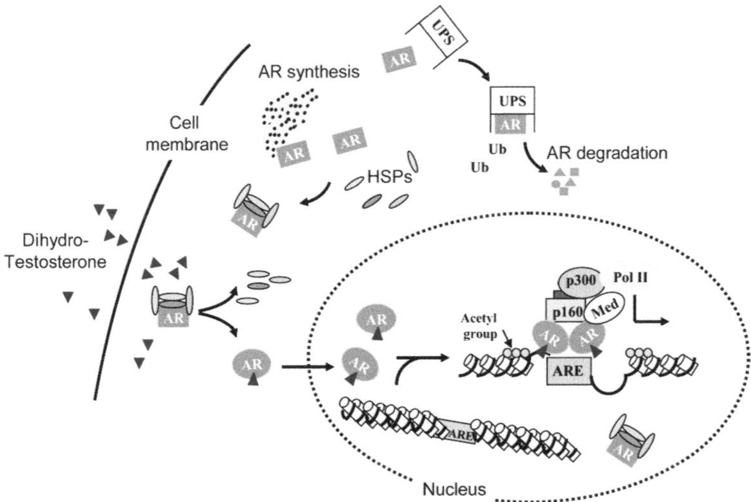

FIGURE 2 (*See color insert*) Ligand-induced AR activation. In the absence of ligand, AR resides mostly in the cytoplasm bound to HSPs in a transcriptionally inactive complex. Androgen binding triggers dissociation of chaperone proteins, AR self-association, and nuclear assembly of the AR transcription factor complex. This complex includes members of the p160 family of coactivator proteins (p160), p300, members of the mediator complex (Med), and RNA Pol II. AR degradation through the UPS is markedly reduced in the presence of dihydrotestosterone. Please see text for details. *Abbreviations*: AR, androgen receptor; HSP, heat shock protein; Pol II, polymerase II; UPS, ubiquition-proteasane system; ARE, androgen response elements.

hormone receptors (AR, GR, PR, and MR) recognize identical DNA response elements which consist of inverted repeats of two hexameric half-sites (5′-AGAACA-3′) with a 3-bp spacer segment (48). In addition to this degenerate set of response elements, AR also binds to selective "androgen response elements" (AREs) which consist of two hexameric half-sites repeating on the same strand (49–52). The ability of AR to bind to a more diverse set of DNA response elements appears to be conferred through the strength of the AR dimer interface (10).

Once bound to target DNA sequences, steroid hormone receptors elicit a hormone-, promoter-, and cell-type-specific transcriptional response through the recruitment of COR which modify chromatin structure and engage components of the basal transcriptional machinery (53,54). Members of the p160 family of coactivators (SRC1, SRC2/TIF2/GRIP1, and SRC3/ACTR/AIB1/RAC3/pCIP) contribute to this process by linking the DNA-bound hormone receptor with histone acetyltransferases (HATs) (e.g., CBP/p300), histone methyltransferases (e.g., CARM1, PRMT1), and ATP-dependent chromatin remodeling enzymatic activities (55–58). Gene repression is accomplished through association of AR with corepressor proteins, such as nuclear receptor corepressor and silencing mediator of retinoid and thyroid receptors which modulate chromatin structure by recruitment of Sin3 and histone deacetylases (HDACs). Unlike retinoic acid receptor and thyroid hormone receptor, steroid hormone receptors do not actively repress gene transcription in the absence of hormone.

Chromatin immunoprecipitation (CHIP) experiments have provided a temporal-spatial model for the ligand-induced assembly of the AR transcription complex. Somewhat surprisingly, the binding of AR, associated HAT complexes, and RNA polymerase II (Pol II) appears to occur primarily at distant enhancer elements of AR-regulated genes. Pol II then tracks from the enhancer to the promoter through a loop structure created by the communication between AR transcription factor complexes assembled on the enhancer and—loosely—on the promoter (14,17). Compared to the rapid and cyclical assembly of the ER coactivator complex which is followed by ER degradation (59,60), the formation of the AR transcription complex appears to be more sustained, consistent with the stabilizing effects of androgen on the AR protein. CHIP experiments also suggest some redundancy in the scaffolding role of p160-coactivator proteins (17) which is consistent with results from genetically defined mouse models (61) and may limit the ability to target individual p160 proteins therapeutically. Finally, it should be pointed out that this model of the AR transcription factor complex is largely based on studies of 5′-regulatory regions of the PSA and related KLK-2 genes both of which contain AREs in their promoter and enhancer regions (62–64). It will be important to extend these studies to biologically more relevant AR-target genes most of which are currently unknown.

Intracellular signaling pathways play an important role in modulating the effects of cognate receptor ligands. Phosphorylation events have been shown to affect all aspects of nuclear hormone receptor function, including ligand binding, nuclear translocation, association with DNA target sequences, and assembly of the hormone-receptor transcription complex (65,66). Regulation of ER function by mitogen-activated protein kinase (MAPK), e.g., occurs through phosphorylation of the receptor itself (67) as well as through phosphorylation of the p160 coactivators AIB1 (68) and TIF-2 (69). It is currently unclear which members of the AR signaling axis are recipients of critical phosphorylation events. Likely candidates are the members of the p160 family of coactivator proteins (70,71), other constituents of the AR transcription complex (72), and the AR itself. Sequence analysis predicts over (41) phosphorylation sites within the AR protein (73) of which only seven have been confirmed by mass spectrometry (74–76). All the phosphosites confirmed by mass spectrometry are serine residues (Ser16, Ser 81, Ser 94, Ser 256, Ser 308, Ser 424, and Ser 650). Although mutagenesis of any of these phosphosites failed to impair AR transcriptional activity (75), mutagenesis of both Serine 424 or Serine 515 affected the phosphorylation status of other serine residues (75,76), suggesting a network of interrelated phosphorylation events. The development of phosphosite-specific anti-AR antibodies provides a framework to define the role of AR phosphorylation during prostate cancer progression and identify kinases mediating these phosphorylation events (77,78).

Post-translational modifications of AR by ubiquitination is likely to add further complexity to the current model of AR regulation. There is increasing evidence for a role of the ubiquitin-degradation system in transcriptional regulation (79,80). The p160 coactivator AIB1, e.g., has recently been linked to agonist-induced ER-α degradation by the proteasome (81) and the ubiquitin-ligase E-6-associated protein has been shown to function as a coactivator for the steroid receptor family (82). In contrast to the estrogen and glucocorticoid receptors, however, ligand binding markedly prolongs the half-life of the AR (83) and we have shown that the HER2/ErbB3 kinase positively regulates AR transcriptional activity and protein stability (84). These observations suggest fundamental differences in the regulation of protein stability between these receptors and further studies are required to elucidate how the ubiquitin-proteasome pathway regulates AR function. In addition to phosphorylation and ubiquitination, AR acetylation may provide a further mechanism to modulate AR function (85–88).

MECHANISMS OF HORMONE-REFRACTORY PROSTATE CANCER GROWTH

Several mechanisms have been proposed to explain resistance to androgen ablation therapy, including mechanisms that completely bypass the AR signaling axis (89). Clinical evidence for such AR-independent mechanisms, however, is sparse and proof of their functional significance difficult in the setting of active AR signaling. The subsequent discussion will therefore focus on mechanisms that either directly involve the AR gene (mutations, amplification) or indirectly enhance AR function.

Gain-of-function mutations in the AR gene are found in 10% to 20% of patients with castration-resistant prostate cancer (90–96) with some variations between studies depending on the extent of AR sequence coverage, mutation detection method, and tissue source. Mutations appear to be more common in hormone-refractory tumors than in hormone-naïve advanced tumors or early-stage disease. The first identified (97) and also most frequently reported mutation results in an amino acid change from threonine to arginine (T877A) in the LBD of AR. This mutation alters the conformation of the ligand-binding pocket (6,7), allows access for bulkier ligands, and explains AR inducibility not only by its natural ligand dihydrotestosterone, but also by progesterone, 17-β-estradiol, adrenal androgens, and even the anti-androgen hydroxyflutamide (98). Altered ligand-binding properties have also been documented for the AR LBD mutants L701H, V715M, H874Y, and T877S (99–103). Somatic missense mutations outside the AR LBD are structurally less well defined, but appear to cluster to regions known to be involved in coregulator binding and/or trans activation (101). Missense mutations in AR thus provide a compelling mechanism for antiandrogen resistance and might explain why some men whose disease progresses during antiandrogen therapy experience an improvement following discontinuation of these agents (104). The overall frequency of AR mutations, however, cannot account for most cases of hormone-refractory prostate cancer.

Increases in AR protein levels may provide a more common mechanism to alter the ligand sensitivity and specificity of AR. It has long been noted that failure of androgen ablation therapy is only rarely associated with the loss of AR expression in prostate cancer cells (105). In fact, a number of studies reported increased AR levels in clinical samples from patients with castration-resistant prostate cancer. These studies include (i) immunohistochemical examinations of large patient cohorts showing AR protein levels in hormone-refractory samples which are comparable or higher than AR levels in hormone-sensitive samples (106), (ii) examinations of AR RNA levels which show up to sixfold higher AR transcript levels in locally recurrent hormone-refractory tumors compared to androgen-dependent tumors or benign prostate hyperplasias (107), and (iii) studies of the AR gene locus using comparative genome hybridization or fluorescence in situ hybridization which report AR amplification in 20% to30% of tumor samples from patients with recurrent prostate cancer, but not in matched pretreatment samples (108) or unrelated hormone-naïve prostate cancer samples (109,110). More conclusive evidence for a role of increased AR levels in hormone-refractory prostate cancer has emerged from the analysis of matched hormone-sensitive and hormone-refractory prostate cancer xenograft pairs. Using microarray-based gene expression profiling, only one out of 12,559 probe sets—directed against the AR cDNA—was found to be differentially expressed in all seven hormone-sensitive/hormone-refractory pairs. The second most consistent probe, upregulated in five of seven pairs, was also directed against the AR. The magnitude of AR overexpression was only about two- to four-fold and this modest increase in AR levels appears to be sufficient to confer hormone-refractory growth (5). Knockdown of endogenous AR levels using mRNA hammerhead ribozyme (111), antisense oligodeoxynucleotides (112), or shRNA (5) confirms the requirement of AR for hormone-refractory growth. Interestingly, an increase in AR levels also appears to be sufficient to convert the AR antagonist bicalutamide into an AR agonists by enhancing the recruitment of p160-AR coactivators (5).

Assembly of steroid hormone receptor transcription complexes is influenced by the relative concentrations of coactivator and corepressor proteins (113,114). Both increased levels of the p160 coactivator AIB1 (115) and decreased levels of the corepressor NCoR (116), e.g., have been associated with the resistance breast cancer to tamoxifen. It appears likely that the ratio of CORs similarly affects the response to AR ligands and overexpression of the p160 coactivators SRC-1 and TIF-2 has been found in subsets of clinical prostate cancer samples (117).

Perhaps the most diverse mechanism to enhance AR function is through AR crosstalk with other signaling pathways. A number of oncogenic kinase pathways have been shown to augment AR transcriptional function at ligand concentrations found intratumorally during androgen ablation therapy (Fig. 3). These include the epidermal growth factor (EGF) and insulin-like growth factor (IGF-1) pathways, protein kinase A, the tumor suppressor PTEN and its effector kinase Akt, interleukin-6, and Ras (118–122). The HER-2/neu kinase, a member of the EGFR-receptor family, has received particular attention due to its well-established role in breast

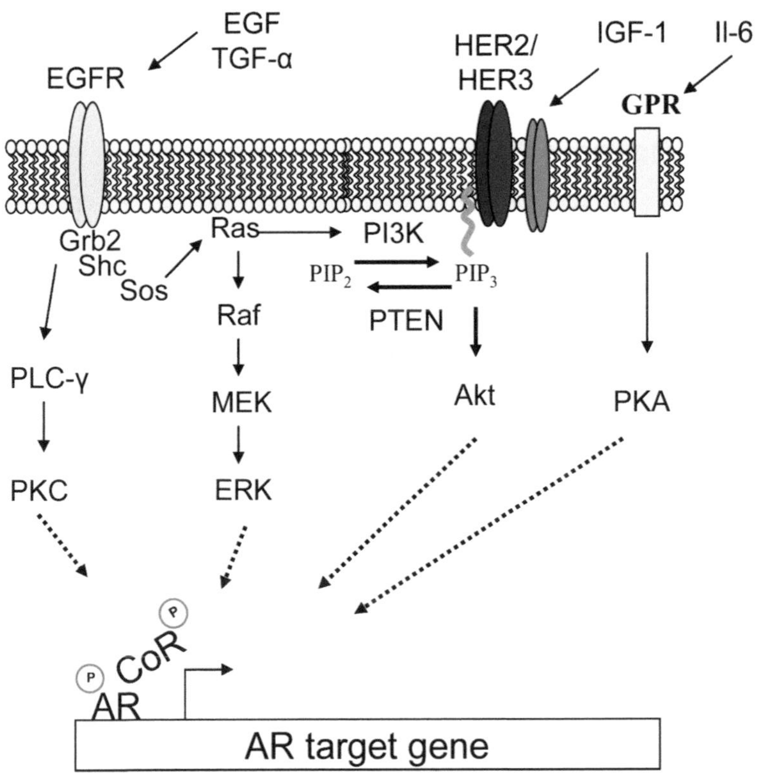

FIGURE 3 Modulation of AR function through kinase pathways. Activation of cell membrane receptors through extracellular ligands (e.g., TGF-α, IL-6) results in activation of downstream signaling pathways which phosphorylate the AR and/or AR-CoR. Pathway activation can also result from oncogenic mutations, such as deletion of the tumor suppressor phosphatase PTEN. Please see text for details. *Abbreviations*: AR, androgen receptor; CoR, coregulator proteins; EGF, epidermal growth factor; TGF, transforming growth factor; EGFR, epidermal growth factor receptor; HER, human EGFR-related; IGF, insulin-like growth factor; Grb2, growth factor receptor-bound protein 2; PIP, phosphatidylinositol phosphate; PTEN, phosphatase and tensin homolog deleted on chromosome ten; PLC, phospholipase C; MEK, MAP kinase kinase; PKC, protein kinase C; PKA, protein kinase A; ERK, extracellular-signal regulated kinase; AkT, protein kinase B, cellular hololog of Akt-8 retrovirus; HER2, human EGFR-related 2 kinase; Sos, son of seveless 1 protein; Shc, SH2 domain containing sequence.

cancer (123). Preclinical data indicate that overexpression of HER2 is sufficient to promote hormone-refractory growth (124,125), inhibition of endogenous HER2 impairs prostate cancer growth (126,127), and HER2 augments AR function (124–128). Interestingly, ErbB3 rather than EGFR appears to be the critical heterodimerization partner for HER2 in this process (84), perhaps accounting for the disappointing clinical activity of EGFR kinase inhibitors (129) or Trastuzumab (130) which does not block HER2/ErbB3 heterodimerization (127). The role of the serine–threonine kinase Akt in AR function has also been of great interest given the solid genetic evidence for PTEN inactivation in human prostate cancer (131). These studies have yielded controversial and perhaps cell-line-specific results as to whether Akt enhances (84,132–134) or impairs (135) AR function.

Genetically defined cancer models using primary prostatic epithelial cells (136,137) may prove particularly useful to validate functional synergism between the AR axis and cellular signaling pathways.

THERAPEUTIC IMPLICATIONS

Therapeutic strategies that interfere with the AR signaling axis can be separated into three broad categories (Table 1). The first includes drugs that lower the concentration of testosterone and its metabolite dihydrotestosterone (DHT). The newest members in this group of drugs are inhibitors of the P450 monooxygenase 17-α-hydroxylase/(17,20)-lyase, the last step in the testicular and adrenal biosynthesis of testosterone. One of these inhibitors, Abiraterone,™Cougar Biotechnology, Los Angeles, CA. has been shown to further lower androgen concentrations in men receiving standard androgen ablation therapy (138) and is under clinical development. The second category comprises of agents which lower AR protein levels in preclinical models and are in various stages of clinical development. They include inhibitors of HSP (91,139–141), inhibitors of the ErbB signaling network (84,142), and inhibitors of HDACs (143,144). HER2 kinase inhibitors (84,128) and HDAC inhibitors (12,143,145) appear to have pleiotropic effects on the AR signaling axis and the results of early clinical trials with these agents are described elsewhere in this book. The third category includes agents that regulate the formation of the AR transcription complex, such as the widely used AR antagonists bicalutamide, flutamide, and nilutamide.

Selective ER modulation has transformed the treatment of breast cancer (114) and provides important lessons for targeting of AR. AR-antagonists have traditionally been viewed as agents that compete with dihydrotestosterone for the AR LBD

TABLE 1 Strategies to Target the Androgen Receptor Signaling Axis

Targeted process	Drug examples	Molecular target
Androgen	DES, PC-SPES	Estrogen receptor (in hypothalamus)
	Leuprolide, Goserelin, Buserelin, Nafarelin	LHRH receptor (agonism)
	Abarelix	LHRH receptor (antagonism)
	Aminoglutethimide	Aromatase, 20-α-hydroxycholesterol synthetase
	Ketoconazole	P450 enzymes
	Finasteride, Dilutamide	5-α-reductase
	Abiraterone	17-α-hydoxylase/ 17,20 lysase
AR levels	17-AAG, DMAG	HSP90
	mAb 2-C4, AEE-788, scFv(FRP5)-ETA	HER2 kinase
	SAHA, sodium phenylbutyrate, LAQ824	HDACs
AR transcription complex	Flutamide, Bicalutamide, Nilutamide	AR LBD
	Cyproterone acetate, Mifepristone	AR LBD
	mAb 2-C4, AEE-788, scFv(FRP5)-ETA	HER2 kinase
	SAHA, sodium phenylbutyrate, LAQ824	HDACs

Abbreviations: AR, Androgen receptors; HDAC, histone deacetylases LBD, ligand binding domain; HSP, heat shock proteins; HER2, human EGFR-related 2 kinase; LHRH, luteinizing hormone-releasing hormone.

and induce a receptor conformation incompatible with coactivator binding. Recent data suggest that conformational changes associated with antagonist binding not only impair coactivator recruitment, but actively repress target genes through the recruitment of corepressor proteins and HDACs (12,59,146). The chemical structure of the ligand has profound effects on the conformation of the ligand-binding pocket, cofactor recruitment, and ultimate transcriptional output. The partial steroidal agonist mifepristone (RU486), e.g., appears to enhance the interaction between AR and the corepressor NCoR to a much greater degree than other AR ligands (18). X-ray crystallography of antagonist-bound receptor has been very productive for the ER field (147–150) and will likely contribute critical insights for AR-antagonist drug-discovery programs (11,26,151,152).

The well-documented effects of clinically relevant AR missense mutations on antagonist binding have raised the question whether AR surfaces outside the binding pocket might be preferable targets for novel AR antagonists. Combinatorial peptide phage libraries have successfully been used to identify LxxLL-containing peptides that interact with the AF-2 domain of the ER and inhibit estradiol-mediated transcriptional activation (153). Similar approaches are currently used to identify peptides that interfere with coactivator binding to AR and/or formation of the AR N/C interaction (9,154).

The use of kinase inhibitors to block AR function and prostate cancer growth is very appealing based on tolerability and efficacy of these agents for other human malignancies (155). Their deployment for hormone-refractory prostate cancer, however, is currently hampered by the lack of understanding which kinases phosphorylate AR and/or critical AR CoRs. Ongoing genome-wide efforts to ascertain gene copy number alterations and mutations in clinical samples from hormone-refractory tumors will likely provide important leads for the clinical testing of signal transduction inhibitors.

The last five years have provided us with a wealth of evidence to pursue more potent and durable strategies of AR-blockade. This includes the structure-based design of novel antagonists and the rational combination of agents that block different steps during AR activation. Similar to other molecularly targeted agents, the optimal clinical deployment of AR inhibitors will likely require repeated measurements of the molecular target (expression, activity, and mutation) in tumor tissue during the course of therapy (156,157). These efforts will be cumbersome, but are likely of lasting impact for the treatment of hormone-sensitive human cancers.

ACKNOWLEDGMENTS

I am grateful to Dr. Charles Sawyers for many helpful discussion regarding prostate cancer biology and the development of targeted cancer therapeutics. This work is supported by a Department of Defense Physician Research Training Award and the UCLA Prostate Cancer Specialized Program of Research Excellence (SPORE).

REFERENCES

1. Denmeade SR, Isaacs JT. A history of prostate cancer treatment. Nat Rev Cancer 2002; 2:389–396.
2. Loblaw DA, et al. American Society of Clinical Oncology recommendations for the initial hormonal management of androgen-sensitive metastatic, recurrent, or progressive prostate cancer. J Clin Oncol 2004; 22:2927–2941.

3. Isaacs W, De Marzo A, Nelson WG. Focus on prostate cancer. Cancer Cell 2002; 2:113–116.
4. Mohler JL, et al. The androgen axis in recurrent prostate cancer. Clin Cancer Res 2004; 10:440–448.
5. Chen CD, et al. Molecular determinants of resistance to antiandrogen therapy. Nat Med 2004; 10:33–39.
6. Matias PM, et al. Structural evidence for ligand specificity in the binding domain of the human androgen receptor: implications for pathogenic gene mutations. J Biol Chem 2000; 275:26164–26171.
7. Sack JS, et al. Crystallographic structures of the ligand-binding domains of the androgen receptor and its T877A mutant complexed with the natural agonist dihydrotestosterone. Proc Natl Acad Sci USA 2001; 98:4904–4909.
8. He B, et al. Structural basis for androgen receptor interdomain and coactivator interactions suggests a transition in nuclear receptor activation function dominance. Mol Cell 2004; 16:425–438.
9. Hur E, et al. Recognition and accommodation at the androgen receptor coactivator binding interface. PLoS Biol 2004; 2:E274.
10. Shaffer PL, Jivan A, Dollins DE, Claessens F, Gewirth DT. Structural basis of androgen receptor binding to selective androgen response elements. Proc Natl Acad Sci USA 2004; 101:4758–4763.
11. Bohl CE, Gao W, Miller DD, Bell CE, Dalton JT. Structural basis for antagonism and resistance of bicalutamide in prostate cancer. Proc Natl Acad Sci USA 2005; 102:6201–6206.
12. Shang Y, Myers M, Brown M. Formation of the androgen receptor transcription complex. Mol Cell 2002; 9:601–610.
13. Wang Q, Sharma D, Ren Y, Fondell JD. A coregulatory role for the TRAP-mediator complex in androgen receptor-mediated gene expression. J Biol Chem 2002; 277:42852–42858.
14. Louie MC, et al. Androgen-induced recruitment of RNA polymerase II to a nuclear receptor-p160 coactivator complex. Proc Natl Acad Sci USA 2003; 100:2226–2230.
15. Kang Z, Janne OA, Palvimo JJ. Coregulator recruitment and histone modifications in transcriptional regulation by the androgen receptor. Mol Endocrinol 2004; 18:2633–2648.
16. Jia L, et al. Androgen receptor signaling: mechanism of interleukin-6 inhibition. Cancer Res 2004; 64:2619–2626.
17. Wang Q, Carroll JS, Brown M. Spatial and temporal recruitment of androgen receptor and its coactivators involves chromosomal looping and polymerase tracking. Mol Cell 2005; 19:631–642.
18. Hodgson MC, et al. The androgen receptor recruits nuclear receptor CoRepressor (N-CoR) in the presence of mifepristone via its N and C termini revealing a novel molecular mechanism for androgen receptor antagonists. J Biol Chem 2005; 280:6511–6519.
19. Schaufele F, et al. The structural basis of androgen receptor activation: intramolecular and intermolecular amino-carboxy interactions. Proc Natl Acad Sci USA 2005; 102:9802–9807.
20. Lubahn DB, et al. Cloning of human androgen receptor complementary DNA and localization to the X chromosome. Science 1988; 240:327–330.
21. Chang CS, Kokontis J, Liao ST. Molecular cloning of human and rat complementary DNA encoding androgen receptors. Science 1988; 240:324–326.
22. Trapman J, et al. Cloning, structure and expression of a cDNA encoding the human androgen receptor. Biochem Biophys Res Commun 1988; 153:241–248.
23. Mangelsdorf DJ, et al. The nuclear receptor superfamily: the second decade. Cell 1995; 83:835–839.
24. Simental JA, Sar M, Lane MV, French FS, Wilson EM. Transcriptional activation and nuclear targeting signals of the human androgen receptor. J Biol Chem 1991; 266:510–518.
25. Gerber HP, et al. Transcriptional activation modulated by homopolymeric glutamine and proline stretches. Science 1994; 263:808–811.
26. Gronemeyer H, Gustafsson JA, Laudet V. Principles for modulation of the nuclear receptor superfamily. Nat Rev Drug Discov 2004; 3:950–964.

27. Wong CI, Zhou ZX, Sar M, Wilson EM. Steroid requirement for androgen receptor dimerization and DNA binding: modulation by intramolecular interactions between the NH2-terminal and steroid-binding domains. J Biol Chem 1993; 268:19004–19012.
28. Schoenmakers, et al. Differential DNA binding by the androgen and glucocorticoid receptors involves the second Zn-finger and a C-terminal extension of the DNA-binding domains. Biochem J 1999; 341(pt 3):515–521.
29. Gast A, Neuschmid-Kaspar F, Klocker H, Cato AC. A single amino acid exchange abolishes dimerization of the androgen receptor and causes Reifenstein syndrome. Mol Cell Endocrinol 1995; 111:93–98.
30. Zhou ZX, Sar M, Simental JA, Lane MV, Wilson EM. A ligand-dependent bipartite nuclear targeting signal in the human androgen receptor: requirement for the DNA-binding domain and modulation by NH2-terminal and carboxyl-terminal sequences. J Biol Chem 1994; 269:13115–13123.
31. Fawell SE, Lees JA, White R, Parker MG. Characterization and colocalization of steroid binding and dimerization activities in the mouse estrogen receptor. Cell 1990; 60: 953–962.
32. Nemoto T, Ohara-Nemoto Y, Shimazaki S, Ota M. Dimerization characteristics of the DNA- and steroid-binding domains of the androgen receptor. J Steroid Biochem Mol Biol 1994; 50:225–233.
33. Heery DM, Kalkhoven E, Hoare S, Parker MG. A signature motif in transcriptional co-activators mediates binding to nuclear receptors. Nature 1997; 387:733–736.
34. Darimont BD, et al. Structure and specificity of nuclear receptor-coactivator interactions. Genes Dev 1998; 12:3343–3356.
35. Feng W, et al. Hormone-dependent coactivator binding to a hydrophobic cleft on nuclear receptors. Science 1998; 280:1747–1749.
36. Quigley CA, et al. Androgen receptor defects: historical, clinical, and molecular perspectives. Endocr Rev 1995; 16:271–321.
37. Gottlieb B, Beitel LK, Wu JH, Trifiro M. The androgen receptor gene mutations database (ARDB): 2004 update. Hum Mutat 2004; 23:527–533.
38. Langley E, Zhou ZX, Wilson EM. Evidence for an anti-parallel orientation of the ligand-activated human androgen receptor dimer. J Biol Chem 1995; 270:29983–29990.
39. Doesburg P, et al. Functional in vivo interaction between the amino-terminal, trans activation domain and the ligand binding domain of the androgen receptor. Biochemistry 1997; 36:1052–1064.
40. He B, Kemppainen JA, Wilson EM. FXXLF and WXXLF sequences mediate the NH2-terminal interaction with the ligand binding domain of the androgen receptor. J Biol Chem 2000; 275:22986–22994.
41. Heinlein CA, Chang C. Androgen receptor (AR) coregulators: an overview. Endocr Rev 2002; 23:175–200.
42. Sathya G, Chang CY, Kazmin D, Cook CE, McDonnell DP. Pharmacological uncoupling of androgen receptor-mediated prostate cancer cell proliferation and prostate-specific antigen secretion. Cancer Res 2003; 63:8029–8036.
43. Veldscholte J, et al. Hormone-induced dissociation of the androgen receptor-heat-shock protein complex: use of a new monoclonal antibody to distinguish transformed from nontransformed receptors. Biochemistry 1992; 31:7422–7430.
44. Marivoet S, Van Dijck P, Verhoeven G, Heyns W. Interaction of the 90-kDa heat shock protein with native and in vitro translated androgen receptor and receptor fragments. Mol Cell Endocrinol 1992; 88:165–174.
45. Bohen SP, Kralli A, Yamamoto KR. Hold 'em and fold 'em: chaperones and signal transduction. Science 1995; 268:1303–1304.
46. Kuil CW, Berrevoets CA, Mulder E. Ligand-induced conformational alterations of the androgen receptor analyzed by limited trypsinization: studies on the mechanism of antiandrogen action. J Biol Chem 1995; 270:27569–27576.
47. Fang Y, Fliss AE, Robins DM, Caplan AJ. Hsp90 regulates androgen receptor hormone binding affinity in vivo. J Biol Chem 1996; 271:28697–28702.
48. Beato M, Herrlich P, Schutz G. Steroid hormone receptors: many actors in search of a plot. Cell 1995; 83:851–857.

49. Claessens F, et al. Functional characterization of an androgen response element in the first intron of the C3(1) gene of prostatic binding protein. Biochem Biophys Res Commun 1989; 164:833–840.
50. Rundlett SE, Wu XP, Miesfeld RL. Functional characterizations of the androgen receptor confirm that the molecular basis of androgen action is transcriptional regulation. Mol Endocrinol 1990; 4:708–714.
51. Tan JA, et al. Response elements of the androgen-regulated C3 gene. J Biol Chem 1992; 267:4456–4466.
52. Ho KC, et al. A complex response element in intron 1 of the androgen-regulated 20-kDa protein gene displays cell type-dependent androgen receptor specificity. J Biol Chem 1993; 268:27226–27235.
53. McKenna NJ, O'Malley BW. Combinatorial control of gene expression by nuclear receptors and coregulators. Cell 2002; 108:465–474.
54. Metzger E, et al. LSD1 demethylates repressive histone marks to promote androgen-receptor-dependent transcription. Nature 2005; 437:436–439.
55. Chen D, et al. Regulation of transcription by a protein methyltransferase. Science 1999; 284:2174–2177.
56. Demarest SJ, et al. Mutual synergistic folding in recruitment of CBP/p300 by p160 nuclear receptor coactivators. Nature 2002; 415:549–553.
57. Huang ZQ, Li J, Sachs LM, Cole PA, Wong J. A role for cofactor–cofactor and cofactor–histone interactions in targeting p300, SWI/SNF and mediator for transcription. EMBO J 2003; 22:2146–2155.
58. Xu W, et al. A methylation–mediator complex in hormone signaling. Genes Dev 2004; 18:144–156.
59. Shang Y, Hu X, DiRenzo J, Lazar MA, Brown M. Cofactor dynamics and sufficiency in estrogen receptor-regulated transcription. Cell 2000; 103:843–852.
60. Metivier R, et al. Estrogen receptor-alpha directs ordered, cyclical, and combinatorial recruitment of cofactors on a natural target promoter. Cell 2003; 115:751–763.
61. Xu J, et al. Partial hormone resistance in mice with disruption of the steroid receptor coactivator-1 (SRC-1) gene. Science 1998; 279:1922–1925.
62. Cleutjens KB, van Eekelen CC, van der Korput HA, Brinkmann AO, Trapman J. Two androgen response regions cooperate in steroid hormone regulated activity of the prostate-specific antigen promoter. J Biol Chem 1996; 271:6379–6388.
63. Cleutjens KB, et al. An androgen response element in a far upstream enhancer region is essential for high, androgen-regulated activity of the prostate-specific antigen promoter. Mol Endocrinol 1997; 11:148–161.
64. Mitchell SH, Murtha PE, Zhang S, Zhu W, Young CY. An androgen response element mediates LNCaP cell dependent androgen induction of the hK2 gene. Mol Cell Endocrinol 2000; 168:89–99.
65. Shao D, Lazar MA. Modulating nuclear receptor function: may the phos be with you. J Clin Invest 1999; 103:1617–1618.
66. Rochette-Egly C. Nuclear receptors: integration of multiple signalling pathways through phosphorylation. Cell Signal 2003; 15:355–366.
67. Kato S, et al. Activation of the estrogen receptor through phosphorylation by mitogen-activated protein kinase. Science 1995; 270:1491–1494.
68. Font de Mora J, Brown M. AIB1 is a conduit for kinase-mediated growth factor signaling to the estrogen receptor. Mol Cell Biol 2000; 20:5041–5047.
69. Lopez GN, Turck CW, Schaufele F, Stallcup MR, Kushner PJ. Growth factors signal to steroid receptors through mitogen-activated protein kinase regulation of p160 coactivator activity. J Biol Chem 2001; 276:22177–22182.
70. Gregory CW, et al. Epidermal growth factor increases coactivation of the androgen receptor in recurrent prostate cancer. J Biol Chem 2004; 279:7119–7130.
71. Wu RC, et al. Selective phosphorylations of the SRC-3/AIB1 coactivator integrate genomic responses to multiple cellular signaling pathways. Mol Cell 2004; 15:937–949.
72. Hong SH, Privalsky ML. The SMRT corepressor is regulated by a MEK-1 kinase pathway: inhibition of corepressor function is associated with SMRT phosphorylation and nuclear export. Mol Cell Biol 2000; 20:6612–6625.

73. Blom N, Gammeltoft S, Brunak S. Sequence and structure-based prediction of eukaryotic protein phosphorylation sites. J Mol Biol 1999; 294:1351–1362.
74. Zhu Z, Becklin RR, Desiderio DM, Dalton JT. Identification of a novel phosphorylation site in human androgen receptor by mass spectrometry. Biochem Biophys Res Commun 2001; 284:836–844.
75. Gioeli D, et al. Androgen receptor phosphorylation: regulation and identification of the phosphorylation sites. J Biol Chem 2002; 277:29304–29314.
76. Wong HY, et al. Phosphorylation of androgen receptor isoforms. Biochem J 2004; 383:267–276.
77. Taneja SS, et al. Cell-specific regulation of androgen receptor phosphorylation in vivo. J Biol Chem 2005; 280:40916–40924.
78. Gioeli D, Black BE, Gordon V, et al. Stress kinase signaling regulates androgen receptor phosphorylation, transcription, and localization. Mol Endocrinol 2005; 20:503–515.
79. Muratani M, Tansey WP. How the ubiquitin-proteasome system controls transcription. Nat Rev Mol Cell Biol 2003; 4:192–201.
80. Lipford JR, Deshaies RJ. Diverse roles for ubiquitin-dependent proteolysis in transcriptional activation. Nat Cell Biol 2003; 5:845–850.
81. Shao W, Keeton EK, McDonnell DP, Brown M. Coactivator AIB1 links estrogen receptor transcriptional activity and stability. Proc Natl Acad Sci USA 2004; 101:11599–11604.
82. Nawaz Z, et al. The Angelman syndrome-associated protein, E6-AP, is a coactivator for the nuclear hormone receptor superfamily. Mol Cell Biol 1999; 19:1182–1189.
83. Kemppainen JA, Lane MV, Sar M, Wilson EM. Androgen receptor phosphorylation, turnover, nuclear transport, and transcriptional activation: specificity for steroids and antihormones. J Biol Chem 1992; 267:968–974.
84. Mellinghoff IK, et al. HER2/neu kinase-dependent modulation of androgen receptor function through effects on DNA binding and stability. Cancer Cell 2004; 6:517–527.
85. Fu M, et al. p300 and p300/cAMP-response element-binding protein-associated factor acetylate the androgen receptor at sites governing hormone-dependent trans activation. J Biol Chem 2000; 275:20853–20860.
86. Gaughan L, Logan IR, Cook S, Neal DE, Robson CN. Tip60 and histone deacetylase 1 regulate androgen receptor activity through changes to the acetylation status of the receptor. J Biol Chem 2002; 277:25904–25913.
87. Thomas M, et al. Androgen receptor acetylation site mutations cause trafficking defects, misfolding, and aggregation similar to expanded glutamine tracts. J Biol Chem 2004; 279:8389–8395.
88. Fu M, et al. Acetylation of androgen receptor enhances coactivator binding and promotes prostate cancer cell growth. Mol Cell Biol 2003; 23:8563–8575.
89. Feldman BJ, Feldman D. The development of androgen-independent prostate cancer. Nat Rev Cancer 2001; 1:34–45.
90. Newmark JR, et al. Androgen receptor gene mutations in human prostate cancer. Proc Natl Acad Sci USA 1992; 89:6319–6323.
91. Gaddipati JP, et al. Frequent detection of codon 877 mutation in the androgen receptor gene in advanced prostate cancers. Cancer Res 1994; 54:2861–2864.
92. Taplin ME, et al. Mutation of the androgen-receptor gene in metastatic androgen-independent prostate cancer. N Engl J Med 1995; 332:1393–1398.
93. Tilley WD, Buchanan G, Hickey TE, Bentel JM. Mutations in the androgen receptor gene are associated with progression of human prostate cancer to androgen independence. Clin Cancer Res 1996; 2:277–285.
94. Suzuki H, et al. Codon 877 mutation in the androgen receptor gene in advanced prostate cancer: relation to antiandrogen withdrawal syndrome. Prostate 1996; 29:153–158.
95. Marcelli M, et al. Androgen receptor mutations in prostate cancer. Cancer Res 2000; 60:944–949.
96. Taplin ME, et al. Androgen receptor mutations in androgen-independent prostate cancer: Cancer and Leukemia Group B Study 9663. J Clin Oncol 2003; 21:2673–2678.
97. Veldscholte J, et al. A mutation in the ligand binding domain of the androgen receptor of human LNCaP cells affects steroid binding characteristics and response to antiandrogens. Biochem Biophys Res Commun 1990; 173:534–540.

98. Veldscholte J, et al. Unusual specificity of the androgen receptor in the human prostate tumor cell line LNCaP: high affinity for progestagenic and estrogenic steroids. Biochem Biophys Acta 1990; 1052:187–194.
99. Fenton MA, et al. Functional characterization of mutant androgen receptors from androgen-independent prostate cancer. Clin Cancer Res 1997; 3:1383–1388.
100. Zhao XY, et al. Glucocorticoids can promote androgen-independent growth of prostate cancer cells through a mutated androgen receptor. Nat Med 2000; 6:703–706.
101. Buchanan G, et al. Collocation of androgen receptor gene mutations in prostate cancer. Clin Cancer Res 2001; 7:1273–1281.
102. Shi XB, Ma AH, Xia L, Kung HJ, de Vere White RW. Functional analysis of 44 mutant androgen receptors from human prostate cancer. Cancer Res 2002; 62:1496–1502.
103. Duff J, McEwan IJ. Mutation of histidine 874 in the androgen receptor ligand-binding domain leads to promiscuous ligand activation and altered p160 coactivator interactions. Mol Endocrinol 2005; 19:2943–2954.
104. Scher HI, Zhang ZF, Nanus D, Kelly WK. Hormone and antihormone withdrawal: implications for the management of androgen-independent prostate cancer. Urology 1996; 47:61–69.
105. Ruizeveld de Winter JA, et al. Androgen receptor status in localized and locally progressive hormone refractory human prostate cancer. Am J Pathol 1994; 144:735–746.
106. Edwards J, Krishna NS, Grigor KM, Bartlett JM. Androgen receptor gene amplification and protein expression in hormone refractory prostate cancer. Br J Cancer 2003; 89: 552–556.
107. Linja MJ, et al. Amplification and overexpression of androgen receptor gene in hormone-refractory prostate cancer. Cancer Res 2001; 61:3550–3555.
108. Visakorpi T, et al. In vivo amplification of the androgen receptor gene and progression of human prostate cancer. Nat Genet 1995; 9:401–406.
109. Koivisto P, et al. Androgen receptor gene amplification: a possible molecular mechanism for androgen deprivation therapy failure in prostate cancer. Cancer Res 1997; 57:314–319.
110. Miyoshi Y, et al. Fluorescence in situ hybridization evaluation of c-myc and androgen receptor gene amplification and chromosomal anomalies in prostate cancer in Japanese patients. Prostate 2000; 43:225–232.
111. Zegarra-Moro OL, Schmidt LJ, Huang H, Tindall DJ. Disruption of androgen receptor function inhibits proliferation of androgen-refractory prostate cancer cells. Cancer Res 2002; 62:1008–1013.
112. Eder IE, et al. Inhibition of LNCaP prostate tumor growth in vivo by an antisense oligonucleotide directed against the human androgen receptor. Cancer Gene Ther 2002; 9:117–125.
113. Shang Y, Brown M. Molecular determinants for the tissue specificity of SERMs. Science 2002; 295:2465–2468.
114. Jordan VC. Selective estrogen receptor modulation: concept and consequences in cancer. Cancer Cell 2004; 5:207–213.
115. Osborne CK, et al. Role of the estrogen receptor coactivator AIB1 (SRC-3) and HER-2/neu in tamoxifen resistance in breast cancer. J Natl Cancer Inst 2004; 95:353–361.
116. Girault I, et al. Expression analysis of estrogen receptor alpha coregulators in breast carcinoma: evidence that NCOR1 expression is predictive of the response to tamoxifen. Clin Cancer Res 2003; 9:1259–1266.
117. Gregory CW, et al. A mechanism for androgen receptor-mediated prostate cancer recurrence after androgen deprivation therapy. Cancer Res 2001; 61:4315–4319.
118. Culig Z, et al. Androgen receptor activation in prostatic tumor cell lines by insulin-like growth factor-I, keratinocyte growth factor, and epidermal growth factor. Cancer Res 1994; 54:5474–5478.
119. Nazareth LV, Weigel NL. Activation of the human androgen receptor through a protein kinase A signaling pathway. J Biol Chem 1996; 271:19900–19907.
120. Hobisch A, et al. Interleukin-6 regulates prostate-specific protein expression in prostate carcinoma cells by activation of the androgen receptor. Cancer Res 1998; 58:4640–4645.

121. Bakin RE, Gioeli D, Sikes RA, Bissonette EA, Weber MJ. Constitutive activation of the Ras/mitogen-activated protein kinase signaling pathway promotes androgen hypersensitivity in LNCaP prostate cancer cells. Cancer Res 2003; 63:1981–1989.
122. Ueda T, Bruchovsky N, Sadar MD. Activation of the androgen receptor N-terminal domain by interleukin-6 via MAPK and STAT3 signal transduction pathways. J Biol Chem 2002; 277:7076–7085.
123. Slamon DJ, et al. Human breast cancer: correlation of relapse and survival with amplification of the HER-2/neu oncogene. Science 1987; 235:177–182.
124. Craft N, Shostak Y, Carey M, Sawyers CL. A mechanism for hormone-independent prostate cancer through modulation of androgen receptor signaling by the HER-2/neu tyrosine kinase. Nat Med 1999; 5:280–285.
125. Yeh S, et al. From HER2/Neu signal cascade to androgen receptor and its coactivators: a novel pathway by induction of androgen target genes through MAP kinase in prostate cancer cells. Proc Natl Acad Sci USA 1999; 96:5458–5463.
126. Mellinghoff IK, Tran C, Sawyers CL. Growth inhibitory effects of the dual ErbB1/ErbB2 tyrosine kinase inhibitor PKI-166 on human prostate cancer xenografts. Cancer Res 2002; 62:5254–5259.
127. Agus DB, et al. Targeting ligand-activated ErbB2 signaling inhibits breast and prostate tumor growth. Cancer Cell 2002; 2:127–137.
128. Liu Y, et al. Inhibition of HER-2/neu kinase impairs androgen receptor recruitment to the androgen responsive enhancer. Cancer Res 2005; 65:3404–3409.
129. Blackledge G. Growth factor receptor tyrosine kinase inhibitors; clinical development and potential for prostate cancer therapy. J Urol 2003; 170:S77–S83; discussion S83.
130. Ziada A, et al. The use of trastuzumab in the treatment of hormone refractory prostate cancer: phase II trial. Prostate 2004; 60:332–337.
131. Majumder PK, Sellers WR. Akt-regulated pathways in prostate cancer. Oncogene 2005; 24:7465–7474.
132. Wen Y, et al. HER-2/neu promotes androgen-independent survival and growth of prostate cancer cells through the Akt pathway. Cancer Res 2000; 60:6841–6845.
133. Lin HK, et al. Suppression versus induction of androgen receptor functions by the phosphatidylinositol 3-kinase/Akt pathway in prostate cancer LNCaP cells with different passage numbers. J Biol Chem 2003; 278:50902–50907.
134. Nan B, et al. The PTEN tumor suppressor is a negative modulator of androgen receptor transcriptional activity. J Mol Endocrinol 2003; 31:169–183.
135. Lin HK, Wang L, Hu YC, Altuwaijri S, Chang C. Phosphorylation-dependent ubiquitination and degradation of androgen receptor by Akt require Mdm2 E3 ligase. EMBO J 2002; 21:4037–4048.
136. Van Dyke T, Jacks T. Cancer modeling in the modern era: progress and challenges. Cell 2002; 108:135–144.
137. Xin L, Teitell MA, Lawson DA, Kwon A, Mellinghoff IK, Witte ON. Progression of prostate cancer by synergy of AKT with genotropic and nongenotropic actions of the androgen receptor. Proc Natl Acad Sci U.S.A. 2006; 103:7789–7794.
138. O'Donnell A, et al. Hormonal impact of the 17alpha-hydroxylase/C(17,20)-lyase inhibitor abiraterone acetate (CB7630) in patients with prostate cancer. Br J Cancer 2004; 90:2317–2325.
139. Solit DB, Basso AD, Olshen AB, Scher HI, Rosen N. Inhibition of heat shock protein 90 function down-regulates Akt kinase and sensitizes tumors to Taxol. Cancer Res 2003; 63:2139–2144.
140. Sausville EA, Tomaszewski JE, Ivy P. Clinical development of 17-allylamino, 17-demethoxygeldanamycin. Curr Cancer Drug Targets 2003; 3:377–383.
141. Banerji U, et al. Phase I pharmacokinetic and pharmacodynamic study of 17-allylamino, 17-demethoxygeldanamycin in patients with advanced malignancies. J Clin Oncol 2005; 23:4152–4161.
142. von Minckwitz G, et al. Phase I clinical study of the recombinant antibody toxin scFv(FRP5)-ETA specific for the ErbB2/HER2 receptor in patients with advanced solid malignomas. Breast Cancer Res 2005; 7:R617–R626.

143. Chen L, et al. Chemical ablation of androgen receptor in prostate cancer cells by the histone deacetylase inhibitor LAQ824. Mol Cancer Ther 2005; 4:1311–1319.
144. Kelly WK, et al. Phase I study of an oral histone deacetylase inhibitor, suberoylanilide hydroxamic acid, in patients with advanced cancer. J Clin Oncol 2005; 23:3923–3931.
145. Johnstone RW, Licht JD. Histone deacetylase inhibitors in cancer therapy: Is transcription the primary target? Cancer Cell 2003; 4:13–18.
146. Masiello D, Cheng S, Bubley GJ, Lu ML, Balk SP. Bicalutamide functions as an androgen receptor antagonist by assembly of a transcriptionally inactive receptor. J Biol Chem 2002; 277:26321–26326.
147. Brzozowski AM, et al. Molecular basis of agonism and antagonism in the oestrogen receptor. Nature 1997; 389:753–758.
148. Shiau AK, et al. The structural basis of estrogen receptor/coactivator recognition and the antagonism of this interaction by tamoxifen. Cell 1998; 95:927–937.
149. Pike AC, et al. Structure of the ligand-binding domain of oestrogen receptor beta in the presence of a partial agonist and a full antagonist. EMBO J 1999; 18:4608–4618.
150. Pike AC, et al. Structural insights into the mode of action of a pure antiestrogen. Structure 2001; 9:145–153.
151. Balog A, et al. The synthesis and evaluation of [2.2.1]-bicycloazahydantoins as androgen receptor antagonists. Bioorg Med Chem Lett 2004; 14:6107–6111.
152. Salvati ME, et al. Structure based approach to the design of bicyclic-1H-isoindole-1,3(2H)-dione based androgen receptor antagonists. Bioorg Med Chem Lett 2005; 15:271–276.
153. Norris JD, et al. Peptide antagonists of the human estrogen receptor. Science 1999; 285:744–746.
154. Chang CY, Abdo J, Hartney T, McDonnell DP. Development of peptide antagonists for the androgen receptor using combinatorial peptide phage display. Mol Endocrinol 2005; 19:2478–2490.
155. Sawyers CL. Opportunities and challenges in the development of kinase inhibitor therapy for cancer. Genes Dev 2003; 17:2998–3010.
156. Sawyers C. Targeted cancer therapy. Nature 2004; 432:294–297.
157. Larson SM, et al. Tumor localization of 16beta-18F-fluoro-5alpha-dihydrotestosterone versus 18F-FDG in patients with progressive, metastatic prostate cancer. J Nucl Med 2004; 45:366–373.

11 Can Post-Transcription Modifiers Change the Course of Prostate Cancer?

David Z. Qian and Roberto Pili

The Sidney Kimmel Comprehensive Care Center, The Johns Hopkins University School of Medicine, Baltimore, Maryland, U.S.A.

INTRODUCTION

Advances in the understanding of the molecular mechanisms implicated in prostate cancer progression have identified many potential therapeutic gene targets that are involved in apoptosis, growth factors, cell signaling, and the androgen receptor (AR). A critical factor responsible for the malignant progression of prostate cancer is the abnormal expression and function of specific proteins. From the transcription of messenger RNA (mRNA) to the translation of proteins and their function, several steps can be exploited as "drugable" targets.

In this chapter, we will review some of the key molecular targets and post-transcriptional strategies that are currently being tested both preclinically and clinically as targeted therapeutic approach for prostate cancer. Most of the targets mentioned in this review involve the prostate cancer signal transduction cascade, and their functions include prosurvival, anti-apoptosis, and proangiogenesis activities. This review will focus in particular on the emerging role of the "chromatin modifiers" histone deacetylase inhibitors not only in transcriptional gene regulation, but also in post-transcriptional protein modifications as a tool for therapeutic intervention in prostate cancer.

TARGETING MRNA

Post-transcriptional targeting of mRNA has been used extensively to investigate gene and protein functions. More recently, with the advancement in the understanding of the biological mechanisms responsible for gene/protein functions in cancer progression, mRNA inhibition has entered the realm of targeted therapeutics (1). Three forms of mRNA targeting strategies have been exploited: antisense oligonucleotide, small interference RNA (siRNA), and more recently microRNA (miRNA). These three strategies involve the introduction of sequence specific RNA molecules into the target cells, and the subsequent binding with the mRNA of the target protein. As a result, the RNA/RNA heteroduplex causes the degradation of target mRNA and prevent the protein synthesis.

siRNA and miRNA have been recognized as mRNA targeting strategies that have more potential in cancer therapeutics including prostate cancer. Both strategies tap into the natural processes that biological systems use to control gene expression, and may prove to be better tolerated and to have long-lasting effects than standard cytotoxic therapies (1). Both siRNA and miRNA are still primarily in the Phase of preclinical development. The results from a trial with siRNA against vascular endothelial growth factor (VEGF) recently concluded in age-related macular degeneration patients are anticipated to be available this year (2).

Among the mRNA targeting strategies, antisense oligonucleotide therapy is the therapeutic modality that has been tested in clinical trials (1). The antisense approach continues to hold promise as a potential therapy to target genes involved in cancer progression, especially those in which the gene products are not amenable to small molecule inhibition or antibodies. Combinations of antisense oligonucleotides with chemotherapeutic agents may also offer important advantages in cancer treatment and in prostate cancer in particular. Several antisense drugs have shown interesting results in animal experiments, and have entered clinical trials. However, control oligonucleotides must be carefully chosen to separate antisense effects from the many potential nonspecific effects of oligonucleotides. Several genes, including BCL-2, BCL-X(L) (3), clusterin (4–6), the inhibitors of apoptosis (IAP) family (7), MDM2 (8), protein kinase C-alpha, c-raf (9), insulin-like growth factor binding proteins (6), and the AR, have been identified as potential targets for these therapeutic strategies in prostate cancer.

BCL-2/BCL-X(L)

The cytotoxic effect of chemotherapy, radiation therapy, and other molecular-targeted therapies can be overcome by the presence of endogenous anti-apoptotic proteins. In prostate cancer, BCL-2/BCL-X(L) protein family plays a major role in anti-apoptotic signals (3). These proteins are potent suppressors of both caspase- and noncaspase-mediated cell death. Antisense oligonucleotide strategy targeting BCL2 has been tested in several clinical trials in solid and heme-malignancies (5). The toxicity profile from several Phase I trials with Oblimersen (Genasense™, Genta Inc. Berkeley Heights, NJ) appears to be acceptable with fatigue and lymphopenia being the most common side effects. Oblimersen combined with docetaxel has been reported to be an active combination in Hormone refractory prostate cancer (HRPC) patients demonstrating both an encouraging response rate and an overall median survival in a recent Phase II study. The absence of severe toxicities at this recommended dose, evidence of Bcl-2 protein inhibition, and encouraging antitumor activity in HPRC patients have warrant further clinical evaluation of this combination. Oblimersen is currently in Phase III clinical testing and on the Food and Drug Administration (FDA) fast-track approval process.

Clusterin

Expression of clusterin has been reported to be up-regulated after androgen withdrawal and during progression to androgen independence in prostate cancer tissue, but not in untreated prostate tissues both in animal models and human clinical specimens. Overexpression of clusterin gene into human prostate cancer cells confers resistance to several therapeutic stimuli, including androgen ablation, chemotherapy, and radiation. Antisense targeting the translation initiation site of the clusterin gene markedly inhibited clusterin expression in prostate cancer cells in a dose-dependent and sequence-specific manner. Systemic treatment with the antisense clusterin oligodeoxynucleotide enhanced the effects of several conventional therapies in prostate cancer xenograft models by induction of apoptosis. A Phase I clinical trial has been completed using the antisense clusterin oligodeoxynucleotide incorporating 2-*O*-(2-methoxy) ethyl-gapmer backbone (OGX-011), showing up to 90% suppression of clusterin in prostate cancer. Preliminary results suggested that inhibition of clusterin expression using the antisense technology may enhance apoptosis induced by several conventional treatments, resulting in the delay of prostate cancer disease progression and improved survival (10). A Phase II clinical trial in patients with prostate cancer is ongoing.

Protein Kinase C-alpha and Raf-1

Protein kinase C(PKC)-alpha and Raf-1 are important elements of proliferative signal transduction pathways in both normal and malignant cells. Abrogation of either Raf-1 or PKC-alpha function can both inhibit cellular proliferation and induce apoptosis in several experimental cancer models including prostate cancer cell lines. ISIS 3521 (11) and ISIS 5132 are antisense phosphorothioate oligonucleotides that inhibit PKC-alpha and Raf-1 expression, respectively, and induce a broad spectrum of antiproliferative and antitumor effects in several human tumor cell lines. The antisense oligonucleotides ISIS 3521 and ISIS 5132, at these doses and schedule, do not possess clinically significant single-agent antitumor activity in HRPC. However, protracted stable disease in some patients may indicate a cytostatic effect.

p65 and NF-κB Signaling

NF-κB is a critical signaling pathway mediating cellular processes of differentiation, survival, apoptosis, inflammation, and stress response (12). In cancer cells, NF-κB has been linked to its pro-survival properties. There are increasing evidences that drug resistance in cancer cells is due in part to the activation NF-κB pathway. p65 is a major transcription factor mediating the NF-κB activation. Many of the genes regulated by p65 are responsible for the activation of anti-apoptosis and pro-survival survival pathways. In a recent report (13), siRNA against p65 effectively attenuated the survival signal in cancer cells including the prostate cancer cell line PC-3. Combination of p65 siRNA and chemotherapeutic agents significantly enhanced the cytotoxic effect.

DNA Repair Proteins

Radiation therapy represents a definitive treatment for localized prostate cancer and effective treatment modality for symptomatic bone metastases. However, radiation-induced cytotoxicity can be inhibited by the DNA repair process (14). To enhance the radiation sensitivity in prostate cancer cells, siRNA against DNA repair protein ATM and DNA-PK has been developed (15). In vitro experiments indicated that siRNA reduced 90% of the target proteins. At the clinically relevant radiation doses, siRNA gave rise to a reduction repair gene expression as compared to control. The radiosensitivity achieved was greater than with PI3K/AKT inhibitors.

Polycomb Group Protein EZH2

Besides NF-κB transcription factor p65, many other transcription factors involved in the prostate cancer progression are being evaluated as "drugable" targets. Polycomb group proteins have been implicated in the maintenance of homeotic gene expression that ensures proper cell proliferation. The Polycomb protein enhancer of zeste homolog 2 (EZH2) has been found to be overexpressed in hormonal refractory metastatic prostate cancer (16). In addition, clinically localized prostate cancer that overexpresses EZH2 has poorer prognosis and lethal phenotype. Thus, inhibition EZH2 mechanistically may improve prostate cancer therapeutics. Indeed, siRNA against EZH2 has been shown to inhibit prostate cancer cell proliferation in vitro (16,17).

Polo-Like Kinase 1

Polo-like kinase 1 has elevated activity in prostate cancer cells, and being evaluated as a prognostic marker. SiRNA inhibition on this enzyme in prostate cancer cell lines significantly reduced cell proliferation, and increased apoptosis (18). The phenotypes associated were mitotic cell-cycle arrest, failure of cytokinesis, and defects in centrosome integrity. In contrast, siRNA inhibition in normal prostate epithelial cells produced no significant effects. This observation suggests that PLK-1 maybe a tumor specific drug target.

Vascular Endothelial Growth Factor

Several evidences support a role for angiogenesis in prostate cancer progression. Circulating VEGF levels have been reported to be elevated in the plasma of patients with malignancies, and plasma VEGF level is an independent prognostic marker for survival in patients with advanced, hormone-refractory prostate cancer (19). Animal studies have demonstrated that VEGF promotes the growth and proliferation of both normal prostatic epithelium and prostate carcinoma cells (20). The prostate gland is regulated by vascular endothelial cells, which themselves respond to angiogenic activity elaborated by prostate epithelium under testosterone stimulation. Castration decreases and testosterone increases VEGF expression in the prostate (21). Microvessel density, a surrogate marker for angiogenesis, is an independent prognostic marker for disease progression in patients with clinically localized prostate cancer (22). Prostatic fluid is a rich source of VEGF production that is regulated by androgen, and radical prostatectomy lowers plasma VEGF levels in patients with prostate cancer (23,24). In a preclinical animal model, siRNA on VEGF significantly inhibited the subcutaneous growth of human prostate cancer xenografts and angiogenesis (25).

TARGETING PROTEIN SYNTHESIS

Protein synthesis can also represent a target for prostate cancer therapeutics. Depending on the half-life and physiological requirement, some cellular proteins need to be constitutively expressed and synthesized to maintain normal or malignant phenotype. Many naturally occurring or synthetic compound may serve as protein synthesis inhibitors. For example, the marine natural product Pateamine A has been shown to inhibit eukaryotic translation initiation through the stalling of initiation complexes on mRNA in vitro, and inducing stress granule formation in vivo (26). The drawback of such strategy is that there is no tumor-specific targeting mechanism because most of the protein synthesis machinery is shared between the normal protein and oncoprotein synthesis. As a result, significant toxic side effects may be anticipated. To date, there have been few human-related clinical development associated with this approach.

Specamycin Derivative (KRN5500)

A Phase I clinical study in solid tumor patients using the specamycin derivative KRN5500, a protein synthesis inhibitor, has been reported (27). In this study,

18 patients were administrated with the inhibitor in the format of 2 hr intravenous infusion every four week at the dosage of 3, 6, 5, 10, and 21 mg/m^2. The major toxicities were nausea, vomiting, diarrhea, fatigue, and a mild reversible prolongation of prothrombin time. The Maximum tolerated dose (MTD) was determined at 21 mg/m^2, and frequent and prolonged nausea and vomiting prevented future increasing of dose. No objective antitumor response was observed.

mRNA Cap-Binding Protein

The contribution of the mRNA cap-binding protein, eIF-4E, to malignant transformation and progression has been demonstrated over the past decade. eIF-4E overexpression has been reported in several human tumors including prostate, and has been related to disease progression. Overexpression of eIF-4E in experimental models significantly alters cellular morphology, enhances proliferation, and increase tumorigenesis. Blocking eIF-4E function by expression of antisense RNA, or overexpression of the inhibitory eIF-4E binding proteins (4E-BPs), suppresses tumor growth. Although eIF-4E regulates the recruitment of mRNA to ribosomes, and thereby globally regulates cap-dependent protein synthesis, eIF-4E contributes to malignancy by selectively enabling the translation of a limited pool of mRNAs—those that generally encode key proteins involved in cellular growth, angiogenesis, survival, and malignancy.

Although there is increased focus and research interest in developing specific protein translation initiation inhibitors, to date there has not been any clinical testing of this therapeutic strategy. Signal transduction pathways regulate protein translation initiation. For example, functional S6 ribosomal proteins are needed for the translation of certain mRNA including hypoxia inducible factor (HIF), and mTOR and/or PI3K/AKT pathways regulate the activation of S6 ribosomal protein by S6 kinase. Therefore, the translational inhibition of HIF-1α has been proposed as a part of the anticancer mechanism induced by inhibitors of mTOR or PI3K/AKT pathways (28,29). Many inhibitors of signal transduction are currently in clinical trials, HIF-1α inhibition may represent an important mechanism for the in vivo anticancer efficacy.

TARGETING PROTEIN MODIFICATION

Prostate cancer cell proliferation is regulated by different patterns of gene expression. Gene transcription depends on the capability of transcription activators and repressors to access chromatin at specific promoters. Increasing evidence supports aberrant transcription regulation as a contributing factor to the development of human cancers. Transcription regulatory proteins are often identified in oncogenic chromosomal rearrangements and are overexpressed in a variety of malignancies including prostate cancer. Most transcription regulators are large proteins, containing multiple structural and functional domains some with enzymatic activity. These activities modify the structure of the chromatin, occluding certain DNA regions and exposing others for interaction with the transcription machinery. Thus, chromatin modifiers represent an additional level of transcription regulation. Several families of transcription activators and repressors have been to show to catalyze histone and nonhistone post-translational modifications (acetylation, methylation, phosphorylation, ubiquitination, and SUMOylation), and alter the correct cell proliferation program, leading to cancer. Our review will focus on the role of the chromatin remodeling agents histone deacetylase inhibitors.

Histone Deacetylase Inhibitors

An emerging body of literature supports the role of the chromatin structure in regulating cell-cycle progression, differentiation, and apoptosis in normal and malignant cells (30). In general, increased DNA–histone interactions condense chromatin and repress transcription, whereas decreased DNA–histone interactions relax chromatin and enhance gene expression.

The steady-state level of acetylation of core histones is governed by the opposing actions of histone acetyltransferases (HATs) and histone deacetylases (HDACs). Several families of HATs have been identified, including p300/CBP, and at least 11 structurally related HDACs have been described and divided in different classes. HDACs have been shown to be involved in oncogenic transformation by mediating the transcriptional regulation of genes that are involved in cell-cycle progression, proliferation, and apoptosis. Several cancer-associated mutations and chromosomal translocations result in repression of transcription through abnormal recruitment or overexpression of HDACs. This is the rationale for the development of HDAC inhibitors as a new class of anticancer therapy. Currently, HDACs are molecular targets for the development of enzymatic inhibitors to treat human cancer, and structurally distinct drug classes have been identified with in vivo bioavailability and intracellular capability to inhibit many of the known mammalian HDACs. They can be categorized into four groups, hydroxamic acids, cyclic peptides, aliphatic acids, and benzamides. HDAC inhibitors have a wide range of antitumor activities including induction of cell-cycle arrest and apoptosis, stimulation of differentiation, and inhibition of angiogenesis (31). An explanation of these effects is that HDAC inhibitors target both transcriptional and nontranscriptional mechanisms to induce their biological effects (Fig. 1) (32).

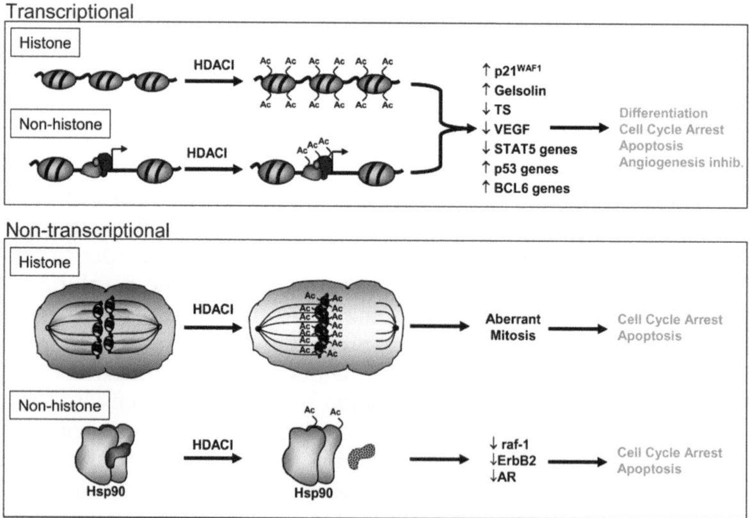

FIGURE 1 Mechanisms of action of histone deacetylases inhibitor: transcriptional and nontranscriptional activity. *Abbreviations*: AR, androgen receptor; HDACI, histone deacetylase inihibitor; VEGF, vascular endothelial growth factor; TS, Thymidylate Synthetase; P21, ; raf-1, ; Erb B2, . *Source*: From Ref. 32.

Up to date, none of the HDAC inhibitors has been shown to selectively inhibit individual HDAC isozymes. Hydroxamic HDAC inhibitors such as TSA, LAQ824, and LBH589 are pan-HDAC inhibitors target both class I and II HDACs. Cyclic peptides, aliphatic acids, and benzamides have significant inhibitory activity against class I HDACs, but have limited activities against class II HDACs at higher concentrations. Although the growth-inhibitory effects of HDAC inhibitors in cancer cell lines including prostate cancer have been observed, their mechanisms of action are highly variable. Depending on the cell line, the type of inhibitor, and the drug concentration, the inhibitory effect can vary from primarily cell-cycle arrest to cell death. Currently, the intrinsic factor determining the pathways of cell death or cell-cycle arrest in prostate cancer cells after HDAC inhibition has yet to be elucidated. p21 induction has been reported as a biomarker for HDAC inhibition, but the functional significance of p21 within this context is unclear.

A common set of genes are induced or repressed in a variety of transformed cell lines treated with HDAC inhibitors of different classes, suggesting that HDAC inhibitors may be a potential treatment for many tumor types (33). The mechanism of selectivity of gene expression is currently not understood. The selectivity of the HDAC inhibitors may be determined by the various classes of HDACs, as well as by the underlying "Histone Code" which may be responsible for cellular memory (34). In addition to histones, many nonhistone proteins are also reversibly acetylated on lysine residues and may also play important roles in the antitumor effects of HDAC inhibitors.

Chemosensitizing Effects of HDAC Inhibitors

Although the molecular basis for their anticancer selectivity remains obscure to date, HDAC inhibitors have the potential to modulate additively or synergistically the activity of other therapeutic agents. Thus HDAC inhibitors, in combination with chemical drugs or radiotherapy, can reduce uncontrolled cell proliferation and apoptosis. Although HDAC inhibitor as single agent exhibited growth-inhibitory effects in many several preclinical studies against human prostrate cancer, the potential use of this type of inhibitors may indeed reside in the combination with other therapeutic means. When combined with radiation, HDAC inhibitors such as Suberoylanilide hydroxamic acid (SAHA) and MS-275 enhanced radiation-induced cytotoxicity (35).

Another rational combination strategy is with differentiation therapy. Retinoic acids have shown to promote tumor cell differentiation and apoptosis. However, there is a subset of prostate tumors that are resistant to retinoic acid (RA) as consequence of the epigenetic silencing of retinoic receptor beta (RARβ) genes. HDAC inhibitors such as MS-275 have shown to upregulate RARβ expression in RA-resistant cell lines PC-3 and DU-145. Combination of MS-275 with 13-*cis* retinoic acid enhanced the antitumor activity both in vitro and in vivo (36).

Synergistic combination of HDAC inhibitors by sensitizing cancer cells to apoptosis has been reported not only with chemotherapy drugs (i.e., topoisomerase inhibitors), but also with many molecularly targeted therapeutic agents, including the Bcr-Abl kinase inhibitor imatinib, the Her-2 antibody trastuzumab, the receptor tyrosine kinase FLT-3 inhibitor PKC412,45 TNF-related apoptosis inducing ligand (TRAIL), the proteasome inhibitors Bortezomib, the purine analog fludarabine, and the Hsp90 antagonist 17-AAG (37–44). Mechanistically, this chemo-/radio-sensitizing effect may be mediated through both histone acetylation-dependent and -independent effects of HDAC inhibitors, of which the underlying mechanism warrants further investigation.

Nonepigenetic Mechanisms of HDAC Inhibitors Antitumor Activity

Protein modification by acetylation at the lysine residue plays important roles in protein functions. The acetylation status at the histone proteins have been linked to the compactness of chromatin structures and gene expression. Nontranscriptional gene regulation by HDAC inhibitors has been reported by several investigators. For example, tumor-associated proteins that mediate proliferation and cell-cycle progression, including p53, Ku70, Hsp90, RelA, and Stats, have been identified as substrates for various HDAC isoforms (45). Targeting the acetylation status of these signal transduction mediators may contribute to the antiproliferative activities of HDAC inhibitors in cancer cells. A recent report indicates that HDAC inhibitors induced cell-cycle arrest/apoptosis in prostate cancer cells through the stabilization of acetylated p53. Increased p53 acetylation diminishes Mdm2-mediated ubiquitination and the subsequent proteasome-facilitated degradation (46).

Furthermore, Hsp90 represents a target of HDAC 6, and inhibition of HDAC 6 resulted in the hyperacetylation and loss of the chaperone activity of Hsp90, suggesting reversible acetylation as a unique mechanism to regulate Hsp90 activity (47). Hsp90 has been reported to play an important role in the regulation of critical protein such as for example the AR. HDAC inhibitor LAQ824 has been recently shown to target the AR, promoting its degradation, and blocking androgen-induced PSA production in human prostate cancer cell line LNCaP (48).

Various HDACs have been also shown to form complexes with a series of cellular proteins including a-tubulin, ubiquitin, and the phosphatase PP1. For example, recent evidence shows that HDACs 1 and 6 formed complexes with PP1 (49). The selective action of HDAC inhibitors on cellular HDAC/PP1 complexes deactivates Akt through the reorganization of PP1 complexes. From a clinical perspective, this unique function provides a molecular basis to use HDAC inhibitors to sensitize cancer cells to the apoptotic effect of molecularly targeted agents by lowering apoptosis threshold.

Rationale for Combining HDAC Inhibitors With Anti-VEGF Therapy in Prostate Cancer

Over the past three decades, the field of angiogenesis has being flourished following the initial observation by Folkman (50). Uncontrolled tumor cell proliferation and new blood vessel formation (angiogenesis) are the two major targets of cancer therapeutics. Accumulated evidences have proved the importance of neovascularization or angiogenesis in tumor progression, and confirmed that inhibition of the VEGF is a promising therapeutic antiangiogenesis and anticancer strategy in epithelial tumors, including prostate cancer. During this multistep angiogenesis process, endothelial cells also require the expression of various proteins such as survivin for cytoprotection and inhibition of apoptosis, angiopoietin-1, and angiopoietin-2 along with their receptor Tie-2 for blood vessel stabilization and sprouting (51). Low oxygen tension or hypoxia, a common feature of malignant tumors, can be detected in central regions of solid tumors. Hypoxia regulates many transcription factors including hypoxia-inducible factor (HIF)-1α, which controls hypoxia-inducible angiogenic factors such as VEGF (52). Thus, enhancement of angiogenesis by hypoxia is a prerequisite for progressive growth and metastasis of solid tumors.

More than 75 angiogenesis inhibitors have entered clinical evaluation in cancer patients (53). At least 12 agents entered or completed Phase III trials. Given the pivotal role of VEGF in angiogenesis and tumor growth, targeting the VEGF system is an attractive and promising therapeutic approach. On the basis of the positive results of the Phase III clinical trial in patients with colon carcinoma, bevacizumab has been the first antiangiogenic compound approved by the U.S. Food and Drug (54). Agents targeting the VEGF pathway by inhibiting the VEGF receptors such as and Sunitinib (pfizer) have been reported to have induce a 5–40% response rate and increased progression free survival in patients with metastatic renal cell carcinoma (55,56). The final results from the Phase III clinical trials are pending but based on the preliminary analyses Sorafenib and Sunitinib have been recently approved by FDA for the treatment of advanced renal cell cancer.

On the basis of the reported antiangiogenesis activity of HDAC inhibitors, our group has investigated the biological effect of the HDAC inhibitor LAQ824 in combination with the VEGF receptor tyrosine kinase inhibitor PTK787 on tumor growth and angiogenesis in a prostate cancer model (57). LAQ824 treatment inhibited the expression of angiogenesis-related genes such as angiopoietin-2, Tie-2, and survivin in ECs, and induced a significant downregulation of HIF-1α and VEGF expression in prostate tumor cells. Combination treatment with LAQ824 and PTK787 was more effective than single agents in inhibiting in vitro and in vivo VEGF-induced angiogenesis. The greater in vivo antitumor effect of this drug combination, as compared to single agents, was the result of the simultaneous targeting of multiple independent and converging pathways.

The molecular mechanism underlying the HDAC inhibitor induced HIF-1α degradation remains unclear. However, some preliminary results from our lab suggest that the molecular mechanism involves post-transcriptional modification of HIF-1α. Class II HDACs appear to be involved in HIF-1α stabilization and hydroxyamic derivative HDAC inhibitors induce HIF-1α acetylation and consequent degradation via a VHL-independent but proteosomal dependent mechanism. On the basis of these and other preclinical data, there are evidences supporting that a "vertical" blockade of the HIF-1α/VEGF pathway in prostate tumor cells and inhibition of survival pathways in endothelial cells by an HDAC inhibitor will enhance the angiogenesis-inhibitory activity of either VEGF blocking agents (i.e., Avastin) or a VEGF receptor tyrosine kinase inhibitor (i.e., Nexavar, Sutent) (Fig. 2).

The combination of HDAC inhibitors with anti-VEGF therapies is of particular interest. There are preclinical and clinical evidences that tumor "escape" to anti-VEGF therapy occurs. It is conceivable that angiogenesis-related gene modulation by HDAC inhibitors may affect tumor cell and endothelial cell adaptation to anti-VEGF therapies, and prevent or delay the escape.

HDAC inhibitors may have the dual function of targeting both tumor cells and proliferating endothelial cells, and to inhibit tumor angiogenesis by gene modulation. Rational clinical testing of these anticancer agents as single agents or in combination with angiogenesis inhibitors in patients with prostate cancer is warranted, and should include angiogenesis-related correlative studies as potential markers of drug efficacy. On the basis of the preclinical results an NCI-CTEP sponsored Phase I/II study with the combination of the HDAC inhibitor SAHA and the anti-VEGF Bevacizumab in patients with metastatic renal cell carcinoma has been initiated. A Phase I/II study of combination with an HDAC inhibitor

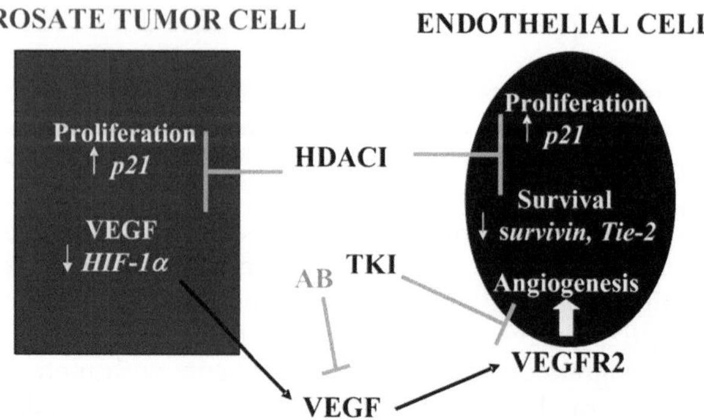

FIGURE 2 Schema of the integrated inhibitory activity on both prostate tumor and endothelial cells by histone deacetylase inhibitors and anti-vascular endothelial growth factor therapy. *Abbreviations*: HDACI, histone deacetylase inhibitor; AB, antibody/blocking agent; TKI, tyrosine kinase inhibitor; VEGF, vascular endothelial growth factor; HIF, hypoxia inducible factor.

and anti-VEGF therapy has been planned in patients with hormone-refractory prostate cancer.

HDAC Inhibitors in Clinical Testing

Initial clinical trials indicate that HDAC inhibitors from several different structural classes are relatively well tolerated and exhibit clinical activity against a variety of human malignancies. Phase I and II clinical trials are ongoing to evaluate these agents as an antitumor agent. The expanding list of HDACIs includes SAHA, MS-275, depsipeptide, LAQ824, LBH589, and PDX-101 (Table 1).

1. Suberoylanilide hydroxamic acid: SAHA is a potent inhibitor of class I and II HDAC activities with broad-spectrum antitumor activity in preclinical studies including prostate cancer (58). A Phase I study of SAHA administered by daily intravenous infusion has shown that this agent can be given at doses that cause an accumulation of acetylated histones in peripheral blood mononuclear (PBM) cells and in tumors, with tolerable adverse effects (59). A clinical trial of oral SAHA was initiated to define the maximal tolerated dose and the pharmacokinetic profile and oral bioavailability of oral SAHA in patients with refractory solid tumors, lymphomas, and leukemias (60). The dose of oral

TABLE 1 Histone decetylase inhibitors currently in clinical development

Agent	Class	Company	Developmental status
VORINOSTAT (SAHA)	Class I/II	Merck	Phase II/III
MS-275	Class I	Schering AG	Phase I
LAQB24	Class I/II	Novartis	Phase I
LBH589	Class I/II	Novartis	Phase I
Depsipeptide	Class I	Fujisawa	Phase II/III
PXD101	Class I/II	CuraGena	Phase I
Valproic acid	Class I	Abbott	Phase II
MGCD0103	Class I/II	Methylgence	Phase I

SAHA was independently escalated in each group of patients with planned doses levels of 200 and 400 mg daily, and 400, 800, and 1200 mg q12. Pharmacokinetic studies were performed on day 1 (identical dose given intravenously), day 8 (oral dose fasting), day 9 (oral dose nonfasting), and day 29 (oral fasting). Western blot analyses of histones isolated from PBM cells obtained pre- and post-SAHA dosing were performed. Twenty-five patients have been entered into three dose levels. Myelosuppression and fatigue were dose-limiting toxicities at 400 mg q12 for solid tumor and lymphoma patients. Mean SAHA oral bioavailability among patients receiving the 200 and 400 mg doses was 56% and 48%, respectively. A dose proportional increase in AUC and Cmax was observed when comparing the 200 and 400 mg dose levels. The half-life ranged from 92 to 150 min. A prolonged duration of acetylated histone accumulation was observed following oral SAHA administration compared to the same dose administered intravenously. Reduction in measurable disease has been observed in refractory papillary thyroid cancer (one patient), squamous cell carcinoma of the larynx (one patient), renal cell carcinoma (one patient), and B-cell lymphoma (one patient). The preliminary results of this Phase I study of oral SAHA demonstrate that this formulation is readily bioavailable and results in prolongation of acetylated histone accumulation in peripheral blood mononuclear (PBM) cells. Dose limiting toxicities (DLTs) were nonhematologic and included anorexia, dehydration, diarrhea, and fatigue. These toxicities were rapidly reversible after interruption of dosing (median duration 3–5 days). Preliminary results with SAHA in patients with refractory cutaneous T-cell lymphoma (CTCL), included partial objective response to therapy in a number of patients (61,62). There are multiple Phase II studies ongoing with SAHA as a single agent and in combination with other biologic or chemotherapeutic drug for different tumor types including prostate cancer.

2. The MS-275 oral formulation on the q14-day schedule is reasonably well tolerated. Histone deacetylase inhibition has been observed in peripheral-blood mononuclear cells. On the basis of PK data from the q14-day schedule, a more frequent dosing schedule, weekly four times, repeated every 6 wk is presently being evaluated. Preliminary data suggest clinical activity in lymphomas and melanoma (63).
3. Depsipeptide completed Phase I evaluation. Phase II studies alone or in combination with other anticancer agents are ongoing to determine the clinical efficacy in a range of solid and hematological malignancies. Preliminary results of Phase II study in cutaneous T-cell and relapsed peripheral T-cell lymphoma reported significant responses in relapsed patients at well-tolerated doses. Other Phase II trials in solid and hematological tumors are continuing to explore the spectrum of clinical activity of this agent (64).
4. LAQ824: LAQ824, a novel cinnamic acid hydroxamate, inhibits HDAC activity (IC_{50}, 0.03 μM) and has antitumor activity in several tumor models including prostate cancer. In three Phase I studies, LAQ824 was administered as a 3-hr intravenous infusion on several dosing schedules, principally days 1–3 of a 21-day cycle, to adult pts with advanced solid or hematologic malignancies (65). Patients with impaired cardiac function were excluded; drugs known to prolong QT interval were prohibited. Serial digital ECGs were performed at baseline, on days of dosing and post-dose each cycle. LAQ824 was found to induce dose-related increases in QTcF of < 20 m/sec at doses up to 200 mg/m^2.

5. LBH589B: LBH589B is a novel, orally administered histone deacetylase inhibitor structurally similar to LAQ284, which inhibits HDAC enzyme activity, activates p21, and inhibits proliferation of tumor cell lines at nanomolar concentrations. A recent Phase I study has tested the safety and tolerability of oral LBH589B in patients with advanced solid tumors or lymphoma (66). LBH589B given orally appeared to be well tolerated with consistent pharmacodynamic (PD) effects and pharmacokinetic (PK). No cardiac toxicity was observed. Additional evaluation is continuing with further dose escalations are planned.

Issues of Clinical Development of Therapies With HDAC Inhibitors in Prostate Cancer

Despite the recent clinical trials reporting clinical activity for HDAC inhibitors, several issues are still unresolved including the optimal dose and schedule, the duration of treatment, long-term side effects of chronic administration, integration with other biological and cytotoxic therapies, the specific tumor phenotypes more suitable for this approach, and potential cross-resistance among different agents.

In regards to clinical end points, it may be difficult to demonstrate a conventional antitumor response (i.e., objective response) with HDAC inhibitors in cohorts of patients with advanced disease resistant to conventional therapy. Probably the more appropriate clinical setting is chemopreventive, adjuvant, or maintenance therapy, once satisfactory tolerability and activity has been proven by Phase I studies in patients with advanced disease.

A rational testing of "epigenetic" therapy will require the use of critical correlative studies. While developing the clinical testing of these novel agents, we will need to determine whether the drug hits the target and whether the modulation of the target translates into an antitumor effect. Surrogate markers of tumor response to HDAC inhibitors and predictors of clinical outcome are still lacking. HADC inhibitors have shown preliminary results in the clinic but identifying the optimal dose, schedule, and duration of therapy remains an unmet task. The implementation of animal models to better select dose and schedule for clinical studies should be encouraged.

It is reasonable to predict that the clinical testing of HDAC inhibitors will occur at different stages of the prostate cancer progression. However, in early disease (biochemical relapse before or after hormone therapy) where the only potential surrogate marker of tumor response is prostate-specific antigen (PSA) levels, the use of HDAC inhibitors may be challenging. The potential modulation of PSA by "differentiation"-inducing agents such as HDAC inhibitors is still not clear, but early study with PB showed a transient induction of PSA (67). Sustained changes in PSA doubling time/velocity rather than PSA response may be a reasonable clinical end point with this strategy. The optimal clinical setting for testing this combination strategy with HDAC inhibitors remains to be elucidated but future Phase II clinical trials will provide critical information.

CONCLUSIONS AND FUTURE PERSPECTIVES

As driven by the translational potential of post-transcriptional modifiers including HDAC inhibitors in cancer therapy, how these agents mediate their anticancer effects is still the focus of current and future investigations. A major challenge is represented by lack of in-depth understanding of the biological function of targeted proteins and their involvement in tumorigenesis. Emerging evidence indicates that HDACs target nonhistone substrates both in the nucleus and the cytoplasm, which provides transcription-independent mechanisms to regulate intracellular signaling and cytoskeleton integrity. For example, disruption of complexes between specific HDAC and phosphorylases (i.e., PP1) by HDAC inhibitors alters the dynamics of phosphorylase complex formation, leading to deactivation of Akt and other signaling kinases.

Transcriptional and post-transcriptional dependent mechanisms can be both targeted to exploit the potency of HDAC inhibitors in suppressing tumor cell growth. These agents will likely not be developed as single agent and the potential combination of HDAC inhibitors with existing therapeutic agents to reduce drug doses or to overcome drug-resistant phenotypes is yet another strategy that warrants clinical evaluation. Although a clinical role of HDAC inhibitors is already a reality, their general clinical utility will likely depend greatly on the future development of molecular or cellular predictors of their antitumor activity (68).

Molecular targeted combination therapies of post-transcription modifiers such as HDAC inhibitors with standard therapies (chemotherapy and radiation therapy) and novel biologics including angiogenesis inhibitor represent an exciting challenge. Understanding of the nature of the molecular basis of the selectivity of HDACs and designing specific HDACs inhibitors will be critical to further exploit the potential of this novel class of agents in the treatment of prostate cancer.

REFERENCES

1. Coppelli FM, Grandis JR. Oligonucleotides as anticancer agents: from the benchside to the clinic and beyond. Curr Pharmaceut Des 2005; 11:2825–2840.
2. Hede K. Blocking cancer with RNA interference moves toward the clinic news. J Natl Cancer Inst 2005; 97(9):626–628.
3. Pienta KJ. Preclinical mechanisms of action of docetaxel and docetaxel combinations in prostate cancer. Semin Oncol 2001; 28(4, suppl 15):3–7.
4. Zhang H, Kim JK, Edwards CA, Xu Z, Taichman R, Wang CY. Clusterin inhibits apoptosis by interacting with activated bax. Nat Cell Biol 2005; 7(9):909–915.
5. Bruchovsky N, Snoek R, Rennie PS, Akakura K, Goldenberg LS, Gleave M. Control of tumor progression by maintenance of apoptosis. Prostate Suppl 1996; 6:13–21.
6. Gleave M, Jansen B. Clusterin and IGFBPs as antisense targets in prostate cancer. Ann NY Acad Sci 2003; 1002:95–104.
7. Devi GR. XIAP as target for therapeutic apoptosis in prostate cancer. Drug News Perspect 2004; 17(2):127–134.
8. Bianco R, Ciardiello F, Tortora G. Chemosensitization by antisense oligonucleotides targeting MDM2. Curr Cancer Drug Targets 2005; 5(1):51–56.
9. Keller ET, Fu Z, Brennan M. The role of Raf kinase inhibitor protein (RKIP) in health and disease. Biochem Pharmacol 2004; 68(6):1049–1053.
10. Chi KN, Eisenhauer E, Fazli L, et al. A phase I pharmacokinetic and pharmacodynamic study of OGX-011, a 2′-methoxyethyl antisense oligonucleotide to clusterin, in patients with localized prostate cancer. J Natl Cancer Inst 2005; 97(17):1287–1296.
11. Advani R, Lum BL, Fisher GA, et al. A phase I trial of aprinocarsen (ISIS 3521/LY900003), an antisense inhibitor of protein kinase C-alpha administered as a 24-hour weekly infusion schedule in patients with advanced cancer. Invest New Drugs 2005; 23(5):467–477.
12. Suh J, Rabson AB. NF-kappaB activation in human prostate cancer: important mediator or epiphenomenon? J Cell Biochem 2004; 91(1):100–117.
13. Li Y, Ahmed F, Ali S, Philip PA, Kucuk O, Sarkar FH. Inactivation of nuclear factor kappaB by soy isoflavone genistein contributes to increased apoptosis induced by chemotherapeutic agents in human cancer cells. Cancer Res 2005; 65(15):6934–6942.

14. Howell SB. Resistance to apoptosis in prostate cancer cells. Mol Urol 2000; 4(3):225–229.
15. Collis SJ, Swartz MJ, Nelson WG, DeWeese TL. Enhanced radiation and chemotherapy-mediated cell killing of human cancer cells by small inhibitory RNA silencing of DNA repair factors. Cancer Res 2003; 63(7):1550–1554.
16. Varambally S, Dhanasekaran SM, Zhou M, et al. The polycomb group protein EZH2 is involved in progression of prostate cancer. Nature 2002; 419(6907):624–629.
17. Takeshita F, Minakuchi Y, Nagahara S, et al. Efficient delivery of small interfering RNA to bone-metastatic tumors by using atelocollagen in vivo. Proc Natl Acad Sci USA 2005; 102(34):12177–12182.
18. Reagan-Shaw S, Ahmad N. Silencing of polo-like kinase (Plk) 1 via siRNA causes induction of apoptosis and impairment of mitosis machinery in human prostate cancer cells: implications for the treatment of prostate cancer. FASEB J. 2005; 19(6):611–613.
19. George DJ, Halabi S, Shepard TF, et al. Prognostic significance of plasma vascular endothelial growth factor levels in patients with hormone-refractory prostate cancer treated on Cancer and Leukemia Group B 9480. Clin Cancer Res 2001; 7:1932–1936.
20. Benjamin LE, Golijanin D, Itin A, et al. Selective ablation of immature blood vessels in established human tumors follows vascular endothelial growth factor withdrawal. J Clin Invest 1999; 103:159–165.
21. Franck-Lissbrant I, Häggström S, Damber J-E, Bergh A. Testosterone has been shown to stimulate angiogenesis and vascular regrowth in the ventral prostate in castrated rats. Endocrinology 1998; 139:451–456.
22. Silberman MA, Partin AW, Veltri RW, et al. Tumor angiogenesis correlates with progression after radical prostatectomy but not with pathologic stage in Gleason sum 5 to 7 adenocarcinoma of the prostate. Cancer 1997; 79:772–779.
23. Brown LF, Yeo KT, Berse B, et al. Vascular permeability factor (vascular endothelial growth factor) is strongly expressed in the normal male genital tract and is present in substantial quantities in semen. J Urol 1995; 154:576–579.
24. George DJ, Regan MM, Oh WK, Tay M, Manola J, et al. Radical prostatectomy lowers plasma vascular endothelial growth factor levels in patients with prostate cancer. Urology 2004; 63(2):327–332.
25. Takei Y, Kadomatsu K, Yuzawa Y, Matsuo S, Muramatsu T. A small interfering RNA targeting vascular endothelial growth factor as cancer therapeutics. Cancer Res 2004; 64(10):3365–3370.
26. Low WK, Dang Y, Schneider-Poetsch T, et al. Inhibition of eukaryotic translation initiation by the marine natural product pateamine A. Mol Cell 2005; 20(5):709–722.
27. Yamamoto N, Tamura T, Kamiya Y, et al. Phase I and pharmacokinetic study of KRN5500, a spicamycin derivative, for patients with advanced solid tumors. Jpn J Clin Oncol 2003; 33(6):302–308.
28. Wullschleger S, Loewith R, Hall MN. TOR signaling in growth and metabolism. Cell 2006; 124(3):471–484.
29. Zhong H, Chiles K, Feldser D, et al. Modulation of hypoxia-inducible factor 1alpha expression by the epidermal growth factor/phosphatidylinositol 3-kinase/PTEN/AKT/FRAP pathway in human prostate cancer cells: implications for tumor angiogenesis and therapeutics. Cancer Res 2000; 60(6):1541–1545.
30. Kouzarides T. Histone acetylases and deacetylases in cell proliferation. Curr Opn Genet Dev 1999; 9:40–48.
31. Johnstone RW, Licht JD. Histone deacetylase inhibitors in cancer therapy: is transcription the primary target? Cancer Cell 2003; 4:13–18.
32. Marks PA, Richon VM, Miller T, Kelly WK. Histone deacetylases inhibitors. Adv Cancer Res 2004; 91:137–168.
33. Marks OA, Rifkind RA, Richon VM, Breslow R, Miller T, Kelly WK. Histone deacetylases and cancer: causes and therapies. Nature Rev Cancer 2001; 1:194–202.
34. Agalioti T, Chen G, Thanos D. Deciphering the transcriptional histone acetylation code for a human gene. Cell 2002; 111:381–392.
35. Jung M, Velena A, Chen B, Petukhov PA, Kozikowski AP, Dritschilo A. Novel HDAC inhibitors with radiosensitizing properties. Radiat Res 2005; 163(5):488–493.

36. Qian DZ, Ren M, Wei Y, et al. In vivo imaging of retinoic acid receptor beta2 transcriptional activation by the histone deacetylase inhibitor MS-275 in retinoid-resistant prostate cancer cells. Prostate 2005; 64(1):20–28.
37. Marchion DC, Bicaku E, Daud AI, Richon V, Sullivan DM, Munster PN. Sequence-specific potentiation of topoisomerase II inhibitors by the histone deacetylase inhibitor suberoylanilide hydroxamic acid. J Cell Biochem 2004; 92(2):223–237.
38. Nimmanapalli R, Fuino L, Bali P, et al. Histone deacetylase inhibitor LAQ824 both lowers expression and promotes proteosomal degradation of Bcr-Abl and induces apoptosis of imatinib mesylate-sensitive or -refractory chronic myelogenous leukemia-blast crisis cells. Cancer Res 2003; 63(16):5126–5135.
39. Fuino L, Bali P, Wittmann S, et al. Histone deacetylase inhibitor LAQ824 down-regulates Her-2 and sensitizes human breast cancer cells to trastuzumab, taxotere, gemcitabine, and epothilone B. Mol Cancer Ther 2003; 2(10):971–984.
40. Bali P, George P, Cohen P, et al. Superior activity of the combination of histone deacetylase inhibitor LAQ824 and the FLT-3 kinase inhibitor PKC412 against human acute myelogenous leukemia cells with mutant FLT-3. Clin Cancer Res 2004; 10(15):4991–4997.
41. Rosato RR, Almenara JA, Dai Y, Grant S. Simultaneous activation of the intrinsic and extrinsic pathways by histone deacetylase (HDAC) inhibitors and tumor necrosis factor-related apoptosis-inducing ligand (TRAIL) synergistically induces mitochondrial damage and apoptosis in human leukemia cells. Mol Cancer Ther 2003; 2(12):1273–1284.
42. Yu C, Rahmani M, Conrad D, Subler M, Dent P, Grant S. The proteasome inhibitor bortezomib interacts synergistically with histone deacetylase inhibitors to induce apoptosis in Bcr/Abl+ cells sensitive and resistant to STI571. Blood 2003; 102(10):3765–3774.
43. Maggio SC, Rosato RR, Kramer LB, et al. The histone deacetylase inhibitor MS-275 interacts synergistically with fludarabine to induce apoptosis in human leukemia cells. Cancer Res 2004; 64(7):2590–2600.
44. Rahmani M, Reese E, Dai Y, et al. Cotreatment with suberanoylanilide hydroxamic acid and 17-allylamino 17-demethoxygeldanamycin synergistically induces apoptosis in Bcr-Abl+ cells sensitive and resistant to STI571 (imatinib mesylate) in association with down-regulation of Bcr-Abl, abrogation of signal transducer and activator of transcription 5 activity, and Bax conformational change. Mol Pharmacol 2005; 67(4):1166–1176.
45. Glozak MA, Sengupta N, Zhang X, Seto E. Acetylation and deacetylation of non-histone proteins. Gene 2005; 363:15–23.
46. Blagosklonny MV, Trostel S, Kayastha G, et al. Depletion of mutant p53 and cytotoxicity of histone deacetylase inhibitors. Cancer Res 2005; 65(16):7386–7392.
47. Aoyagi S, Archer TK. Modulating molecular chaperone Hsp90 functions through reversible acetylation. Trends Cell Biol 2005; 15(11):565–567.
48. Chen L, Meng S, Wang H, et al. Chemical ablation of androgen receptor in prostate cancer cells by the histone deacetylase inhibitor LAQ824. Mol Cancer Ther 2005; 4(9):1311–1319.
49. Chen CS, Weng SC, Tseng PH, Lin HP, Chen CS. Histone acetylation-independent effect of histone deacetylase inhibitors on Akt through the reshuffling of protein phosphatase 1 complexes. J Biol Chem 2005; 280(46):38879–38887.
50. Folkman J. Tumor angiogenesis: therapeutic implications. N Engl J Med 1971; 285: 1182–1186.
51. Holash J, Wiegand SJ, Yancopoulos GD. New model of tumor angiogenesis: dynamic balance between vessel regression and growth mediated by angiopoietins and VEGF. Oncogene 1999; 18:5356–5362.
52. Semenza GL. Targeting HIF-1 for cancer therapy. Nat Rev Cancer 2003; (10):721–732.
53. Ferrara N, Kerbel RS. Angiogenesis as a therapeutic target. Nature 2005; 438(7070): 967–974.
54. Hurwitz H, Fehrenbacher L, Cartwright T, et al. Bevacizumab plus irinotecan, fluorouracil, and leucovorin for metastatic colorectal cancer. N Engl J Med 2004; 350:2335–2342.
55. Escudier B, Szczylik C, Eisen T, et al. Randomized phase III trial of the Raf kinase and VEGFR inhibitor sorafenib (BAY 43–9006) in patients with advanced renal cell carcinoma (RCC). Abstract #4510 Proc ASCO 2005, Abstract# 4510.

56. Motzer RJ, Rini BI, Michaelson MD, et al. The SU11248 Study Group phase 2 trials of SU11248 show antitumor activity in second-line therapy for patients with metastatic renal cell carcinoma (RCC). Proc ASCO 2005 [abstr 4508].
57. Qian DZ, Wang X, Kachhap SK, et al. The histone deacetylase inhibitor NVP-LAQ824 inhibits angiogenesis and has a greater antitumor effect in combination with the vascular endothelial growth factor receptor tyrosine kinase inhibitor PTK787/ZK222584. Cancer Res 2004; 64(18):6626–6634.
58. Kelly WK, Marks PA. Drug insight: histone deacetylase inhibitors—development of the new targeted anticancer agent suberoylanilide hydroxamic acid. Nat Clin Pract Oncol 2005(3):150–157.
59. Kelly WK, Richon VM, O'Connor O, et al. Phase I clinical trial of histone deacetylase inhibitor: suberoylanilide hydroxamic acid administered intravenously. Clin Cancer Res 2003; 9(10.1):3578–3588.
60. Kelly WK, O'Connor OA, Krug LM, et al. Phase I study of an oral histone deacetylase inhibitor, suberoylanilide hydroxamic acid, in patients with advanced cancer. J Clin Oncol 2005; 23(17):3923–3931.
61. O'Connor OA, Heaney ML, Schwartz L, et al. Clinical experience with intravenous and oral formulations of the novel histone deacetylase inhibitor suberoylanilide hydroxamic acid in patients with advanced hematologic malignancies. J Clin Oncol 2006; 24(1):166–173.
62. Talpur C, Zhang A, Goy V, et al. Phase II trial of oral suberoylanilide hydroxamic acid (SAHA) for cutaneous T-cell lymphoma (CTCL) unresponsive to conventional therapy. Proc ASCO 2005 [abstr #6571].
63. Ryan QC, Headlee D, Acharya M, et al. Phase I and pharmacokinetic study of MS-275, a histone deacetylase inhibitor, in patients with advanced and refractory solid tumors or lymphoma. J Clin Oncol 2005; 23(17):3912–3922.
64. Piekarz RL, Robey RW, Zhan Z, et al. T-cell lymphoma as a model for the use of histone deacetylase inhibitors in cancer therapy: impact of depsipeptide on molecular markers, therapeutic targets, and mechanisms of resistance. Blood 2004; 103(12):4636–4643.
65. Beck J, Fischer T, George D, et al. Phase I pharmacokinetic (PK) and pharmacodynamic (PD) study of oral LBH589B: a novel histone deacetylase (HDAC) inhibitor. Proc ASCO 2005 [abstr #3148].
66. Rowinsky EK, Pacey S, Patnaik A, et al. A phase I, pharmacokinetic (PK) and pharmacodynamic (PD) study of a novel histone deacetylase (HDAC) inhibitor LAQ824 in patients with advanced solid tumors. Proc ASCO 2005 [abstr #3022].
67. Carducci MA, Gilbert J, Bowling MK, et al. A Phase I clinical and pharmacological evaluation of sodium phenylbutyrate on an 120-h infusion schedule. Clin Cancer Res 2001; 7(10):3047–3055.
68. Minucci S, Pelicci PG. Histone deacetylase inhibitors and the promise of epigenetic (and more) treatments for cancer. Nat Rev Cancer 2006(1):38–51.

12 Telomere Targeting Agents

Angelika M. Burger

Department of Pharmacology and Experimental Therapeutics, Marlene and Stewart Greenebaum Cancer Center, University of Maryland School of Medicine, Baltimore, Maryland, U.S.A.

Lloyd R. Kelland

Antisoma Research Laboratories, St. Georges Hospital Medical School, Cranmer Terrace, London, U.K.

INTRODUCTION

Telomeres

Human telomeres are noncoding DNA sequences at the end of chromosomes, which are composed of $(TTAGGG)_n$ hexanucleotide repeats. During each cell division, telomeric DNA (30–100 bp) is lost because of the so-called end-replication problem. Telomeres maintain chromosomal integrity and prevent replication of defective genes (1,2). As all chromosomes begin life with a limited amount of telomeric DNA, there is a finite number of cell divisions that a cell can undergo before it reaches an irreducible lower limit of telomeres (1–3). Without this minimal amount of telomeric DNA, the cell is no longer capable of supporting chromosomal replication or cell division. When normal cells reach a critical telomere length, they exit the cell cycle, enter M2 (mortality stage 2) crisis, and undergo senescence. This mechanism is thought to be the clock that determines human lifespan (3,4).

Different cell types have different telomere dynamics. For example, the average available telomere length in normal somatic cells is 10 kb, it erodes over time and normal cells enter replicative senescence. Stem cells of renewal tissues have an average telomere length of 12 kb which shortens at reduced rates, whereas germ cells and fetal tissues have approximately 15–20 kb and maintain their telomeres through expression of low levels of telomerase, and they can undergo reproductive senescence. However, the average telomere length of cancer cells is only 5 kb. During early tumorigenesis from normal to malignant cells, telomeres erode, but are then maintained at a stable length through, in the great majority of cases, the reactivation of the enzyme telomerase (4–7).

Telomerase

Telomerase is a ribonucleoprotein reverse transcriptase and its activity can be reconstituted in vitro by two essential components, namely the RNA component hTERC (human telomerase RNA component), which acts as the template for addition of new telomeric repeats, and the catalytic subunit hTERT (human telomerase reverse transcriptase) (6,8–11). Telomerase permits cells to overcome one of the fundamental limitations to mammalian cell immortality, namely the progressive loss of telomeric DNA.

Cell populations that continue dividing throughout life, such as germ cells, gastrointestinal mucosal cells, and hematopoietic stem cells require the addition of new telomeres to their chromosomes to replace the sequences lost during repeated rounds of cell division (12,13). The latter and cancer cells, which have also acquired a high proliferative potential, surpass replicative senescence by activation of the enzyme telomerase. As telomerase is reactivated, it can *de novo* synthesize TTAGGG hexanucleotide repeats onto shortened telomeres, thus maintaining the protective cap of chromosomes at a stable length. Cancer and stem cells have therefore an infinite capacity to proliferate and are immortal (6,11).

Virtually all human tumor cell lines and approximately 90% of human cancer tissues have been shown to possess telomerase activity. In contrast, normal tissues adjacent to tumor and human somatic tissues, other than stem cells, do not possess detectable levels of telomerase (11,13).

Telomere Maintenance and Uncapping

Telomere length is maintained by a balance between processes that lengthen (telomere synthesis by telomerase) and those that shorten telomeres (cell division/ DNA replication). In the majority of human cells, telomere length is not maintained and they are destined to undergo senescence. In tumors, however, telomerase is active and maintains telomeres at a short but stable length (14). The telomere length set point and its regulation involve telomere-binding proteins and other members of the telomere/telomerase complex (Fig. 1). Telomeres and the associated binding protein complex provide protective capping for chromosome ends.

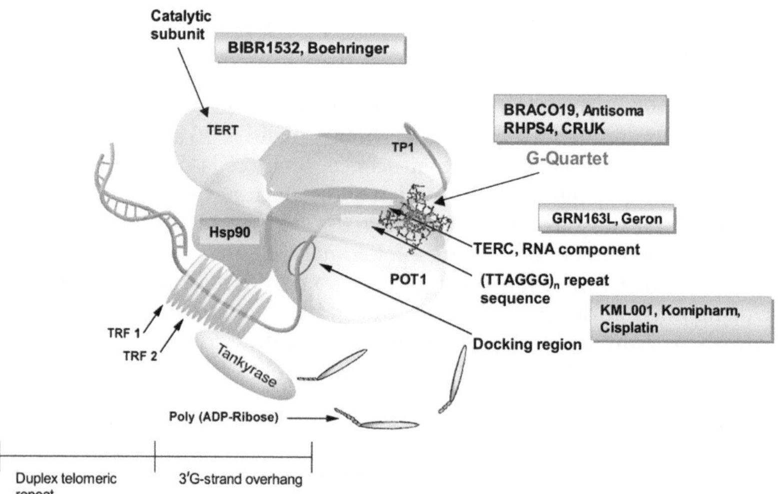

FIGURE 1 (*See color insert*) The human telomere/telomerase complex: Telomere structure, telomerase components, and associated proteins with possible points of therapeutic intervention. *Abbreviations*: TERT, telomerase reverse transcriptase = catalytic subunit; TERC, telomerase RNA component; CRUK, Cancer Reasearch United Kingdom; TP1, telomerase associated protein 1; Hsp90, heat shock protein 90; POT1, protection of telomerase 1; TRF1, telomeric repeat binding factor 1; TRF2, telomeric repeat binding factor 2; CRT, cancer research technology. The G-quartet structure at the single-stranded 3′-end was adopted from Ref. 25.

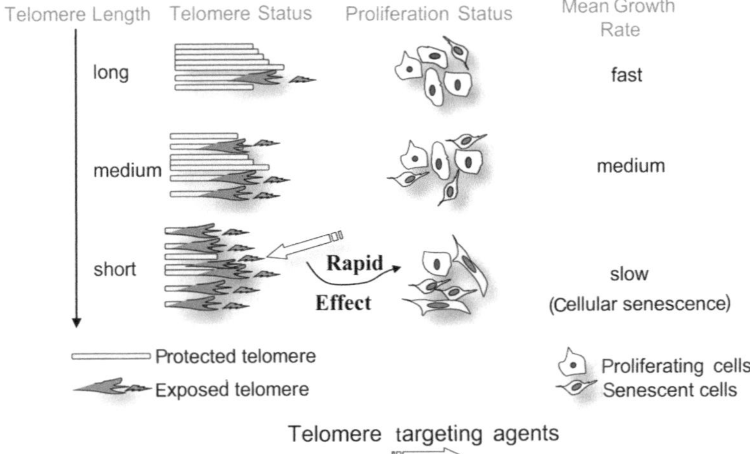

FIGURE 2 (*See color insert*) Uncapping of telomeres and cellular senescence. Cells with capped telomeres are functional and cycling. Uncapped telomeres cause exit from the cell cycle and at a certain rate of uncapped telomeres, net growth of the cell population ceases, and cells senesce. Cell growth rate and proliferation depend on telomere length and capping status. Gray arrow, telomere targeting agents have an uncapping effect and can rapidly induce cellular senescence.

Analyses of uncapped and capped telomeres in budding yeast have recently revealed that deregulation that is associated with DNA aberrations and morphological defects results from telomere uncapping rather than telomere length *per se*, thus challenging the paradigm that telomeres have to critically shorten in order to cause telomere dysfunction and senescence (Fig. 2) (15). According to the telomere capping/uncapping hypothesis proposed by Blackburn, capping is functionally defined as preserving the physical integrity of the telomere, allowing cell division to proceed. Regulated uncapping would occur normally in dividing cells with the crucial property that a functional telomere would rapidly switch back to a capped state. Left uncorrected for too long, the uncapped state will elicit cell-cycle arrest or other responses (Fig. 2) (1,15).

The Telomere/Telomerase Complex

In vitro, TERC and hTERT are sufficient to bestow telomerase activity (8,9). In vivo, these core subunits are augmented by additional factors that comprise the functional telomere/telomerase complex, the telomerase-associated proteins, and the telomere-binding proteins, which play a role in equilibrium length establishment by affecting the localization and activity of the enzyme. Telomerase-associated protein 1 (TP1) and the molecular chaperones Hsp90/p23 are physically associated with the telomerase catalytic subunit protein hTERT. hTERT requires Hsp90-mediated chaperone conformational folding for maturation and functional activation (Fig. 1) (16,17). Telomere-binding proteins include but are not limited to the telomeric repeat binding factors 1 and 2 (TRF1 and TRF2), protection of telomeres 1 (POT1) as well as tankyrase [TRF1-inactivating ankyrin-related adenosine diphosphate (ADP)-ribose polymerase] (Fig. 1) (18–20).

TRF1 acts by inhibiting telomerase at the telomere termini and is a negative regulator of telomere length. Its over-expression leads to telomere shortening, whereas inhibition increases telomere length (18). TRF2 maintains telomere integrity and telomeres lacking TRF2 directly signal apoptosis in cells with functional p53 or DNA damage response (19). Tankyrase is an enzyme that binds to TRF1 and removes this protein, which otherwise would block telomerase access to chromosome ends from its telomere-binding site by poly (ADP)-ribosylation, thus enabling telomerase to work (Fig. 1) (20). Pot 1 is a single-stranded DNA telomere-binding protein, and has been shown to interact with the G-strand overhang (Fig. 1).

Key components of the homologous recombination (HR) and non-homologous end joining (NHEJ) pathways for DNA double-strand break repair are also found at mammalian telomeres, in particular, the NHEJ DNA-dependent protein kinase (DNA-PK) complex. DNA-PK is composed of Ku70 and Ku86 proteins, and of DNA-PKcs. The study of Ku86 and DNA-PKcs-deficient mice indicated that these proteins have essential roles at the mammalian telomeres (21).

Telomeres consist predominantly of double-stranded telomeric repeats with only the extreme terminus containing some single-stranded G-rich sequences (G-strand or 3′ single-stranded overhang). Telomerase adds the single-strand TTAGGG extension, whereas double-stranded regions are replicated by conventional polymerases (Fig. 1) (10).

Two structures of the 3′ single-stranded $(TTAGGG)_n$ overhang have been proposed. One suggesting the presence of a T-loop, which would result from a foldback of the 3′ overhang into a loop of duplex DNA, the other proposes the formation of dimers and tetramers involving G-quartets (22–24). G-quartet formation seems to be accelerated in the presence of telomere-binding proteins, which appear to act as chaperones (23). The G-quartet was recently crystallized and seems to confer an energetically preferable conformation (Fig. 1) (25). However, both structures of the 3′-end overhang might coexist (22). Nonetheless, the existence of a folding of the G-strand overhang into a G-quartet has to be considered most plausible in human cells, based on the available experimental evidence (25,26).

Targets for Anticancer Therapy

Targeting telomerase and telomeres has evolved as a very attractive strategy to treat cancer because (i) telomerase activation is an early event during tumorigenesis, (ii) more than 90% of human tumors express the enzyme telomerase, which maintains their telomere length, and (iii) tumors have relatively shorter telomeres compared to normal cell types (2,6,7,27). The telomere/telomerase complex provides multiple possibilities for the development of inhibitors; various approaches are currently under advanced preclinical investigations and are summarized in Figure 1 (27,28). The essential RNA component has been targeted by anti-sense oligonucleotides (28–30). The first template antagonist targeting hTERC, termed GRN163L (Geron Corporation, California, U.S.A.), which is a 13-mer oligonucleotide N3′→P5′ thio-phosphoramidate, has just entered clinical trials (Fig. 1). GRN163L has shown preclinical activity against breast and lung cancer cell lines and was effective in preventing lung metastases in xenograft animal models (30,31).

Despite significant efforts made by pharmaceutical industries to identify inhibitors of the telomerase catalytic subunit hTERT, only one small molecular inhibitor, namely BIBR1532 (Boehringer Ingelheim, Ingelheim, Germany) has been identified and has undergone preclinical studies (28,32).

Agents that target telomeric repeat sequences are cisplatin, KML001, and G-quartet interactive compounds (BRACO19, RHPS4), respectively (7,33–35). The clinically used cytotoxic agent cisplatin was shown to form cross-links at the G-rich single-strand telomeric overhang, which cannot be repaired by the DNA excision repair system. As a consequence, telomerase is inhibited and telomeres are "uncapped" and shortened. The mechanism has been postulated to contribute to cisplatin's curative activity in germ cell tumors (33,34,36,37).

KML001 is an orally bioavailable, novel arsenic compound (KOMINOX, Komipharm, Shihenung-Shi, Kyonggi-Do, Korea; Fig. 1). Effects by arsenic trioxide on telomerase and telomeres have been well established. It was shown that KML001 treatment leads to direct telomere shortening in a dose- and concentration-dependent manner without inhibiting telomerase activity, thus indicating telomere poisoning (35). KML001 has shown preclinical activity in solid tumors and leukemias, and has just entered a Phase I/II clinical trial (35).

Compounds that have been rationally designed to interact with the G-rich telomeric overhang by inducing it to form and stabilize the G-quartet structure (RHPS4, Cancer Research Technology—Cancer Research U.K.; BRACO19 analogs, Antisoma, London, U.K.) are also being developed, and will be described in detail in the following paragraphs (Fig. 1) (28,38,39).

Additional "less specific" targets in the telomere/telomerase complex are telomerase-associated and telomere-binding proteins, respectively. Several drugs from the latter categories are in early clinical trials. They include the heat shock protein 90 inhibitor, 17-allylaminogeldanamycin, which was shown to down-regulate telomerase activity as a result of loss of Hsp90 chaperone function (28,40), and poly-(ADP-ribose) polymerase (PARP) inhibitory compounds (41,42). The telomere-binding protein tankyrase is a PARP family member (Fig. 1), which can be inhibited by broad-spectrum PARP inhibitory compounds such as 3-aminobenzamide (41,42).

Targeting the Telomere vs. the Holoenzyme

After the catalytic subunit hTERT had been identified as the key component of the telomerase holoenzyme (8,43), experiments were performed to overexpress hTERT in telomerase-deficient, normal cells and to inhibit hTERT by expression of dominant negative (DN) hTERT in cancer cells (43–45). The expression of a catalytically inactive form of the human TERT subunit in cancer-derived cell lines disrupted telomerase activity and was coincident with a decrease in telomere length (38,45). This resulted in proliferative defects with successive population doublings. Time to growth arrest correlated with initial telomere length. A cell line that maintained its telomeres independent of telomerase by the so-called alternative telomere lengthening (ALT) mechanism was resistant to growth-inhibitory effects of DN-hTERT transfection (45). Genetic hTERT inhibition together with the data resulting from studying the synthetic hTERT inhibitor BIBR1532 and hTERC template antagonists such as GRN163L clearly indicate that enzyme inhibition requires a substantial lag time—dependent on the initial length of telomeres—before replicative senescence occurs (30,32,45). If this scenario is operable in vivo in patients, telomerase inhibition alone is probably insufficient for effective tumor growth inhibition and would require combination with other targeted or cytotoxic agents.

Most recently, however, evidence is emerging that the potential cellular outcome in cancer cells after treatment with "telomerase inhibitors" should not only be expected to lead to induction of cellular senescence after successive telomere shortening. Experimental data have accumulated indicating that telomere uncapping will lead to more rapid cell killing. DNA damage signals at the G-strand overhang and the corresponding lagging strand could lead to uncapping of the chromosome and rapidly occurring apoptosis or genomic instability. In addition, telomere-based senescence and premature senescence due to static telomere conditions can also contribute to a much reduced lag time as compared to telomere shortening by telomerase enzyme inhibition alone (1,24,46).

Thus, agents that directly target telomeres are likely to be more effective as a monotherapy and can act faster as compared to pure enzyme inhibitors.

The research efforts of our laboratories are therefore focused on the development of telomere targeting agents (TTAs) and their combinations with molecules that can act at other components of the telomere/telomerase complex such as Hsp90 inhibitors. This chapter will in the following sections focus on the development of TTAs and their usefulness for the treatment of prostate cancer.

TELOMERASE AND TELOMERES IN PROSTATE CANCER DEVELOPMENT

Telomerase reactivation and telomere dynamics during prostate cancer development and progression have been evaluated (47–49). We have previously studied telomerase activity and telomere length status during the stepwise transformation of normal human prostate epithelial cells and fibroblasts to tumor cells using viral oncogenes (Table 1). Transfection with SV40 virus leads to expression of the SV40 T large antigen, which degrades the tumor suppressor proteins Rb and p53, whereas transformation with the human papilloma virus (HPV) 16 leads to E7 oncoprotein expression and degradation of p53. v-Ki-ras transfection leads to expression of oncogenic ras (Table 1) (47). Similar to the findings reported by Weinberg *et al.* on the creation of a tumor cell, we found that transformation of human primary prostate epithelial cells and fibroblasts with one oncogenic virus (SV40 or HPV 18) alone led to telomere shortening and reactivation of telomerase, but did not make these cells tumorigenic (44,47). However, after a second oncogenic hit, using either viral Ki-ras or X-ray treatment, all transformed prostate cell lines did form tumors in immunodeficient mice (47).

In agreement with our prostate carcinogenesis model, the three commonly available permanent prostate cancer cell lines PC3, DU145, and LNCaP have high levels of endogenous telomerase activity, an average telomere length between 2.5 and 4 kb, and they can form tumors in nude mice (Table 1) (47,48). These data indicate that telomere shortening and telomerase activation is an early event during prostate carcinogenesis and that the telomere/telomerase complex might be a good target for therapeutic intervention.

Telomerase Activity and Telomere Length in Prostate Cancer

A survey of the average telomere length and telomerase activity in 25 matched normal, benign prostate hyperplasia (BPH) and prostate cancer tissues revealed that high levels of telomerase activity are present in primary prostate cancer, but not in adjacent normal and benign prostate tissues. Lymph node metastases were also strongly positive for telomerase (Table 1) (48). When telomere length was compared in normal, BPH, and cancer tissues from the same patients, gradual losses of telomeric sequences between 0.3 and 0.5 kb from normal to BPH, and 1.0 kb in

TABLE 1 Telomerase Activity and Telomere Length in Human Normal and Malignant Prostate Cells and Tissues

Origin[a]	Transformation status	Tumorigenic	Telomerase	TRF (kb)
BPH	Senescent	No	−	Not done
Fetal prostate epithelial cells	SV40 immortalized	No	+	5.2
SV40 immortalized fetal PE	v-Ki-ras transformed	Yes	+	4.0
SV40 immortalized fetal PE	X-ray transformed	Yes	+	3.7
Adult prostate epithelial cells	SV40 immortalized	No	+	3.5
Adult prostate epithelial cells	HPV18 immortalized	No	+	3.5
HPV18 immortalized adult PE	v-Ki-ras transformed	Yes	+	4.0
Adult prostate fibroblast	SV40 immortalized	No	+	3.5
PC3 prostate cancer cell line	Patient derived, immortal	Yes	+	2.5–3.0
LNCaP prostate cancer line	Patient derived, immortal	Yes	+	2.5
DU145 prostate cancer line	Patient derived, immortal	Yes	+	3.5–3.7
Origin[b]	Number of Samples Analyzed	Telomerase(+/+)		
Normal prostate (adjacent to cancer)	25	25−		5.9–7.7
BPH (from patients with BPH only)	10	10−		5.8–7.5
BPH (adjacent to cancer)	25	3+/22−		5.8–7.5
Prostate cancer	25	21+/4−		5.8–6.0
Lymph node metastases	4	4+/0−		Not done

[a]In vitro prostate tumorigenesis model.
[b]Distribution of telomerase activity and telomere length in human prostate tissues.
Abbreviations: BPH, benign prostate hyperplasia; PE, prostate epithelial cells; SV40, simian virus 40; HPV18, human papillloma virus 18; TRF, mean telomere restriction fragment length; +, positive; −, negative.
Source: From Refs. 38, 47 and 48.

cancers were seen (48). However, the average telomere (TRF) length between all normal and BPH samples was not significantly different; in contrast, tumor tissues showed a marked average telomere shortening (Table1) (48).

A recent study, which employed more sensitive and single-cell-based telomere length measurement methods, namely fluorescent in situ hybridization instead of Southern blotting, examined telomere length in high-grade prostatic intraepithelial neoplasia (HGPIN) in comparison to adjacent normal tissues. Telomeres of luminal cells of HGPIN lesions, a putative preinvasive precursor of prostatic adenocarcinoma, were on average approximately fourfold shorter than their normal counterparts (49). Specimens that contained foci of invasive cancer showed that cancer cells exhibited shortened telomeres similar to the corresponding HGPIN lesions. Stromal cells generally exhibited telomere lengths similar to, or slightly longer than, adjacent benign normal-appearing prostatic epithelium (49). These results together with our in vitro prostate carcinogenesis model data suggest that telomere shortening occurs early, at or before the PIN stage, and is likely to contribute to chromosomal instability, hence neoplastic transformation during prostate tumorigenesis (47–49).

TTA AND PROSTATE CANCER

Based on the differential telomere equilibrium in normal, benign, pre-cancerous, and cancerous prostate tissues and high telomerase activity levels in primary and metastatic prostate cancers, TTAs that aim to uncap the relatively short telomeres of malignant prostate cells might offer very effective treatment strategies (Table 1). Several first- and second-generation G-quartet interactive/TTAs have been evaluated by others and us in prostate cancer model systems in vitro and in vivo and are described in the following sections (Table 2) (38,50,51).

G-Quartet-Interactive Agents

Human TTAGGG telomere sequences can form intramolecular quadruplex structures. Both human telomeric repeats forming a quadruplex structure in solution and the G-quartet crystal structure have been resolved (25,52,53).

TABLE 2 First- and Second-Generation G-Quartet-Interactive Agents

Chemical classification	Lead compound	Prostate cancer activity	References
First generation compounds			
Porphyrins	TMPyP4	Yes (in vivo)	(50)
Amidoanthracene-9, 10-diones	Not specified	Not evaluated	(61)
Ethidium derivatives	Compound 4	Not evaluated	(62)
Second-generation compounds			
Pentacyclic acridines	RHPS4	Yes (in vitro)	(38, 58)
Trisubstituted acridines	BRACO19/AS1410	Yes (in vitro/vivo)	(28, 39, 51)
2,6-Pyridine-dicarboxamide	307A	Not evaluated	(63)
Triazine derivatives	12459	Not evaluated	(57,64)
Natural product (*Streptomyces anulatus*)	Telomestatin	Not evaluated	(65)

The unique nature of the 3′-end telomeric overhang, which facilitates T-loop and G-quartet formation as reviewed above, has emerged as an attractive anticancer target (Fig. 1) (27,28,54). In particular, G-quartet-interactive agents have been rationally designed, to bind to these G-rich telomeric regions, and were found to inhibit telomerase activity (27,28,54–58).

First-Generation vs. Second-Generation TTAs

G-quartet-interactive compounds as telomerase-inhibitory agents were first described in 1997 by Sun et al. (59,60) who found that a 2,6-diamidoanthraquinone and cationic phorphyrin derivatives were able to disrupt G-quadruplex formation of telomeres during telomerase-dependent telomere extension. In addition, these drugs were capable of reducing telomerase activity in cancer cells and showed target effects at concentrations that were not generally cytotoxic (60). Other classes of early G-quartet-interactive agents include amidoanthracene-9,10-diones and ethidium derivatives (61,62). The development of most of the latter agents was stopped because of a marginal or no differential between cytotoxicity and telomerase inhibition owing to nonspecific DNA intercalation (duplex-DNA) and inhibition of DNA polymerases. In the case of the porphyrin analogs, their properties as photosensitizers may have further impeded their use as chronically administered tumor therapies. Nonetheless, the cationic porphyrin TMPyP4 was tested in animal tumor models, namely the prostate cancer xenograft PC3 and the breast cancer xenograft MX1 (50). TMPyP4 treatment led to increased survival of mice bearing MX-1 breast cancers in an adjuvant setting (after debulking of tumor with cyclophosphamide). It was also able to produce tumor growth inhibition in early-stage PC3 prostate cancer xenografts when given as monotherapy (50). Interestingly, PC3 prostate cancer cells have short telomeres (2.5–3 kb, Table 1) suggesting that prostate cancers owing to their relatively short telomere length status might respond to G-quadruplex-stabilizing anticancer drugs.

Because of such encouraging preclinical antitumor activity of G-quartet-interactive compounds, the second generation of G-quadruplex ligands were developed according to three criteria: (i) to display a strong inhibition of telomerase and to possess a large differential (at least one log-fold) between telomerase inhibition and induction of acute cell death; (ii) to selectively interact with/bind to G4 structures; and (iii) to lack nonspecific inhibition of *Taq* polymerases (27). As a result, small molecule pentacyclic acridines, trisubstituted acridines, triazines, 2,6-pyridine-dicarboxamide derivatives, and the natural product telomestatin have been designed or discovered by screening and found to fulfil these criteria (27,28,56–58,63–65,.

First- and second-generation G-quartet-interactive agents are summerized in Table 2.

Clinical Candidate Compounds with Activity in Prostate Cancer

Our laboratories have been involved in the preclinical development of two of the most promising lead compounds representative of the second generation G-quartet interactive agents, namely RHPS4 and BRACO19 (Table 2) (27,28,38,39,56,58). Both agents were evaluated in a panel of human tumor cell lines of variable telomere length and showed enhanced activity against tumors with shorter telomeres in vitro and in vivo (38,56,58,66). We could further demonstrate that RHPS4 and BRACO19 treatment leads to telomere shortening in the order of 0.5–1 kb before tumor cells "rapidly" enter replicative senescence (after ~15 days under continuous exposure to drug) and completely cease growth (38,39). This is consistent with a telomere uncapping mechanism caused by DNA-damaging signals at the telomeric G-strand after inducing it to fold into a 4-stranded guanine quadruplex structure (Fig. 2). We therefore proposed that RHPS4 and BRACO19 are TTAs that also inhibit telomerase by enforcing its displacement from the telomere, its translocation out of the nucleus and its rapid degradation into the cytoplasm (28,38,39).

For BRACO19, we could show single agent activity in an early-stage human uterus carcinoma xenograft model with short telomeres (2.7 kb) and that this activity was related to telomerase inhibition/lack of telomerase expression in responsive tumor tissues (39). Moreover, BRACO19 inhibited tumor re-growth after debulking of a short telomere vulval tumor with taxol (56). BRACO19 was therefore also evaluated for antitumor activity in vitro and in vivo in the human prostate cancer cell line DU145 with an average telomere length of 3.5 kb (Table 1). Consistent with the uterus and vulval carcinoma data, BRACO19 induced senescence more rapidly than would be expected solely by the inhibition of the catalytic function of telomerase. Occurrence of senescence was accompanied by an initial up-regulation of the tumor suppressor cyclin-dependent kinase inhibitor

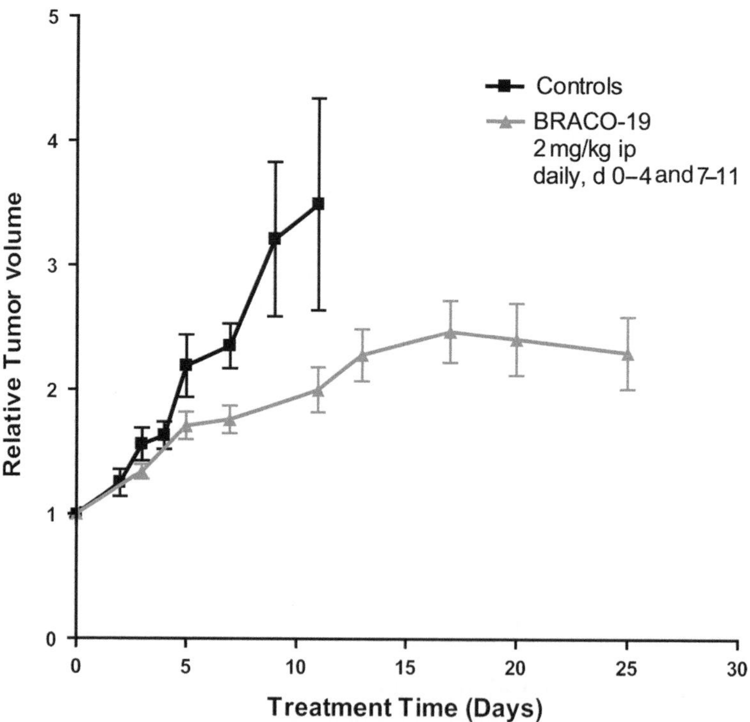

FIGURE 3 In vivo activity of BRACO19 in the DU145 prostate cancer xenograft model. Tumors were grown subcutaneous in nude mice and treatment initiated when they reached a size of 6–8 mm diameter ($n = 8$ mice/group). BRACO19 was administered at 2 mg/kg/day intraperitoneally once daily for five days and two consecutive cycles (on days 0–4 and 7–11). Tumor growth was followed by biweekly serial calliper measurements and calculated using the formula: $(\text{width}^2 \times \text{length})/2$.

p21 and extensive end-to-end chromosomal fusions indicative of telomere uncapping (51). This in vitro activity translates into marked in vivo antitumor efficacy (Fig. 3) (28). When BRACO19 was administered at 2 mg/kg/day intraperitoneally to DU145 tumor bearing nude mice for two consecutive weeks (on days 0–4 and 7–11), static tumor growth in the order of 90% to 100% inhibition compared to vehicle treated control tumors was observed. Notably antitumor activity was evident from only seven days after the start of treatment (d0) (Fig. 3).

RHPS4 has been evaluated for growth-inhibitory potential in 36 patient derived explants and xenografts of human tumor cell lines in a long-term (15 day) clonogenic assay in vitro (38). The mean 50% growth-inhibitory concentration (IC_{50}) over all 36 tumors was 11.4 μM. When the response to RHPS4 was compared to telomere length of the tumor lines, a positive correlation was found ($r = 0.75$) for enhanced sensitivity of tumors with shorter telomeres. The prostate cancer xenografts derived from PC3 and DU145 cell lines were among the five most sensitive tumors with IC_{50} of 23 nM and 1.9 μM, respectively, and were among the five tumors with the shortest telomeres (38).

Both, BRACO19 and RHPS4 are small molecule TTAs, which have very promising properties and potential for clinical development. They (or close relatives thereof) are currently undergoing lead optimization and toxicological evaluation and are anticipated to enter clinical trials in the near future (28).

FUTURE AND CLINICAL PERSPECTIVES

Clinically relevant agents targeting telomerase are eagerly awaited ever since the discovery of telomerase as a cancer-associated enzyme and our understanding of the differential telomere dynamics in normal and cancer cells (6,11,54). TTAs accomplish both that is the shortening and uncapping of telomeres as well as the inhibition of telomerase activity (39). This might in part explain their single agent and relatively rapid onset of activity against in vivo human tumor models with relatively short telomeres such as prostate cancers. G-quartet-based TTAs have an additional positive feature compared to template or catalytic subunit telomerase inhibitors in that they were shown to be active in human tumor cells that do not maintain telomere length by expression of telomerase. A very small portion of tumors maintain telomere length by an alternative lengthening (ALT) mechanism that is based on HR. G-quartet ligands can be effective against ALT tumor cells (56,58,63). This is of potential importance in the clinical applicability of TTAs as it is possible that ALT of telomeres might occur upon chronic enzyme inhibitor treatment as a mechanism of resistance. Thus, TTAs might not be susceptable to the development of drug resistance *via* this mechanism.

Because of the importance of telomerase reactivation and telomere length equilibrium at an early stage during tumorigenesis and prostate carcinogenesis in particular, it seems very plausible that the inhibition of the enzyme telomerase or one of its components and the proteins involved in the telomere/telomerase complex by targeted therapeutics or other telomerase directed approaches, will lead to inhibition of malignant transformation and tumor growth (Fig. 1). Thus, the telomerase inhibitors and specific TTAs highlighted in this chapter have the potential to become very valuable components in future prostate cancer treatment regimens and could therefore add to the rather limited current armamentarium of active drugs for the treatment of hormone-refractory prostate cancer.

Although a range of exciting and effective molecular therapeutics are being currently developed for the treatment of prostate and other cancers, it is clear that combination therapies will be required to ultimately combat multigenic cancers. Sophisticated drug cocktails or single drugs acting on multiple downstream targets will be needed for successful individualized and curative cancer therapy. We have found that the TTAs BRACO19 and RHPS4 can act additive to synergistic in combination with taxol and molecularly targeted agents such as the Hsp90 inhibitor 17-allylaminogeldanamycin or the cyclin-dependent kinase inhibitor flavopiridol (38,67).

TTAs hold therefore great promise for clinical activity and would be a valuable addition to our available anticancer agents.

REFERENCES

1. Blackburn EH. Telomere states and cell fates. Nature 2000; 408:53–56.
2. Keith NW, Evans JTR, Glasspool RM. Telomerase and cancer: time to move from a promising target to a clinical trial. J Pathol 2001; 195:404–414.
3. Hayflick L. Aging, longevity, and immortality in vitro. Exper Gerontol 1992; 27:363–368.
4. Harley CB, Fuchter BA, Greider CW. Telomeres shorten during ageing of human fibroblasts. Nature 1990; 345:458–460.
5. Hastie ND, Dempster M, Dunlop MC, et al. Telomere reduction in human colorectal carcinoma and with ageing. Nature 1990; 346:866–868.
6. Holt SE, Shay JW, Wright WE. Refining the telomere–telomerase hypothesis of aging and cancer. Nature Biotechnol 1996; 14:1734–1741.
7. Burger AM. Telomerase in cancer diagnosis and therapy. BioDrugs 1999; 12:413–422.
8. Feng J, Funk WD, Wang SS, et al. The RNA component of human telomerase. Science 1995; 269:1236–1241.
9. Nakamura TM, Morin GB, Chapman KB, et al. Telomerase catalytic subunit homologs from fission yeast and human. Science 1997; 277:955–959.
10. Greider CW. Chromosome first aid. Cell 1991; 67:645–647.
11. Kim NW, Piatyszek MA, Prowse KR, et al. Specific association of telomerase activity with immortal cells and cancer. Science 1994; 266:2011–2015.
12. Burger AM, Bibby MC, Double JA. Telomerase activity in normal and malignant mammalian tissues: feasibility of telomerase as target for cancer chemotherapy. Br J Cancer 1997; 75:516–522.
13. Shay JW, Bacchetti S. A survey of telomerase activity in human cancer. Eur J Cancer 1997; 33:787–791.
14. Greider CW. Telomere length regulation. Ann Rev Biochem 1996; 65:337–365.
15. Smith CD, Blackburn EH. Uncapping and deregulation of telomeres lead to detrimental cellular consequences in yeast. J Cell Biol 1999; 145:203–214.
16. Holt SE, Aisner DL, Baur J, et al. Functional requirement of p23 and Hsp90 in telomerase complexes. Genes Dev 1999; 13:817–826.
17. Forsythe HL, Jarvis JL, Turner JW, et al. Stable association of hsp90 and p23, but not hsp70, with active human telomerase. J Biol Chem 2001; 276:15,571–15,574.
18. Van Steensel B, de Lange T. Control of telomere length by the human telomeric binding protein TRF1. Nature 1997; 385:740–743.
19. Karlseder J, Broccoli D, Dai Y, et al. P53 and ATM-dependent apoptosis induced by telomeres lacking TRF2. Science 1999; 283:1321–1325.
20. Smith S, Giriat I, Schmitt A, et al. Tankyrase, a poly (ADP-ribose) polymerase at human telomeres. Science 1998; 282; 1484–1487.
21. Blasco MA. Telomeres in cancer and aging: lessons from the mouse. Cancer Lett 2003; 194:183–188.
22. Murti KG, Prescott DM. Telomeres of polytene chromosomes in a ciliated protozoan terminate in duplex DNA loops. Proc Natl Acad Sci USA 1999; 96:14,436–14,439.

23. Fang G, Cech TR. Characterization of a G-quartet formation reaction promoted by the beta-subunit of the Oxytricha telomere-binding protein. Biochemistry 1993; 32:11,646–11,657.
24. de Lange T. Protection of mammalian telomeres. Oncogene 2002; 21:532–540.
25. Parkinson GN, Lee MP, Neidle S. Crystal structure of parallel quadruplexes from human telomeric DNA. Nature 2002; 417:876–880.
26. Neidle S, Parkinson GN. The structure of telomeric DNA. Curr Opin Struct Biol 2003; 13:275–283.
27. Kelland RL. Telomerase: biology and Phase I trials. Lancet Oncol 2001; 2:95–102.
28. Kelland LR. Overcoming the immortality of tumour cells by telomere and telomerase based cancer therapeutics—current status and future prospects. Eur J Cancer 2005; 41:971–979.
29. Norton JC, Piatyszek MA, Wright WE, et al. Inhibition of human telomerase activity by peptide nucleic-acids. Nat Biotechnol 1996;14:615–619.
30. Dikmen ZG, Gellert GC, Jackson S, et al. In vivo inhibition of lung cancer by GRN163L: a novel human telomerase inhibitor. Cancer Res 2005; 65:7866–7873.
31. Gellert GC, Dikmen ZG, Wright WE, et al. Effects of a novel telomerase inhibitor, GRN163L, in human breast cancer. Breast Cancer Res Treat 2005; 96: 73–81. Epub ahead of print.
32. Damm K, Hemmann U, Garin-Chesa P, et al. A highly selective telomerase inhibitor limiting human cancer cell proliferation. EMBO J 2001; 20:6958–6968.
33. Burger AM, Double JA, Newell DR. Inhibition of telomerase activity by cisplatin in human testicular cancer cells. Eur J Cancer 1997; 33:638–644.
34. Ishibashi T, Lippard SJ. Telomere loss in cells treated with cisplatin. Proc Natl Acad Sci USA 1998; 95:4219–4223.
35. Hendriks H, Dai F, Rademaker B, et al. The novel compound KML001 induces telomere attrition, senescence and chromosomal instability in tumor cell lines with short telomeres. Eur J Cancer 2004; S2(8):130.
36. Schrader M, Burger AM, Müller M, et al. The differentiation status of primary gonadal germ cell tumors correlates inversely with telomerase activity and the expression level of the gene encoding the catalytic subunit of telomerase. BMC Cancer 2002; 2. www.biomedcentral.com/1471–2407/2/32.
37. Burger AM, Harnden, P. Telomerase in germ cell tumours: inhibition of telomerase activity after cisplatin-based therapy. In: Jones I, Appelyard I, Harnden P, Joffe J, eds. Germ Cell Tumours IV. London: John Libbey & Co. Ltd., 1998:73–80.
38. Cookson JC, Dai F, Smith V, et al. Pharmacodynamics of the G-quadruplex-stabilizing telomerase inhibitor 3,11-difluoro-6,8,13-trimethyl-8H-quino(4,3,2-kl) acridinium methosulfate (RHPS4) in vitro: activity in human tumor cells correlates with telomere length and can be enhanced, or antagonized, with cytotoxic agents. Mol Pharmacol 2005; 68: 1551–1558.
39. Burger AM, Dai F, Schultes CM, et al. The G-quadruplex interactive molecule BRACO19 inhibits tumor growth, consistent with telomere binding and interference with telomerase function. Cancer Res 2005; 65:1489–1496.
40. Villa R, Folini M, Porta CD, et al. Inhibition of telomerase activity by geldanamycin and 17-allylamino, 17-demethoxygeldanamycin in human melanoma cells. Carcinogenesis 2003; 24:851–859.
41. Seimiya H, Muramatsu Y, Tomokazu O, et al. Tankyrase 1 as a target for telomere-directed molecular cancer therapeutics. Cancer Cell 2005; 7:25–37.
42. Wright WE, Shay JW. Mechanism-based combination telomerase inhibition therapy. Cancer Cell 2005; 7:1–2.
43. Bodnar AG, Ouellette M, Frolkis M, et al. Extension of life-span by introduction of telomerase into normal human cells. Science 1998; 279:349–352.
44. Hahn WC, Counter CM, Lundberg AS, et al. Creation of human tumour cells with defined genetic elements. Nature 1999; 400:464–468.
45. Hahn WC, Stewart SA, Brooks MW, et al. Inhibition of telomerase limits the growth of human cancer cells. Nat Med 1999; 5:1164–1170.
46. Shay JW. Telomerase therapeutics: telomeres recognized as a DNA damage signal. Clin Cancer Res 2003; 9:3521–3525.

47. Burger AM, Fiebig HH, Kuettel MR, et al. Effect of oncogene expression on telomerase activation and telomere length in human endothelial, fibroblast and prostate epithelial cells. Int J Oncol 1998; 13:1043–1048.
48. Sommerfeld JH, Meeker AK, Piatyszek MA, et al. Telomerase activity: a prevalent marker of malignant human prostate tissue. Cancer Res 1996; 56:218–222.
49. Meeker AK, Hicks JL, Platz EA, et al. Telomere shortening is an early somatic DNA alteration in human prostate tumorigenesis. Cancer Res 2002; 62:6405–6409.
50. Grand LC, Han H, Munoz RM, et al. The cationic porphyrin TMPyP4 down-regulates c-myc and human telomerase reverse transcriptase expression and inhibits tumor growth in vivo. Mol Cancer Ther 2002;1:566–573.
51. Incles CM, Schultes CM, Kempski H, et al. A G-quadruplex telomere targeting agent produces p16-associated senescence and chromosomal fusions in human prostate cancer cells. Mol Cancer Ther 2004; 3:1201–1206.
52. Wellinger RJ, Sen D. The DNA structures at the ends of eukaryotic chromosomes. Eur J Cancer 1997; 33:735–749.
53. Wang Y, Patel DJ. Solution structure of the human telomeric repeat d[AG3(T2AG3)3] G-tetraplex. Structure 1993; 1:263–282.
54. D'Incalci M, Zupi G. Are we close to the clinical development of novel drugs targeting telomeres and telomerase?. Eur J Cancer 2005; 41:970.
55. Sharma S, Raymond E, Soda H, et al. Preclinical and clinical strategies for development of telomerase and telomere inhibitors. Ann Oncol 1997; 8:1063–1074.
56. Read M, Harrison RJ, Romagnoli B, et al. Structure-based design of selective and potent G quadruplex-mediated telomerase inhibitors. Proc Natl Acad Sci USA 2001; 98:4844–4849.
57. Riou JF, Guittat L, Mailliet P, et al. Cell senescence and telomere shortening induced by a new series of specific G-quadruplex DNA ligands. Proc Natl Acad Sci USA 2002; 99:2672–2677.
58. Gowan S, Heald R, Stevens MFG, et al. Potent inhibition of telomerase by small-molecule pentacyclic acridines capable of interacting with G-quadruplexes. Mol Pharmacol 2001; 60:981–968.
59. Sun D, Thompson B, Cathers BE, et al. Inhibition of human telomerase by a G-quadruplex-interactive compound. J Med Chem 1997; 40:2113–2116.
60. Izbicka E, Wheelhouse RT, Raymond E, et al. Effects of cationic prophyrins as G-quarduplex interactive agents in human tumour cells. Cancer Res 1999; 59:639–644.
61. Perry PJ, Reszka AP, Wood AA, et al. Human telomerase inhibition by regioisomeric disubstituted amidoanthracene-9–10-diones. J Med Chem 1998; 41:4873–4884.
62. Koeppel F, Riou JF, Laoui A, et al. Ethidium derivatives bind to G-quartets, inhibit telomerase and act as fluorescent probes for quadruplexes. Nucl Acids Res 2001; 29(5):1087–1096.
63. Pennarun G, Granotier C, Gauthier LR, et al. Apoptosis related to telomere instability and cell-cycle alterations in human glioma cells treated by new highly selective G-quadruplex ligands. Oncogene 2005; 24:2917–2928.
64. Gomez D, Aouali N, Londono-Vallejo A, et al. Resistance to the short term antiproliferative activity of the G-quadruplex ligand 12459 is associated with telomerase overexpression and telomere capping alteration. J Biol Chem 2003; 278:50,554–50,562.
65. Kim MY, Gleason-Guzman M, Izbicka E, et al. The different biological effects of telomestatin and TMPyP4 can be attributed to their selectivity for interaction with intramolecular or intermolecular G-quadruplex structures. Cancer Res 2003; 63: 3247–3256.
66. Gowan SM, Harrison JR, Patterson L, et al. A G-quadruplex-interactive potent small-molecule inhibitor of telomerase exhibiting in vitro and in vivo antitumour activity. Mol Pharmacol 2002; 61:1154–1156.
67. Incles CM, Schultes CM, Kelland LR, et al. Acquired cellular resistance to flavopiridol in a human colon carcinoma cell line involves up-regulation of the telomerase catalytic subunit and telomere elongation: sensitivity of resistant cells to combination treatment with a telomerase inhibitor. Mol Pharmacol 2003; 64:1101–1108.

13 Expanding the Role of EGFR Inhibitors in Prostate Cancer

Srikala S. Sridhar
Department of Medicine, Juravinski Cancer Center, McMaster University, Hamilton, Ontario, Canada

Malcolm J. Moore
Department of Medicine and Pharmacology, Princess Margaret Hospital, University of Toronto, Toronto, Ontario, Canada

INTRODUCTION

Prostate cancer is the most frequently diagnosed malignancy in North American men and the second leading cause of cancer-related death, accounting for an estimated 33,000 deaths annually (1). The standard first-line therapy for advanced prostate cancer is androgen deprivation therapy and although initially effective in controlling the disease progression to androgen-independent prostate cancer (AIPC) is inevitable. This critical step is associated with an increased expression of growth factors and receptors capable of establishing autocrine and/or paracrine growth stimulatory loops. The epidermal growth factor receptor (EGFR) family and its ligands which promote cell-cycle progression, inhibition of apoptosis, angiogenesis, tumor cell motility, metastases, and is involved in the pathogenesis and progression of several human cancers have been implicated in this process (2). During progression to androgen independence, EGFR expression increases which correlates with a worse overall prognosis, making the EGFR a relevant therapeutic target in prostate cancer (3). A novel class of anti-cancer agents that specifically inhibit EGFR signaling have recently entered clinical trials in a wide range of cancer types. In prostate cancer, they are being evaluated as monotherapy and in combination with hormonal therapy, radiation therapy, chemotherapy, and other targeted agents at various stages of the disease.

EGFRs AND THEIR LIGANDS

The EGFR family consists of four distinct, but structurally similar, tyrosine kinase receptors, which are encoded by the proto-oncogenes c-erbB1/EGFR/EGFR1 (referred to as EGFR), c-erbB2/HER2 (referred to as HER2), c-erbB3/HER3, and c-erbB4/HER4 (4). The EGFR and HER4 receptors have an extracellular ligand binding domain, a transmembrane domain, and an intracellular tyrosine kinase domain. The HER2 receptor has no known cognate ligand but strong tyrosine kinase activity, whereas the HER3 receptor has little or no tyrosine kinase activity (Fig. 1A) (5). Both HER2 and HER3 are therefore dependent on heterodimerization with other members of EGFR family in order to activate downstream signaling pathways (6). The EGFR also exists in a deletion-mutant form, EGFRvIII, which is formed by a 267-amino acid in-frame deletion and insertion of a glycine in the fusion junction of the extracellular domain. This leads to ligand-independent

(A)

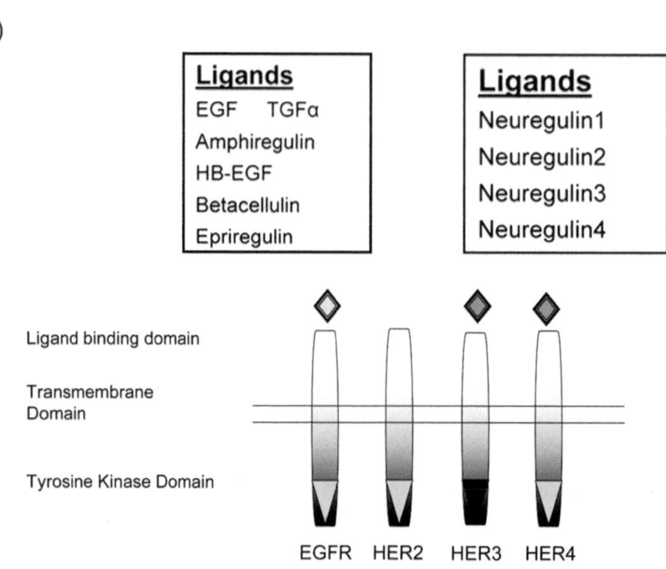

(B)

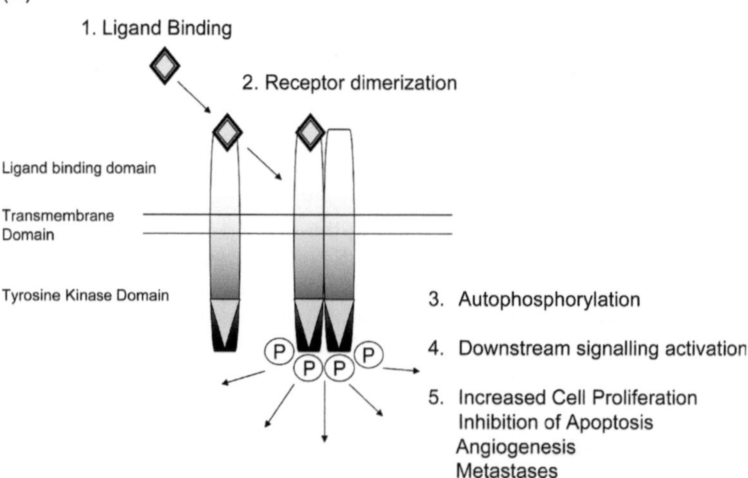

FIGURE 1 (**A**) EGFR family of receptors. Only EGFR, HER2, and HER4 possess intrinsic TK activity. There is no known ligand for HER2. EGF, TGFα are the key stimulatory ligands for EGFR. Amphiregulin, Betacellulin, HB-EGF, Epiregulin, and Neuregulin are other ligands interacting with the EGFR family. (**B**) EGF binding to the receptor, dimerization, autophosphorylation (P), signaling cascade. Dimerization occurs between identical receptors (homodimers), or between two different members of the EGFR family (heterodimers), leading to a range of downstream responses including cell proliferation, inhibition of apoptosis and angiogenesis. *Abbreviations*: EGFR, epidermal growth factor receptor; HB-EGF, heparin-binding EGF-like growth factor; HER, human epidermal growth factor receptor; TGFα, transforming growth factor alpha; TK, tyrosine kinase. *Source*: From Ref. 4.

constitutive EGFR activity signaling via the PI3 kinase cascade which can then result in uncontrolled cell proliferation and growth (7,8).

Several endogenous ligands for EGFR are known, but the most important stimulatory ligands which are overexpressed in some cancers, are the epidermal growth factor (EGF) and transforming growth factor alpha (TGFα). Ligand binding results in receptor homo- or heterodimerization with internalization of the receptor–ligand complex and tyrosine autophosphorylation which activates downstream signaling pathways, such as the ERK and PI3 kinase pathways. This triggers a cascade of physiological responses involved in cell proliferation, cell survival, angiogenesis, and potentially metastasis (Fig. 1B) (9).

EGFRs AND PROSTATE CANCER

Advances in our understanding of cell signaling suggest that the EGFR family of receptors and its ligands may play an important role, not only in the development of prostate cancer, but also in the critical step of progression to androgen independence. Cross-talk between the EGFR and androgen receptor (AR), may result in activation of AR transcriptional function even in the absence of androgens, leading to cell proliferation and survival. EGFR signaling increases AR trans activation by promoting phosphorylation of the p160 family co-activator transcription intermediary factor 2/glucocorticoid receptor interacting protein 1 and increasing its interaction with the AR (10). In terms of EGFR expression in the prostate, the most interesting data comes from Di Lorenzo et al., who have shown that in 41% of patients post-radical prostatectomy, 76% of patients post-radical prostatectomy with preoperative androgen ablation, and 100% patients with hormone-refractory metastatic disease, EGFR expression was detected and correlated significantly with a high Gleason score ($p < 0.01$) and high prostate-specific antigen (PSA, $p < 0.02$). EGFR expression was also an independent prognostic indicator of disease relapse after radical prostatectomy (3). These results are in agreement with a study from Scher et al. (11) that showed a homogeneous staining pattern for EGFR in 17 of 19 AIPC specimens.

Overexpression of HER2, may also activate the AR transcriptional function via the ERK or Akt pathways. In vitro, forced HER2 inhibition leads to impairment of AR-mediated functions, such as androgen-stimulated growth and the induction of endogenous PSA mRNA and protein. Androgen-stimulated recruitment of the AR and histone acetylation at the androgen response enhancer of the PSA gene were also affected by HER2 inhibition. Like EGFR signaling, HER2 signaling may thus regulate the phosphorylation status of co-activator proteins that interact with the AR (12).

Although the HER2 receptor is an important prognostic indicator in breast cancer, the exact role of HER2 expression in the development and progression of prostate cancer remains controversial. In HRPC, recent studies suggest that increased HER2 expression is linked to the development of metastatic disease, and a worse overall prognosis (13,14). Interestingly in hormone-sensitive prostate cancer, the opposite may be true. High levels of both HER2 and HER4 were associated with increased time to biochemical relapse and increased overall survival (13). In contrast, EGFRvIII expression in HRPC is associated with a shorter time to biochemical relapse, and decreased overall survival. This latter finding may be due both to EGFRvIII-mediated constitutive activation of the PI3K/Akt cascade in combination with loss of phosphate and tensin homolog deleted on chromosome ten

(PTEN) a common mutation found in prostate cancer, which results in cell proliferation and growth (15).

The EGF network also consists of a group of ligands, of which EGF and TGFα have been shown to increase both the proliferation and the survival of prostate cancer cells (16,17). Recently, increased expression of two other ligands of the EGFR family, amphiregulin and epiregulin, have been reported in an androgen-sensitive prostate cancer xenograft following castration, which may promote the development of AIPC (18).

Collectively, these results suggest that the EGFR family of receptors and ligands may have multiple roles in prostate cancer, and their expression alone cannot be used to necessarily predict the biological response. This is an important consideration as we move forward with anti-EGFR targeted therapies. Identifying and better understanding the role of EGFR and its ligands in prostate cancer could help to identify subsets of patients that are more likely to benefit from these novel treatment approaches.

TARGETING THE EGFR FAMILY IN PROSTATE CANCER

The EGFR family can be targeted therapeutically using either small molecules, which inhibit the tyrosine kinase domain of the receptor, or monoclonal antibodies. The use of each of these in the setting of prostate cancer will be discussed below.

TYROSINE KINASE INHIBITORS

The tyrosine kinase inhibitors are small molecules that compete with and prevent binding of adenosine triphosphate to the intracellular tyrosine kinase region. These agents cause tumor regression by increasing apoptosis and by inhibiting cellular proliferation and angiogenesis. The two compounds that are the most advanced in development are gefitinib and erlotinib, although several other agents are undergoing both preclinical and clinical evaluation.

Gefitinib (Iressa™, ZD 1839, Astra Zeneca Pharmaceuticals LP, Wilmington, DE 19850-5437)

Gefitinib, is an orally administered quinazoline-based molecule that reversibly inhibits EGFR tyrosine kinase autophosphorylation, resulting in reduced c-fos mRNA, a transcription factor-forming part of the AP-1 complex and a shift of cells from S Phase into G_0/G_1 (19). In the prostate cancer cell lines PC3 and DU145, gefitinib has shown inhibition of EGF-induced activation of the PI3K/AKT pathway. Gefitinib can also induce increased expression of both nuclear and cytoplasmic p27Kip1 and potentiate the anti-proliferative activity of both the anti-androgen flutamide and ionizing radiation suggesting a potential role for gefitinib use in combination with these conventional therapies (20). In prostate cancer xenografts studies, daily gefitinib treatment has been shown to have growth inhibitory effects both as monotherapy and in combination with the anti-androgen, bicalutamide (21).

In Phase I studies of gefitinib (150–1000 mg/day), the most frequent adverse events were nausea, vomiting, an acneiform rash, and diarrhea, the latter two becoming dose-limiting at the maximum tolerated dose (MTD) of 800 mg/day (22). The skin was particularly susceptible to the effects of gefitinib largely because EGFR is highly expressed in both keratinocytes and in cells of eccrine and sebaceous glands (23). Antitumor activity was seen at all dose levels, without evidence of a dose–response relationship. The doses chosen for Phase II/III investigations were 250 and 500 mg/day, doses at which both antitumor activity and pharmacokinetics consistent with preclinical activity were routinely seen (22).

The National Cancer institute of Canada-Clinical Trials Group recently reported a randomized Phase II study of two doses of gefitinib in HRPC. Forty patients with increasing PSA or progression of measurable disease who had not received prior chemotherapy were randomly assigned to 250 mg ($n = 19$) or 500 mg ($n = 21$) oral gefitinib daily continuously. The primary end points were PSA response rate (defined as a 50% decrease from baseline confirmed by a second PSA four weeks later) and objective response in measurable disease (using response evaluation criteria in solid tumors criteria). Quality of life (QOL) assessments were performed at baseline and during treatment. Gefitinib did not result in any PSA responses, or objective responses in either treatment arm. QOL assessments demonstrated symptomatic worsening compared with baseline. The most common drug-related nonhematologic toxicities were grade 1–2 diarrhea, fatigue, and grade 1–2 skin rash (24). Similar findings were also reported by Schroder and Wildhagen, who conducted a placebo-controlled, double-blind randomized Phase II study of gefitinib (500 mg/day) in 58 patients with progressive HRPC. There were no differences seen in clinical progression rates between the two arms (25). Gefitinib also failed to show PSA responses in another Phase II study evaluating a dose of 500 mg/day. Fifty-one patients entered the study. Of 28 patients assessable for a PSA response only one patient had a PSA response (26).

Clearly the clinical experience with gefitinib as monotherapy in HRPC has been disappointing. As yet it is unclear whether this is due to the fact that the EGFR is simply a poor target in HRPC, or if these agents would be more effective if used in earlier stages of the disease where tumor burden is less, or as suggested by recent preclinical data, that these agents may be more effective when used in combination with other agents or radiation. Patient selection may also play an important role, as has been seen in the lung cancer setting, where gefitinib shows increased activity in a distinct subsets of patients.

Clinical trials are currently underway aimed at answering these important questions. In a Phase II study, patients with locally advanced prostate cancer are treated with docetaxel and gefitinib neoadjuvantly, followed by radical prostatectomy. The main outcomes are pathologic complete response, margin positivity, PSA response, clinical response, and toxicity. This study is particularly interesting in that it will allow examination of treatment effect at the tissue level. A second combination study, examines the role of gefitinib 250 mg/day with radiotherapy in nonmetastatic prostate cancer. The primary objectives are safety and tolerability with secondary outcomes being EGFR expression and activation status at diagnosis. In patients with early biochemical failure post-prostatectomy, a Phase II trial is underway to look at the effect of 250 mg/day gefitinib monotherapy on PSA response, partial PSA response rate, and duration of response. These studies, if positive, may suggest a role for gefitinib in earlier stages of the disease or in combination regimens which may serve to delay or prevent the development of AIPC.

The use of gefitinib in combination with targeted therapies is another interesting area. The most advanced in this regard is a Phase I/II trial, which examines the combination of the mTor inhibitor Everolimus and gefitinib in HRPC. This trial is based on the fact that one of the most commonly found mutations in prostate cancer is the loss of the tumor suppressor gene PTEN, which promotes tumorigenesis and may contribute to gefitinib resistance. By treating concurrently with Everolimus, and gefitinib, this resistance could potentially be overcome and gefitinib sensitivity restored. The primary end points of this study are safety and efficacy.

Other combination approaches are at the preclinical stages of development. These include gefitinib with bicalutamide, which in vitro results in dual inhibition of the AR and EGFR/HER2 pathways and preclinically causes a delay in the onset of androgen independence (27). Another approach combines gefitinib with an antisense to the MDM2 gene, which causes synergistic in vitro growth inhibition. MDM2 is a negative p53 regulator which interacts with retinoblastoma, E2F, $p19^{arf}$ and the ERK pathway and has been associated with disease progression and poor prognosis in prostate cancer (28).

In summary, though the initial clinical trial results with gefitinib have been disappointing, the results from the ongoing trials will likely provide us with important information as to how this new class of biologically targeted agents should optimally be used.

Erlotinib (Tarceva™, CP-358774, OSI 774, OSI Pharmaceuticals, Inc., Melville, NY 11747)

Erlotinib, an anilino-quinazoline derivative is an orally active EGFR inhibitor that can induce both cell-cycle arrest in G_1 and apoptosis. It inhibits EGFR autophosphorylation with a selectivity of >1000-fold over other tyrosine kinase inhibitors producing approximately 70% reduction in EGFR-associated phosphotyrosine 24-hour after a single 100 mg/kg dose (29). Erlotinib also interferes with signaling via the variant receptor EGFRvIII (30). Phase I studies showed that diarrhea, rash, nausea, headache, emesis, and fatigue were the most frequent side effects. At 200 mg/day, diarrhea was dose-limiting, but manageable with loperamide therapy or dose reduction to 150 mg/day. The 150 mg/day dose of erlotinib was thus selected for subsequent studies based on its safety and tolerability profile and pharmacokinetic parameters (29). In contrast, the 250 and 500 mg/day doses of gefitinib chosen for clinical trials were much lower than the MTD for gefitinib which is 800 mg/day raising questions about appropriate dosing of anti-EGFR therapies.

There is much less data on the use of erlotinib in the setting of prostate cancer. There are two Phase II trials of erlotinib monotherapy in hormone-refractory, chemotherapy-naïve prostate cancer. The main outcomes of interest being clinical benefit, PSA response rate, overall survival, and toxicity. Two combination studies with erlotinib are also open. In one, erlotinib is combined with docetaxel in older patients with progressive hormone-refractory disease. The main objective of this study is to determine the rate and duration of response. The second study is an early stage study, which combines erlotinib with the anti-angiogenic agent bevacizumab in patients at high risk for early relapse following radical prostatectomy. The primary outcome is time to biochemical failure evidenced by rising PSA, overall survival and safety and tolerability of this regimen. Taken together these trials with erlotinib will provide us with added information regarding the use of this class of agents in prostate cancer. In the lung cancer setting, it is interesting to note that erlotinib, appears to be more effective than gefitinib, although it is unclear whether this is due to the drug itself or issues around dosing, as has been previously discussed.

GW572016 (Tykerb™, Lapatanib, GlaxoSmithKline, Research Triangle Park, North Carolina, 27709)

GW572016 is a 6-thiazolyquinazoline, reversible, dual kinase inhibitor of both EGFR and HER2 kinases. In human xenograft studies, GW572016 has shown dose-dependent kinase inhibition and appears to selectively target tumor cells overexpressing EGFR or HER2 (31). The main toxicities associated with GW572016 were gastrointestinal symptoms, rash, and headache (32). As both EGFR and HER may play a key role in the pathogenesis prostate cancer, GW572016 could prove to be particularly effective. In one Phase II trial, patients with hormone-refractory disease, who have had no prior chemotherapy, are treated with GW572016 orally. The main objectives of this study are PSA response rate, time to progression, and safety. Again it will be interesting to compare with the results from the gefitinib and erlotinib trials. GW572016 is also being evaluated in two trials in early stage disease, following biochemical failure, but prior to initiation of hormonal therapy. The main objectives are PSA response rate and duration, safety and tolerability, and overall survival. One of these studies is expected to complete accrual for the first stage by mid-2006.

PKI166 (Novartis Pharma AG, Basel, Switzerland)

PKI166, a pyrrolo [2,3,-*d*] pyrimidine derivative, is a dual EGFR/HER2 tyrosine kinase inhibitor, that has recently undergone preclinical evaluation in prostate cancer. Mellinghoff et al. have shown that using PKI-166 resulted in EGFR/HER2 pathway inhibition, which in turn caused reduced AR transcriptional activity. Additional genetic and pharmacologic experiments further suggested that this modulation of the AR function is mediated by the HER2/HER3 dimerization pathway and not by EGFR. The HER2/HER3 signal appears to play a critical role in stabilizing the AR protein levels and optimize binding of the AR to promoter/enhancer regions of androgen-regulated genes. Another key finding of this study was that the serine–threonine kinase Akt/protein kinase B (PKB), which lies immediately downstream of the HER2/HER3 dimer appears to not be involved in activation of the AR (33). Overall this data suggest that the HER2/HER3 pathway may be a critical target in hormone-refractory prostate cancer. Phase I trials with PKI166 have found elevations in liver enzymes to be dose-limiting. Other milder toxicities included vomiting, diarrhea, fatigue, and skin rash. The recommended Phase II dose was either 600 or 750 mg in a 2-week on/off scheme as this was well tolerated (34). Based on interesting preclinical data, this compound may warrant further evaluation in the Phase II setting though no trials are currently underway.

MONOCLONAL ANTIBODIES

Another approach to targeting the EGFR is the use of monoclonal antibodies. The compound with which we have the most clinical experience is by far Traztuzumab (Herceptin), which targets the HER2 receptor. Other monoclonal antibodies, such as cetuximab (IMC-C225) directed against the EGFR have also been evaluated in the Phase III clinical setting in various cancer types.

Traztuzumab (Herceptin™, F. Hoffman-La Roche Ltd., Basel, Switzerland)

Traztuzumab is a humanized monoclonal antibody directed against the extracellular HER2 domain. It has clinically proven antitumor activity in breast cancer, where HER2 expression correlates strongly with a worse prognosis (35,36). As discussed, the role of HER2 in prostate cancer remains unclear. In preclinical studies, traztuzumab monotherapy had antitumor activity only in the androgen-dependent xenograft models but not in androgen-independent models. In combination with paclitaxel however antitumor activity was enhanced in both models. In clinical studies, traztuzumab monotherapy is well tolerated, but has failed to show single-agent efficacy in hormone-refractory prostate cancer (37). In combination with docetaxel and estramustine, Small et al. (38) showed traztuzumab was safe, but response data were too preliminary at the time of the report. There are two other studies examining traztuzumab and docetaxel in HRPC. One closed for nonfeasibility due to HER 2-positivity rates of <20% by IHC, and another is ongoing with results pending at this time (39). To date, clinical trials with traztuzumab in prostate cancer have not been particularly encouraging.

Cetuximab (Erbitux™ IMC-C225 ImClone Systems Incorporated, New York, NY 10014, Bristol-Myers Squibb Company, Princeton, NJ 08543)

Cetuximab is a human:murine chimeric anti-EGFR IgG monoclonal antibody that competitively binds to the extracellular ligand-binding domain of EGFR, preventing tyrosine kinase activation, inhibiting cell growth, and in some cases inducing apoptosis (40). It binds to the EGFR with higher affinity than its naturally occurring ligands and has shown preclinical activity alone and in combination in prostate cancer. Prewett et al. initially demonstrated in vitro that cetuximab blocked EGF-induced receptor activation and induced internalization of the receptor in both androgen-sensitive and resistant cell lines. In vivo, cetuximab alone or with doxorubicin significantly inhibited tumor progression of well-established DU145 and PC-3 xenografts in nude mice (41). In vitro the combination of cetuximab and perifosine (an Akt inhibitor) has shown synergistic antitumor effects in PTEN-deficient cells, however perifosine is a poorly tolerated drug, which may limit further development of this combination (42). More exciting, however, is the data from Karashima et al. (43) showing enhanced antitumor activity with the combination of paclitaxel and cetuximab in an androgen-independent xenograft model. As the taxanes are currently the standard of care for HRPC the addition of cetuximab, if well-tolerated could be another therapeutic strategy.

ABX-EGF (Panitumumab, Amgen Inc. Thousand Oaks, CA, 91320–1799)

ABX-EGF is a fully humanized IgG2 monoclonal antibody with a higher binding affinity for EGFR than cetuximab. It inhibits tyrosine phosphorylation in a dose-dependent manner, due to both blockade of the EGF binding site on the receptor, and to rapid internalization of EGFR (44). In preclinical studies, ABX-EGF inhibited prostate tumor proliferation in vitro, and EGF-induced production of angiogenic factors IL8 and VEGF. ABX-EGF monotherapy inhibited PC3 and DU145 cells in xenografts models, and when combined with doxorubicin led to cooperative antitumor activity. At the clinical level, ABX-EGF was generally well tolerated, with only a transient acneiform skin rash (45). Two Phase II studies examining ABX-EGF in hormone resistant prostate cancer have completed accrual with results pending at this time.

Pertuzumab (Omnitarg™, rhuMAb 2C4, F. Hoffman-La Roche Ltd., Basel Switzerland)

2C4 is an antibody against the ectodomain of HER2 at a site distinct from that of traztuzumab. It acts specifically by inhibiting the association of HER2 with other members of the EGFR family, and is noncross-reactive with traztuzumab. Preclinical information suggests that 2C4 will inhibit the growth of both androgen-dependent and androgen-independent prostate tumors grown as xenografts in athymic mice (46). A Phase I study of 2C4 administered every three weeks demonstrated safety and activity in prostate cancer leading to a Phase II study. Although no responses were observed, stabilization of disease was observed in a small number of patients with taxane resistant hormone-refractory prostate cancer (47). Further studies are required to confirm this result.

Combination EGFR Targeted Therapy

Pre-clinical studies suggest that combining distinct classes of EGFR inhibitors may serve to potentiate antitumor effects and overcome inherent or acquired resistance to a single class of EGFR inhibitor. Xenograft studies in prostate cancer using combinations specifically of gefitinib and traztuzumab have unfortunately been disappointing and likely will not be pursued into the clinical setting (48,49).

DISCUSSION

Over the past decade, numerous molecules that contribute to proliferation, invasion, and metastasis of cancer cells have been identified. The EGFR which is overexpressed by many tumors and associated with poor prognosis has become a key target of novel anticancer therapies, especially in the treatment of prostate cancer that remains an incurable disease especially in the advanced stages.

The two major classes of compounds specifically targeting EGFR include the tyrosine kinase inhibitors and the monoclonal antibodies. Gefitinib, a tyrosine kinase inhibitor, has unfortunately shown disappointing results in three Phase II studies in HRPC. Phase II trials are currently underway with the other tyrosine kinase inhibitors namely erlotinib, GW572016, and PKI166, with preliminary results expected in the next year. Among the monoclonal antibodies, traztuzumab, an anti-HER2 antibody, demonstrating significant clinical benefit in breast cancer, has failed to show activity in prostate cancer. Three other monoclonal, cetuximab, ABX-EGF, and pertuzumab, are currently undergoing clinical evaluation.

Although, the anti-EGFR agents have often demonstrated activity in the preclinical models, the negative results of clinical trials in prostate cancer emphasize that preclinical models may not reliably predict clinical response. Potential reasons include the presence of redundancy in the EGFR signaling systems, alternate active signaling cascades, or inherent mutations, such as PTEN which may contribute to resistance. In contrast to conventional therapies, toxicity and antitumor activity of biological therapies may not correlate and specific biological assays and pharmacologically guided studies may be required to determine the most effective dose of these agents. A greater emphasis on generating pre- and posttreatment tumor banks, may further allow us to better understand these therapies at the molecular level and determine why they have not been effective.

Other issues include whether anti-EGFR therapies should be administered as monotherapy or with conventional therapies, such as radiation, hormonal therapy, or chemotherapy as well as the optimal timing and sequencing of their administration with these therapies. It is unclear if anti-EGFR agents may be more effective if used earlier in the time course of the disease, such as in the neoadjuvant or adjuvant settings, where both tumor burden and resistance mechanisms may be less. The issue of combined anti-EGFR therapy, using agents that target more than one member of the EGFR family and combinations of EGFR targeting agents or combinations with other biological agents with different mechanisms of action, has yet to be fully addressed clinically. The negative clinical results of the anti-EGFR therapies as monotherapy in HRPC, force us to address many of these issues and will impact future clinical trial design.

Recent experience with anti-EGFR therapies in lung cancer, has raised issues related to patient selection for these therapies. It is not clear for example, that it is necessary for tumors to express or to overexpress the receptor to derive benefit, and the best method for assaying this expression using either immunohistochemistry or fluorescence in situ hybridization has not been established. In addition, it appears patients with specific mutations in the EGFR receptor may have increased antitumor effects of the anti-EGFR agents. A recent paper has highlighted that in prostate cancer, race contributes significantly to variability of EGFR expression and this may have important implications as we evaluate these agents further (50). Our increasing knowledge into the molecular biology of cell signaling may further help to identify biomarkers that will help predict response or resistance to novel biological agents.

In conclusion, anti-EGFR-directed therapies will continue to be evaluated in prostate cancer. By addressing the issues of dosage, duration, scheduling, sequencing, concurrent therapies, and patient selection the true efficacy will be determined. Considerable research is still required, but the positive results seen in other tumor types justify further evaluation of EGFR as a therapeutic target in prostate cancer.

REFERENCES

1. Jemal A, Murray T, Ward E, et al. Cancer statistics, 2005. CA Cancer J Clin 2005; 55(1):10–30.
2. Mendelsohn J, Baselga J. Status of epidermal growth factor receptor antagonists in the biology and treatment of cancer. J Clin Oncol 2003; 21(14):2787–2799.
3. Di Lorenzo G, Tortora G, D'Armiento FP, et al. Expression of epidermal growth factor receptor correlates with disease relapse and progression to androgen-independence in human prostate cancer. Clin Cancer Res 2002; 8(11):3438–3444.
4. Sridhar SS, Seymour L, Shepherd FA. Inhibitors of epidermal-growth-factor receptors: a review of clinical research with a focus on non-small-cell lung cancer. Lancet Oncol 2003; 4(7):397–406.
5. Barton J, Blackledge G, Wakeling A. Growth factors and their receptors: new targets for prostate cancer therapy. Urology 2001; 58(2 suppl 1):114–122.
6. Sweeney C, Carraway KL III. Negative regulation of ErbB family receptor tyrosine kinases. Br J Cancer 2004; 90(2):289–293.
7. Olapade-Olaopa EO, Moscatello DK, MacKay EH, et al. Evidence for the differential expression of a variant EGF receptor protein in human prostate cancer. Br J Cancer 2000; 82(1):186–194.
8. Olapade-Olaopa EO. The expression of a mutant epidermal growth factor receptor in prostatic tumours. BJU Int 2001; 87(3):224–226.
9. Arteaga CL. Overview of epidermal growth factor receptor biology and its role as a therapeutic target in human neoplasia. Semin Oncol 2002; 29(5 suppl 14):3–9.

10. Gregory CW, Fei X, Ponguta LA, et al. Epidermal growth factor increases coactivation of the androgen receptor in recurrent prostate cancer. J Biol Chem 2004; 279(8):7119–7130.
11. Scher HI, Sarkis A, Reuter V, et al. Changing pattern of expression of the epidermal growth factor receptor and transforming growth factor alpha in the progression of prostatic neoplasms. Clin Cancer Res 1995; 1(5):545–550.
12. Liu Y, Majumder S, McCall W, et al. Inhibition of HER-2/neu kinase impairs androgen receptor recruitment to the androgen responsive enhancer. Cancer Res 2005; 65(8):3404–3409.
13. Edwards J, Traynor P, Munro AF, Pirret CF, Dunne B, Bartlett JM. The role of HER1-HER4 and EGFRvIII in hormone-refractory prostate cancer. Clin Cancer Res 2006; 12(1):123–130.
14. Hernes E, Fossa SD, Berner A, Otnes B, Nesland JM. Expression of the epidermal growth factor receptor family in prostate carcinoma before and during androgen-independence. Br J Cancer 2004; 90(2):449–454.
15. Moscatello DK, Holgado-Madruga M, Emlet DR, Montgomery RB, Wong AJ. Constitutive activation of phosphatidylinositol 3-kinase by a naturally occurring mutant epidermal growth factor receptor. J Biol Chem 1998; 273(1):200–206.
16. Schuurmans AL, Bolt J, Veldscholte J, Mulder E. Regulation of growth of LNCaP human prostate tumor cells by growth factors and steroid hormones. J Steroid Biochem Mol Biol 1991; 40(1–3):193–197.
17. Lin J, Adam RM, Santiestevan E, Freeman MR. The phosphatidylinositol 3′-kinase pathway is a dominant growth factor-activated cell survival pathway in LNCaP human prostate carcinoma cells. Cancer Res 1999; 59(12):2891–2897.
18. Torring N, Hansen FD, Sorensen BS, Orntoft TF, Nexo E. Increase in amphiregulin and epiregulin in prostate cancer xenograft after androgen deprivation-impact of specific HER1 inhibition. Prostate 2005; 64(1):1–8.
19. Wakeling AE, Guy SP, Woodburn JR, et al. ZD1839 (Iressa): An orally active inhibitor of epidermal growth factor signaling with potential for cancer therapy. Cancer Res 2002; 62(20):5749–5754.
20. Sgambato A, Camerini A, Faraglia B, et al. Targeted inhibition of the epidermal growth factor receptor-tyrosine kinase by ZD1839 ('Iressa') induces cell-cycle arrest and inhibits proliferation in prostate cancer cells. J Cell Physiol 2004; 201(1):97–105.
21. Sirotnak FM, She Y, Lee F, Chen J, Scher HI. Studies with CWR22 xenografts in nude mice suggest that ZD1839 may have a role in the treatment of both androgen-dependent and androgen-independent human prostate cancer. Clin Cancer Res 2002; 8(12):3870–3876.
22. Herbst RS, Maddox AM, Rothenberg ML, et al. Selective oral epidermal growth factor receptor tyrosine kinase inhibitor ZD1839 is generally well-tolerated and has activity in non-small-cell lung cancer and other solid tumors: results of a Phase I trial. J Clin Oncol 2002; 20(18):3815–3825.
23. Albanell J, Rojo F, Averbuch S, et al. Pharmacodynamic studies of the epidermal growth factor receptor inhibitor ZD1839 in skin from cancer patients: Histopathologic and molecular consequences of receptor inhibition. J Clin Oncol 2002; 20(1):110–124.
24. Canil CM, Moore MJ, Winquist E, et al. Randomized Phase II study of two doses of gefitinib in hormone-refractory prostate cancer: a trial of the National Cancer Institute of Canada-Clinical Trials Group. J Clin Oncol 2005; 23(3):455–460.
25. Schroder FH, Wildhagen MF. ZD1839 (gefitinib) and hormone resistant (HR) prostate cancer—final results of a double blind randomized placebo-controlled Phase II study [abstr 4698]. Proc Am Soc Clin Oncol 2004; 22:430s.
26. Rosenthal M, Toner GC, Gurney H, et al. Inhibition of the epidermal growth factor receptor (EGFR) in hormone refractory prostate cancer (HRPC): Initial results of a Phase II trial of gefitinib [abstr 1671]. Proc Am Soc Clin Oncol 2003; 21:416.
27. Festuccia C, Gravina GL, Angelucci A, et al. Additive antitumor effects of the epidermal growth factor receptor tyrosine kinase inhibitor, gefitinib (Iressa), and the nonsteroidal antiandrogen, bicalutamide (Casodex), in prostate cancer cells in vitro. Int J Cancer 2005; 115(4):630–640.
28. Bianco R, Caputo R, Damiano V, et al. Combined targeting of epidermal growth factor receptor and MDM2 by gefitinib and antisense MDM2 cooperatively inhibit hormone-independent prostate cancer. Clin Cancer Res 2004; 10(14):4858–4864.

29. Hidalgo M, Siu LL, Nemunaitis J, et al. Phase I and pharmacologic study of OSI-774, an epidermal growth factor receptor tyrosine kinase inhibitor, in patients with advanced solid malignancies. J Clin Oncol 2001; 19(13):3267–3279.
30. Iwata KK, Provoncha K, Gibson N. Inhibition of mutant EGFRvIII transformed cells by tyrosine kinase inhibitor OSI774 (Tarceva) [abstr 79]. Proc Am Soc Clin Oncol 2002; 21:21a.
31. Xia W, Mullin RJ, Keith BR, et al. Anti-tumor activity of GW572016: a dual tyrosine kinase inhibitor blocks EGF activation of EGFR/erbB2 and downstream Erk1/2 and AKT pathways. Oncogene 2002; 21(41):6255–6263.
32. Bence AK, Anderson EB, Halepota MA, et al. Phase I pharmacokinetic studies evaluating single and multiple doses of oral GW572016, a dual EGFR-ErbB2 inhibitor, in healthy subjects. Invest New Drugs 2005; 23(1):39–49.
33. Mellinghoff IK, Vivanco I, Kwon A, Tran C, Wongvipat J, Sawyers CL. HER2/neu kinase-dependent modulation of androgen receptor function through effects on DNA binding and stability. Cancer Cell 2004; 6(5):517–527.
34. Hoekstra R, Dumez H, Eskens FA, et al. Phase I and pharmacologic study of PKI166, an epidermal growth factor receptor tyrosine kinase inhibitor, in patients with advanced solid malignancies. Clin Cancer Res 2005; 11(19 Pt 1):6908–6915.
35. Slamon DJ, Godolphin W, Jones LA, et al. Studies of the HER-2/neu proto-oncogene in human breast and ovarian cancer. Science 1989; 244(4905):707–712.
36. Press MF, Jones LA, Godolphin W, Edwards CL, Slamon DJ. HER-2/neu oncogene amplification and expression in breast and ovarian cancers. Prog Clin Biol Res 1990; 354A:209–221.
37. Ziada A, Barqawi A, Glode LM, et al. The use of traztuzumab in the treatment of hormone refractory prostate cancer; Phase II trial. Prostate 2004; 60(4):332–337.
38. Small EJ, Bok R, Reese DM, Sudilovsky D, Frohlich M. Docetaxel, estramustine, plus traztuzumab in patients with metastatic androgen-independent prostate cancer. Semin Oncol 2001; 28(4 suppl 15):71–76.
39. Lara PN Jr., Chee KG, Longmate J, et al. Traztuzumab plus docetaxel in HER-2/neu-positive prostate carcinoma: final results from the California Cancer Consortium Screening and Phase II Trial. Cancer 2004; 100(10):2125–2131.
40. Herbst RS, Langer CJ. Epidermal growth factor receptors as a target for cancer treatment: the emerging role of IMC-C225 in the treatment of lung and head and neck cancers. Semin Oncol 2002; 29(1 suppl 4):27–36.
41. Prewett M, Rockwell P, Rockwell RF, et al. The biologic effects of C225, a chimeric monoclonal antibody to the EGFR, on human prostate carcinoma. J Immunother Emphasis Tumor Immunol 1996; 19(6):419–427.
42. Li X, Luwor R, Lu Y, Liang K, Fan Z. Enhancement of antitumor activity of the anti-EGF receptor monoclonal antibody cetuximab/C225 by perifosine in PTEN-deficient cancer cells. Oncogene 2005.
43. Karashima T, Sweeney P, Slaton JW, et al. Inhibition of angiogenesis by the antiepidermal growth factor receptor antibody ImClone C225 in androgen-independent prostate cancer growing orthotopically in nude mice. Clin Cancer Res 2002; 8(5):1253–1264.
44. Yang XD, Jia XC, Corvalan JR, Wang P, Davis CG. Development of ABX-EGF, a fully human anti-EGF receptor monoclonal antibody, for cancer therapy. Crit Rev Oncol Hematol 2001; 38(1):17–23.
45. Foon KA, Yang XD, Weiner LM, et al. Preclinical and clinical evaluations of ABX-EGF, a fully human anti-epidermal growth factor receptor antibody. Int J Radiat Oncol Biol Phys 2004; 58(3):984–990.
46. Agus DB, Akita RW, Fox WD, et al. A potential role for activated HER-2 in prostate cancer. Semin Oncol 2000; 27(6 suppl 11):76–83; discussion 92–100.
47. Agus DB, Sweeney CJ, Morris M, et al. Efficacy and safety of single agent pertuzumab (rhuMAB 2C4), a HER dimerization inhibitor, in hormone refractory prostate cancer after failure of taxane based therapy [abstr 4624]. Am Soc Clin Oncol 2005; 23:408s.
48. Formento P, Hannoun-Levi JM, Gerard F, et al. Gefitinib–traztuzumab combination on hormone-refractory prostate cancer xenograft. Eur J Cancer 2005; 41(10):1467–1473.

49. Formento P, Hannoun-Levi JM, Fischel JL, Magne N, Etienne-Grimaldi MC, Milano G. Dual HER 1–2 targeting of hormone-refractory prostate cancer by ZD1839 and traztuzumab. Eur J Cancer 2004; 40(18):2837–2844.
50. Shuch B, Mikhail M, Satagopan J, et al. Racial disparity of epidermal growth factor receptor expression in prostate cancer. J Clin Oncol 2004; 22(23):4725–4729.

14 Bone-Directed Therapy in Prostate Cancer: Rationale and Novel Approaches

Colby L. Eaton, Kate D. Linton, and Freddie C. Hamdy
Academic Urology, University of Sheffield, Royal Hallamshire Hospital, Sheffield, U.K.

"All reasoning from statistics is liable to many errors. The best work in the pathology of cancer is now done by those who are studying the nature of the seed. He who turns over the records of cases of cancer is only a ploughman, but his observation of the properties of the soil may also be useful."

Stephen Paget, 1889

ABSTRACT

The recognition that prostate cancer cells preferentially metastasize to the skeleton in patients with advanced disease has led to the development of new therapies not only directed to the cancer cell, but also specifically targeted towards altering the bone microenvironment into a less favorable "soil" for tumor growth and survival. These new and exciting strategies are based around three key concepts that describe the processes involved in tumor metastasis to bone: the first is that prostate cancer cells preferentially bind to endothelial cells in the marrow sinusoids in a way that allows them to be retained and to enter the bone marrow proper. The second is that once tumor cells have passed through the sinusoid walls into the marrow they benefit from growth and/or survival factors already present in this environment, with the marrow acting as a 'fertile soil.' The third concept is that when established in bone, prostate cancer cells become involved in a so-called "vicious cycle" where they induce modification of bone turnover resulting in the increased production or release of factors that benefit their growth. Suppression of the latter process has been the focus of some of the most recent advances in bone-directed therapies for prostate cancer. This chapter will review these new approaches and their efficacy, but will also discuss developments in other areas that might be exploited to suppress prostate cancer growth in bone.

PRIMARY CONSIDERATIONS IN THE EVALUATION OF NEW TREATMENTS IN PROSTATE CANCER

The design of new treatments for prostate cancer faces challenges on two fronts. Firstly, there is a need to develop new approaches to suppress the growth of established, hormone-refractory metastatic disease in advanced patients. The primary aim of this may not be to provide a cure but more realistically to induce extended remission with good life quality so that patients can complete their natural lives without significant curtailment by their disease. In prostate cancer patients, developments in this area are in the treatment of bone metastases, specifically targeting the proposed "vicious cycle" present in established disease. Secondly, with better detection of early cancer at a pre/perimetastatic stage there is a need to define strategies that will prevent the metastatic process occurring. The aim of the latter would potentially be curative, an objective that would be more likely to be achievable in these patients than those with advanced disease, and that would clearly be more valuable in a potentially younger population of patients.

In patients with advanced disease, recent developments have gone some way to delivering the goal of inhibiting the onset of symptoms associated with extensive skeletal metastases. In this group, measures of success would be suppression of increases in tumor volume associated with relapse from antiandrogen-based treatments, and elimination of the morbidity caused by tumor-induced bone disease, such as pathological fractures and other skeletal-related events (SREs).

TREATMENT OF ESTABLISHED BONE METASTASES: TARGETING THE "VICIOUS CYCLE"

Bisphosphonate Therapy in Patients with Prostate Cancer

Bisphosphonates are organic analogs of pyrophosphate that bind to bone matrix with high affinity (1). Binding to the skeleton is very rapid with blood clearance rates and accumulation in bone taking place within minutes of intravenous injection. This characteristic enables these compounds to be very effectively delivered to the bone microenvironment where they can be concentrated and potentially released by bone resorption. The latter process is the function of osteoclasts. These are specialized cells of macrophage lineage generated by fusion of circulating monocytic cells under the appropriate conditions in locations where bone remodeling is required. When these cells resorb bisphosphonate-containing bony matrices they take up these compounds. At the concentrations available in bone, this inhibits an important metabolic pathway (mevalonate pathway and farnesyl diphosphate synthase) with the effect of inducing programmed cell death or apoptosis in affected osteoclasts (Fig. 1) (2,3).

The nitrogen-containing bisphosphonates, such as zoledronic acid (ZA) have particular potency in suppressing the activity of existing osteoclasts and in inhibiting the recruitment and maturation of osteoclast progentors (3). These compounds have been shown to be very effective in the treatment of osteoporosis and in metabolic bone diseases, such as Paget's disease (3). In the context of the treatment of bone metastases in prostate cancer patients the effects of bisphoshonate treatments are potentially three-fold. First, the suppression of osteoclast action prevents bone lysis and associated weakening of the axial skeleton that could result in fracture. Second, the suppression of resorption would be expected to interfere with the "vicious cycle" proposed to provide established metastases with a continuing supply of factors that aid their survival in bone, and third a direct antitumor effect has been demonstrated in preclinical studies, but has yet to prove its efficacy in patients (4). A summary of the interacting signaling thought to be involved in this cycle is provided in Figure 2.

To date, bisphosphonates have been evaluated most extensively in cancer patients where osteolytic lesions predominate (breast cancer and myeloma) (5,6). However, bone resorption and new bone production are integrated processes

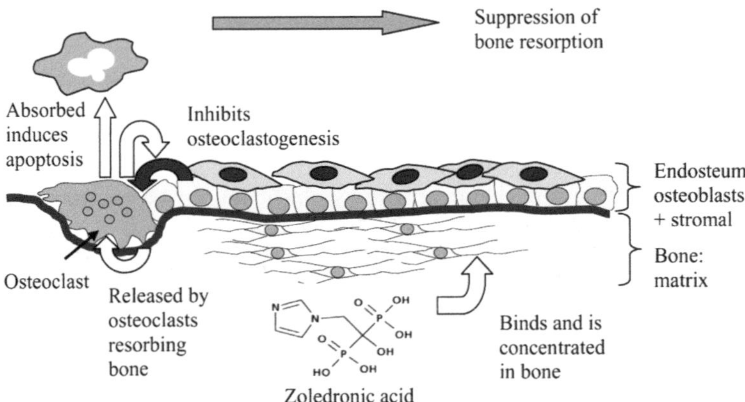

FIGURE 1 Mechanism of action of bisphosphonates. Nitrogen-containing bisphosphonates like zoledronic acid bind with high affinity to bony matrices and are released by the lytic action of osteoclasts. The released bisphosphonates are taken up by osteoclasts and induce apoptosis in these cells leading to suppression of bone remodeling.

and is not surprising that bisphosphonates have also been shown to reduce biochemical markers of bone resorption in patients with osteoblastic bone lesions resulting from advanced prostate cancer (7–9). Again, although these lesions are largely osteoblastic, their generation has a lytic phase and clinical studies assessing effects of bisphosphonate treatment on bone pain and analgesic usage have shown some benefit for this therapy. However until recently randomized, placebo-controlled trials of bisphosphonates had not shown a significant reduction in skeletal complications from bone metastases in prostate cancer patients (8–23).

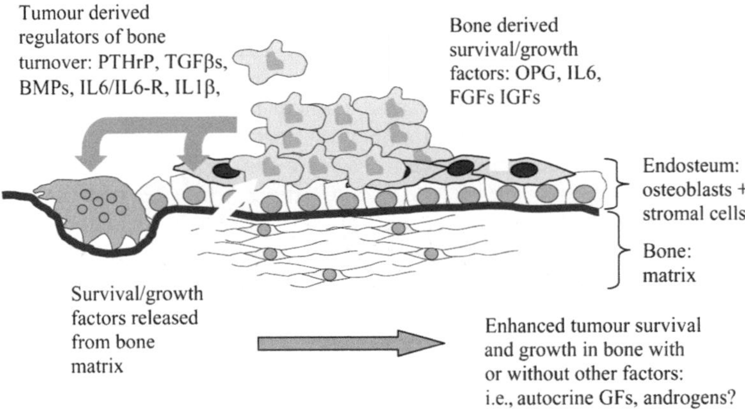

FIGURE 2 The "vicious cycle" in established bone metastases. Tumor-derived factors increase bone turnover and release/produce bone-derived factors that in turn facilitate the growth and survival of tumor cells. These factors include PTHrP, TGFβs, BMPs, IL6/IL6-R, IL1β, OPG, FGFs, and IGFs. *Abbreviations*: PTHrP, parathyroid hormone-related protein; TGFβs, transforming growth factor betas; BMPs, bone morphogenetic proteins; IL6/IL6-R, interleukin 6 and its receptor; IL1β, interleukin 1 beta; OPG, osteoprotegerin; IL6, interleukin 6; FGFs, fibroblast growth factors; IGFs, insulin-like growth factors; GF, growth factor.

The rationale for testing and using bisphosphonates in the management of advanced prostate cancer can be summarized as follows:

1. In hormone-independent metastatic prostate cancer
   a. To improve analgesia from bone pain.
   b. To prevent SREs, such as the need for radiation, pathologic fractures, spinal cord compression, change in antineoplastic therapy, hypercalcemia of malignancy.
   c. To delay the onset of SREs.

2. In hormone-sensitive prostate cancer
   a. To prevent symptomatic disease progression in metastatic disease.
   b. To prevent skeletal metastasis in patient with MO disease.

In early trials with small patient numbers treated with etidronate or clodronate no significant differences between bisphosphonate therapy and placebo control groups were seen.

A meta-analysis of two multicenter randomized controlled trials in a total of 350 patients with androgen-independent prostate cancer receiving intravenous pamidronate versus placebo with end points of relieving pain and reducing SREs showed a reduction in bone resorption markers, but no significant benefit to the patients otherwise (24).

The Medical Research Council in the United Kingdom has performed a Phase Three trial of oral clodronate in 311 men with metastatic bone disease from prostate cancer. Quite a high dose of oral clodronate (Loron™ F. Hoffmann-La Roche Ltd, Basel, Switzerland 1040 mg twice daily) was administered for a median duration of 43 months. The final analysis showed that after a median follow-up of 59 months, the sodium clodronate group showed statistically nonsignificant improvement in bone progression-free survival, but an increase in gastrointestinal side effects attributed to the bisphosphonate-treated group (25).

Despite the failures of other bisphosphonates, ZA was investigated in patients with advanced prostate cancer to determine if the increased potency of this compound would translate into improved clinical benefits for this patient population. Six-hundred and forty-three patients with hormone-refractory prostate cancer (HRPC) and documented bone metastases were randomized to one of the three different treatment groups: 4 mg ZA ($n = 214$), 8 mg ZA ($n = 221$), or placebo ($n = 208$). In the 8 mg arm, the dose was reduced by a protocol amendment to 4 mg because of concerns over renal safety, and conclusions on the efficacy of this cohort are difficult to make. Zoledronic acid or placebo were administered as a 15-minute, 100-ml intravenous infusion every three weeks for 15 months followed by an extension phase of a further 10 months. All patients received daily oral supplements of calcium and vitamin D. The primary end point was the proportion of patients with a skeletal event. Secondary end points included the time to first skeletal complication, an Andersen–Gill multiple-event analysis, levels of bone pain, and biochemical markers of bone resorption.

Zoledronic acid was significantly more effective than placebo across all primary and secondary end points. The ZA 4 mg treatment group achieved significant reductions in the proportion of patients with any skeletal complication (33% vs. 44% with placebo; $P = 0.021$) or pathologic fracture (13% vs. 22% with placebo; $P = 0.015$) compared with the placebo group. Furthermore, there were consistent reductions in the proportion of patients with each type of skeletal complication, including nonvertebral fractures. Zoledronic acid 4 mg was still significantly superior to placebo when fractures were excluded indicating that the beneficial effect was not simply as a result of the prevention of osteoporotic fractures. Zoledronic acid also prolonged the time to first skeletal complication by more than four months ($P = 0.011$). Using the Andersen–Gill multiple-event analysis, it was calculated that ZA 4 mg reduced the overall risk of skeletal complications by 36%.

Zoledronic acid reduced bone pain compared with placebo at all time points, and these differences were significant at three and nine months. Significant reductions in markers of bone resorption were documented for the ZA group compared with the placebo group throughout the duration of the study. These effects were shown to be sustained in an updated follow-up report (26). However, despite the favorable effects on skeletal morbidity, there were no significant effects on disease-related end points, such as time to progression and survival.

These studies focus on the benefits of suppression of tumor-induced bone disease in order to prevent SREs and their associated morbidity. However, the central question remains: Do bisphosphonates reduce/prevent prostate tumor growth and survival in bone by interfering with the vicious cycle? Animal studies using prostate cancer xenografts suggest that although the numbers of lytic lesions and overall tumor volumes are decreased in animals bearing intraosseous tumors, tumor cells are still present in large numbers in these lesions. Suppression of the vicious cycle therefore does not appear to be critical to survival in these models. Figure 3 illustrates this phenomenon, whereby tumors in animals treated with ZA (left panel) retain trabecular bone but also viable tumor cells albeit at lower numbers than in untreated control animals (right panel) (27).

This suggests that targeting the vicious cycle may not be ultimately effective in suppressing tumor growth, but it should be remembered that the cell lines used in these models are poorly differentiated with a capacity for autonomous growth in vitro so that they may not be representative of the comparatively well-differentiated, slow-growing tumors seen in patients at least during the early phase of metastasis. The latter would be more likely to depend on bone marrow-derived factors.

Aside from effects on the vicious cycle and bone turnover, bisphosphonates have been shown to have direct antitumor activity in prostate cancer cells lines grown in vitro (4,28). Specifically, these cells have been shown to be growth

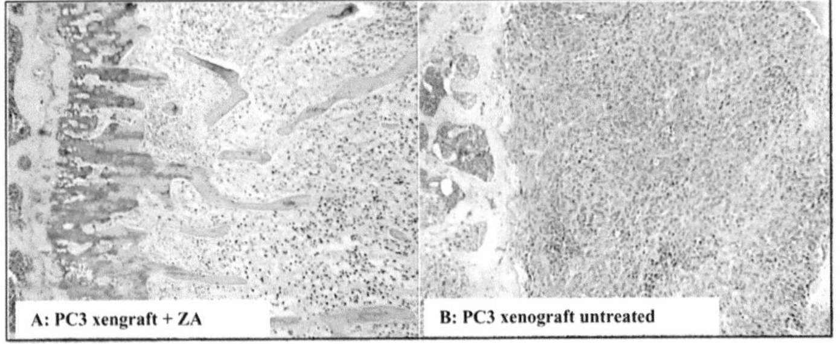

FIGURE 3 (*See color insert*) Prostate cancer xenografts± ZA. Histology (H&E) of prostate tumor (PC3) intratibial xenografts grown in athymic mice with (**A**) or without (**B**) ZA treatment. *Abbreviation*: ZA, zoledronic acid.

inhibited at relatively high doses (in excess of 10 μM) and to be induced to undergo apoptosis at this and higher doses. These effects appear to be mediated via inhibition of the mevalonate pathway with subsequent failure in protein prenylation (2). In the case of apoptosis, this appears to result from inhibition of the Ras translocation/signaling function leading to activation of the intrinsic pathway for caspase and apoptosis activation via mitochondrial release of protein kinase C (2,4,29,30). These effects have only been reported at high concentrations in vitro and it is unlikely that prostate tumor populations would be exposed to such levels in vivo even in bone. Indeed there is no evidence that outside the skeleton, in subcutaneous or orthotopic sites, bisphosphonates have any effect on tumor growth in experimental models (4,29,31). There is some evidence that lower doses of bisphosphonates (submicromolar) can affect tumor attachment to bone matrix which may indicate their usefulness in the inhibition of establishment of metastases as discussed below. The detailed role of bisphosphonates in cancer-induced bone disease has been recently extensively reviewed (4).

Endothelin-Selective Receptor Antagonists in the Treatment of Prostate Cancer

Endothelins are 21 amino-acid peptides first characterized in 1988. Three endothelin subtypes, endothelins 1–3, have been identified that bind to two classes of receptors ET_A and ET_B with the latter binding all three endothelins, mediating clearance, while the former binds ET1/2-mediating activity (32,33). Much of the characterization of activity is based on studies of endothelin1 (ET1). This peptide is a potent vasoconstrictor but has also been shown to mediate pain perception. ET1 is produced by a variety of cell types including vascular endothelial cells and normal and malignant prostatic epithelial cells (34). Plasma concentrations of ET1 have been shown to be raised in the patients with metastatic prostate cancer compared to those with organ-confined disease (35). In vitro, ET1 is a mitogen for prostate cancer cells and enhances the effects of other mitogens (36). In addition to effects on tumor cells themselves, ET1 is also a potential mediator of interactions involved in the "vicious cycle" being shown to contribute to the formation of osteosclerotic bone lesions in prostate cancer in vivo (37). An ET_A receptor-selective antagonist has been recently studied that inhibits ET1-induced growth of prostate cancer cells in vitro and in vivo and reduces the growth of skeletal metastases in vivo (38). Interestingly, the effect was mediated through the effect of $ET1_A$ receptor antagonist on osteoblasts rather that through the cancer cells which did not require to express the receptor: a prime example of the ability to affect tumor growth by altering the bone microenvironment, independently from the cancer cell (39). This agent has been evaluated in Phases I–III clinical trials in prostate cancer patients (37). In the latter, patients with metastatic prostate cancer with signs of biochemical progression following androgen ablation treated with the ET_A receptor antagonist showed significant reduction in bone turnover markers. Effects of this agent on the suppression of tumor burden in bone in these patients require further clinical trials which are currently underway.

Combination Therapies

The aim of combination therapies is to target both the primary cancer cell and the bone microenvironment simultaneously. Recent advances suggest for the first time that systemic chemotherapy using taxanes improves both survival and quality-of-life in patients with HRPC (40,41).

Ideally, treatments could be given simultaneously to target proliferation of the cancer cell directly, its biological behavior through key pathways, and to alter the fertile soil represented by the bone microenvironment in the case of prostate cancer, to prevent tumor growth and survival. Studies in both prostate cancer and other tumor types suggest that there may be advantages in combining bisphosphonate treatments with other small molecules or chemotherapeutic agents. In breast cancer cell lines grown in vitro, sequence-specific combinations of doxorubicin with ZA have been shown to be more effective than either agent alone in inducing apoptosis (42). More complex approaches using agents targeting growth factor signaling (imatinib mesylate, an inhibitor of platelet-derived growth factor signaling) in combination with ZA and the cell cycle inhibitor paclitaxel have recently demonstrated significant suppression of tumor incidence and size with preservation of bone structure in intraosseous xenografts of human prostate cancer cells grown in athymic mice. This study also showed very significant decreases in the frequency of lymph node metastases in animals receiving the three-agent combination treatment compared with control animals or animals receiving single agents or combinations of any two treatments. This study highlights the potential value of targeting heterogenous tumors with a multimodality approach including that focused on bone turnover (43).

PREVENTION OF METASTASIS: TARGETING THE ESTABLISHMENT OF BONE METASTASES

An analysis of 1376 autopsies of patients with advanced disease by Saitoh et al. in 1984 (44) suggested that while most (~83%) had metastases in multiple organs at the time of death (i.e., >2 organs involved), of those who had single or two organs involved, between a third and 50% had bone metastases: the most common distant site in all patients. More recent similar studies have shown that greater than 85% of patients with metastatic prostate cancer have bone metastases (45). These studies underline the established clinical observation that the skeleton is a preferred site of metastasis in prostate cancer at least initially, acting as a "fertile soil" where these tumors can survive and grow. Importantly, the above study also suggests that skeletal metastases may act as a launch pad for further rounds of metastasis of cells that no longer need the bone marrow resulting in the colonization of more vital organ systems. Clearly blockade of the establishment of a foothold in bone would obviate the need for the treatment of advanced disease in bone or potentially elsewhere. Of particular interest in this context are patients with cancer apparently localized to the prostate (stage T1/T2) but in whom micrometastases, undetectable by current methods, may be suspected. Less than 60% of these patients might be expected to be metastasis free 10 years after diagnosis and it would be important to be able to offer this group additional treatment to suppress the development of metastases in addition to the radical surgery many would receive. This is particularly important since early diagnosis initiatives are leading to increasing numbers of patients diagnosed and treated in this category.

Recent studies using animal models of tumor growth in bone have indicated that metabolically active bone may be more susceptible to tumor colonization than quiescent bone (46). In these studies murine melanoma cells were injected into animals that were either intact (control) or in which increased bone turnover had been induced by ovariectomy. Tumor growth and lytic bone disease was shown to be increased in the ovariectomized animals. These studies provide evidence to support the existence of a "vicious cycle" in tumor–bone interactions suggesting that active bone turnover can induce increased tumor growth. To date, there have been no definitive, published studies to support this type of process using prostate cancer models. However, it is possible that castration of prostate cancer patients, while suppressing the growth of androgen-sensitive cancers, could enhance the growth of surviving androgen-insensitive cells in bone, by inducing increased bone turnover. This has yet to be fully explored experimentally but, if shown to be the case, would suggest that bisphosphonate suppression of bone turnover in combination with castration could benefit patients at an early stage in their disease.

Studies investigating the effects of bisphosphonates in preventing skeletal metastasis have failed to date to show any beneficial effects in patients with locally advanced, nonmetastatic disease. The Medical Research Council (MRC) PRO4 study investigated 508 patients with clinical stage T2–4 M0, testing oral clodronate versus placebo for five years. Treatments received included external beam irradiation $\pm$ hormones and hormones alone. End point consisted of time to development of symptomatic bone metastases or prostate cancer-specific death, and median follow-up was seven years. Overall survival was 78% at five years, and there were no significant differences in all end points between the two groups (47). A further study investigated ZA versus placebo in 398 patients with progressing, hormonally escaping nonmetastatic prostate cancer. The primary end point was time to development of metastases. The study however closed before completion of accrual as there were too few events to demonstrate meaningful results, and there was no difference in time to first event between the two groups (48). However, it should be noted that both studies were not focused on patients with early disease with low risk of pre-existing micrometastases.

Potential modifications of the "soil" that appear to induce alterations in metastases rates have been demonstrated in tumor types other than prostate cancer. In particular, strain differences have been shown to provide more than a 10-fold difference in the frequency of metastases in mammary cancer models (49). Together these findings suggest that particular features of the host (genetic predisposition) and the metabolic activity of the preferred site of metastasis could greatly influence the establishment of metastases. Such characteristics could be used to target therapies and if fully understood, could predict susceptibility to metastasis in patients where spread of the tumor is suspected but not currently demonstrable. There are a number of candidate pathways potentially responsible for the favored site status of the skeleton for prostate cancer metastasis.

Survival/Growth Factors Present in Bone at the Time of Metastasis

Osteoprotegerin

Osteoprotegerin (OPG) is an abundant protein in the normal bone microenvironment where it is an important regulator of osteoclastogenesis, acting as a decoy receptor for receptor activation of nuclear factor κ B (RANK) ligand and inhibiting the RANK/receptor activation of nuclear factor κ B ligand (RANKL) interactions between bone marrow cells and osteoclast progenitors. This signaling system is central to the formation of mature osteoclasts so that the presence of OPG acts as a brake on bone lysis where this process requires control. Circulating OPG levels have been shown to be elevated in prostate cancer patients with advanced cancer compared to those with organ-confined disease (50) and it has been suggested that this may be a result of increased bone turnover in an environment favoring osteosclerotic bone disease (51). However, other studies have demonstrated that OPG is produced and secreted by prostate cancer cells (52) so circulating levels of this protein may be a reflection of production by tumor cell themselves rather than a result of cancer-induced bone remodeling.

The effects of OPG on suppression of bone resorption have resulted in its consideration as a potential therapeutic agent targeting the vicious cycle in established bone metastases. However, OPG has additional activities that could aid tumor survival. These are considered here in the context of early colonization of bone. Recent studies have demonstrated that OPG derived from either bone marrow stromal cells or from prostatic cancer cells can protect the latter from apoptosis by acting as a soluble decoy receptor for the proapoptotic cytokine tissue necrosis factor (TNF) related apoptosis-inducing ligand (TRAIL) (52,53). TRAIL is produced by monocytes and potentially other cell types throughout adult tissues and the presence of OPG in the bone marrow, where it is primarily involved in regulating bone turnover, could offer a protective advantage for low numbers of tumor cells arriving in bone (Fig. 4). Once established in high numbers in bony lesions, bone-derived OPG may become less important as tumor-derived OPG becomes sufficient to sustain survival. Targeting bone marrow-derived OPG at the time of metastasis may therefore be a useful strategy for preventing metastasis by increasing their vulnerability to TRAIL before they have the opportunity to form

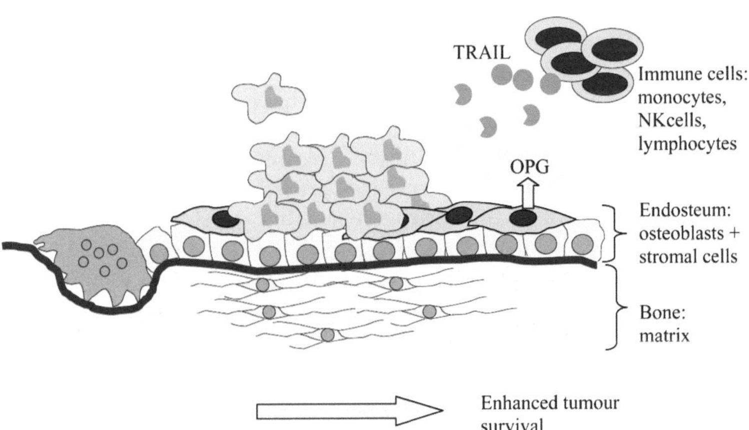

FIGURE 4 Proposed role of OPG in establishment of metastases in bone. OPG produced by bone marrow stromal cells and osteoblasts provide an environment where the effects of TRAIL are suppressed. This provides a relatively safe haven for low numbers of metastasizing tumor cells not yet present at sufficient numbers to generate enough OPG for their own protection. *Abbreviations*: OPG, osteoprotegerin; TRAIL, TNF-related apoptosis-inducing ligand; NK, natural killer.

established foci. Studies to establish proof of principle for this approach are currently underway in our laboratories.

RANKL and the Treatment of Prostate Cancer

Osteoclastogenesis is an important component of tumor-induced bone disease in prostate cancer, and is regulated by a cytokine system consisting of the TNF family member RANKL, its receptor RANK and its decoy receptor OPG. RANKL, a transmembrane molecule located on bone marrow stromal cells and osteoblasts binds to RANK on the surface of osteoclast precursors and stimulates differentiation of these cells to mature osteoclasts. OPG, also produced by osteoblasts/stromal cells, is a soluble decoy receptor in this system that binds to RANKL, preventing binding to RANK and inhibiting osteoclastogenesis. This is an effective method for targeting part of the vicious cycle; however, as discussed previously, OPG has potential antiapoptotic activity that could enhance tumor survival and limit its value as a therapeutic agent. To circumvent the latter disadvantage, a recent study (54) used a soluble form of RANK (sRANK-Fc) as an alternative decoy for RANKL without the antiapoptotic activity of OPG, to treat athymic mice carrying intraosseous human prostate cancer xenografts. This study showed diminished tumor-induced lesions as demonstrated by radiograph, bone mineral density measurement, and bone histomorphometry. sRANK-Fc also reduced systemic markers of bone turnover, including serum osteocalcin, bone-specific alkaline phosphatase and urine *N*-telopeptide of collagen. sRANK-Fc also decreased serum prostate-specific antigen levels and tumor volume in bone. In contrast, sRANK-Fc had no effect on subcutaneous implanted xenografts, suggesting that inhibition of RANKL reduces progression of prostate cancer growth in bone by preventing bone remodeling.

Interleukin-6 and Prostate Cancer

Interleukin-6 (IL6) signaling components have been shown to be integral to the processes regulating bone turnover and are present in the normal bone microenvironment (55,56). Studies using prostate cancer cell lines have indicated that IL6 may function as a growth promoter for prostate cancer. The androgen-insensitive prostate cancer cell lines PC3 and Du145 constitutively express IL6 at high levels and their treatment with anti-IL6 antibodies decreases growth rates of both cell lines (57). Interestingly, IL6 expression in the androgen-sensitive prostate cancer cell line LNCaP has been shown to be induced by androgens (58). PC3, Du145, and LNCaP have all been shown to express IL6 receptors (57,58). These studies suggest that constitutive expression of IL6 may be associated with androgen-insensitive phenotypes and conversely that in androgen-sensitive tumor cells, removal of androgens results in depletion of available IL6. If, as the above studies suggest, IL6 is a growth promoter for prostate cancer cells, an alternative supply of this factor could be provided by the bone microenvironment in androgen-deprived conditions. This concept remains to be examined in detail but again targeting this factor during establishment of metastases may be an effective therapeutic strategy. Recent clinical studies have also shown that elevated serum levels of IL6 in prostate cancer patients correlate strongly with objective markers of prostate cancer morbidity and suggested that this cytokine may be a useful marker of prostate cancer activity, and possibly also of disease progression.

SDF-1 and its Receptor (CXCR4) Signaling and Prostate Cancer Metastasis

Recent studies focused on defining the signaling pathways involved in targeting transplanted stem cells to bone marrow have shown that stromal-derived factor (SDF)-1 and its receptor are key mediators of this process. Endothelial cells and preosteoblasts in bone marrow are abundant producers of SDF-1, an important survival factor for progenitor cells, as well as being involved in induction of hematopoietic differentiation and consolidating cellular attachments (59). Defects in expression of SDF-1/CXCR4 in mice result in loss of hematopoietic function and the inability of transplanted stem cells to recolonize bone. Prostate cancer cells carry CXCR4 receptors and respond to SDF-1 in vitro, increasing migration rates through matrices in response to this factor (60). Recent studies (61) have also shown that blockade of SDF-1/CXCR4 signaling, in a xenograft model of metastasis, inhibited colonization of bone by tumor cells. In these studies, human prostate cancer cells were injected into the circulation of animals in the presence or absence of blocking antibodies to CXCR4. The incidence and growth of tumors in bone was suppressed in animals receiving the antibody treatment. In addition, growth of tumors after direct intratibial injection of tumor cells into these animals was inhibited compared to untreated controls. Interestingly, these studies also showed a positive correlation between SDF-1 production in tissues and sites of colonization following intracardiac injection of prostate cancer cells. These studies provide a basis for the development of completely novel therapeutic approaches directed towards suppression of the establishment of bone metastases.

CONCLUDING REMARKS

An explosion of scientific discoveries in the past decade has revolutionized our understanding of cancer biology. There is now, in clinical practice, a significant paradigm shift in the management of advanced prostate cancer metastasizing to bone, from previously debilitating cytotoxic chemotherapy to more modern agents with some efficacy, such as docetaxel, and to targeted approaches with the promise of early intervention, chronic treatment of earlier disease, fewer, more benign side effects and more effective combination therapy. The latter is becoming a particularly attractive proposition for patients, whereby targeting both the "seed" and the "soil" simultaneously could achieve enhanced effects of therapy. It has become clear over recent years that we no longer require to "cure" advanced prostate cancer, but to convert a debilitating disseminated malignancy into a controlled chronic disease with minimal symptoms and improved quality-of-life—a challenge to clinicians and scientists alike, for the benefit of our patients.

REFERENCES

1. Bisaz S, Jung A, Fleisch H. Uptake by bone of pyrophosphate, diphosphonates and their technetium derivatives. Clin Sci Mol Med 1978; 54:265–272.
2. Luckman SP, Hughes DE, Coxon FP, Graham R, Russell G, Rogers MJ. Nitrogen-containing bisphosphonates inhibit the mevalonate pathway and prevent post-translational prenylation of GTP-binding proteins, including Ras. J Bone Miner Res 1998; 13(4):581–589.
3. Fleisch H. Bisphosphonates: mechanisms of action. Endocr Rev 1998; 19(1):80–100.
4. Clézardin P, Ebetino FH, Fournier PGJ. Bishphosphonates and cancer induced bone disease: beyond their anti resorptive activity. Cancer Res 2005; 65:4971–4973.

5. Luftner D, Richter A, Geppert R, et al. Normalisation of biochemical markers of bone formation correlates with clinical benefit from therapy in metastatic breast cancer. Anticancer Res 2003; 23:1017–1026.
6. Rosen LS, Gordon D, Kaminski M, et al. Long term efficacy and safety of zoledronic acid compared with pamidronate disodium in the treatment of patients with advanced multiple myeloma or breast carcinoma: a randomized, double blind, multicenter, comparative trial. Cancer 2003; 98:1735–1744.
7. Garnero P, Buchs N, Zekri J, et al. Markers of bone turnover for the management of patients with bone metastases from prostate cancer. Br J Cancer 2000; 82:858–864.
8. Adami S, Salvagno G, Guarrera G, et al. Dichloromethylene-diphosphonate in patients with prostatic carcinoma metastatic to the skeleton. J Urol 1985; 134:1152–1154.
9. Adami S, Mian M. Clodronate therapy of metastatic bone disease in patients with prostatic carcinoma. Recent Results Cancer Res 1989; 116:67–72.
10. Vorreuther R. Bisphosphonates as an adjunct to palliative therapy of bone metastases from prostatic carcinoma.A pilot study on clodronate. Br J Urol 1993; 72:792–795.
11. Cresswell SM, English PJ, Hall RR, et al. Pain relief and quality-of-life assessment following intravenous and oral clodronate in hormone-escaped metastatic prostate cancer. Br J Urol 1995; 76:360–365.
12. Papapoulos SE, Hamdy NA, van der Pluijm G. Bisphosphonates in the management of prostate carcinoma metastatic to the skeleton. Cancer 2000; 88(suppl):3047–3053.
13. Coleman RE, Purohit OP, Black C, et al. Double-blind, randomised, placebo-controlled, dose-finding study of oral ibandronate in patients with metastatic bone disease. Ann Oncol 1999; 10:311–316.
14. Pelger RC, Hamdy NA, Zwinderman AH, et al. Effects of the bisphosphonate olpadronate in patients with carcinoma of the prostate metastatic to the skeleton. Bone 1998; 22:403–408.
15. Heidenreich A, Elert A, Hofmann R. Ibandronate in the treatment of prostate cancer associated painful osseus metastases. Prostate Cancer Prostatic Dis 2002; 5:231–235.
16. Kylmala T, Tammela TL, Lindholm TS, et al. The effect of combined intravenous and oral clodronate treatment on bone pain in patients with metastatic prostate cancer. Ann Chir Gynaecol 1994; 83:316–319.
17. Elomaa I, Kylmala T, Tammela T, et al. Effect of oral clodronate on bone pain. A controlled study in patients with metastatic prostate cancer. Int Urol Nephrol 1992; 24:159–166.
18. Kylmala T, Taube T, Tammela TL, et al. Concomitant i.v. and oral clodronate in the relief of bone pain—a double-blind placebo-controlled study in patients with prostate cancer. Br J Cancer 1997; 76:939–942.
19. Strang P, Nilsson S, Brandstedt S, et al. The analgesic efficacy of clodronate compared with placebo in patients with painful bone metastases from prostatic cancer. Anticancer Res 1997; 17:4717–4721.
20. Smith JA Jr. Palliation of painful bone metastases from prostate cancer using sodium etidronate: results of a randomized, prospective, double-blind, placebo-controlled study. J Urol 1989; 141:85–87.
21. Ernst DS, Tannock IF, Venner PM, et al. Randomized placebo controlled trial of mitoxantrone/prednisone and clodronate versus mitoxantrone/prednisone alone in patients with hormone-refractory prostate cancer (HRPC) and pain: National Cancer Institute of Canada Clinical Trials Group study. Proc Am Soc Clin Oncol 2002; 21, abstract 705, 177a.
22. Dearnaley DP, Sydes MR on behalf of the MRC PR05 collaborators. Preliminary evidence that oral clodronate delays symptomatic progression of bone metastases from prostate cancer: first results of the MRC PR05 trial. Proc Am Soc Clin Oncol 2001, 20, abstract 693, 174a.
23. Lipton A, Small E, Saad F, et al. The new bisphosphonate, Zometa (zoledronic acid), decreases skeletal complications in both osteolytic and osteoblastic lesions: a comparison to pamidronate. Cancer Invest 2002; 20(Suppl 2):45–54.
24. Small EJ, Smith MR, Seaman JJ, Petrone S Kowalski MO. Combined analysis of two multicenter, randomized, placebo controlled studies of pamidronate disodium for the

palliation of bone pain in men with metastatic prostate cancer. J Clin Oncol 2003; 21:4277–4284.
25. Dearnaley DP, Sydes MR, Mason MD, et al. A double-blind, placebo-controlled, randomized trial of oral sodium clodronate for metastatic prostate cancer (MRC PR05 Trial). J Natl Cancer Inst 2003; 95:1300–1311.
26. Saad F, Gleason DM, Murray R, et al. Long-term efficacy of zoledronic acid for prevention of skeletal complications in patients with hormone-refractory prostate cancer. J Natl Cancer Inst 2004; 96:879–882.
27. Linton KD, Eaton CL, Croucher PI, et al. The effects of Zoledronic Acid on PC3 cell tumor growth in the bone. Abstracts of the BAUS Annual Meeting: Harrogate, UK, 21–25 June, 2004. BJU International 2004; 93:(s4), 34.
28. Green J. Antitumour effects of bisphosphonates. Cancer 2003; 97:840–847.
29. Clezardin P, Fournier P, Boissier S, et al. In vitro and in vivo antitumour effects of bisphosphonates. Curr Med Chem 2003;10:173–180.
30. Bezzi M, Hasmim M, Bieler G, Dormond O, Ruegg C. Zoledronate sensitizes endothelial cells to tumour necrosis factor-induced programmed cell death. J Biol Chem 2003; 278:43603–43614.
31. Corey E, Brown LG, Quinn JE, et al. Zoledronic acid exhibits inhibitory effects on osteblastic and osteolytic metastases of prostate cancer. Clin Cancer Res 2003; 9:295–306.
32. Yanagisawa M, Kurihara H, Kimura S, et al. A novel potent vasoconstrictor peptide produced by vascular endothelial cells. Nature 1988; 332:411–415.
33. Inoue A, Yanag Isawa M, Kimura S, et al. The human endothelial family: three structurally and pharmacologically distinct isopeptides predicted by three separate genes. Proc Natl Acad Sci USA 1989; 86:2863–2867.
34. Nelson JB, Chan-Tack K, Hedican SP, et al. Endothelin-1 production and decreased endothelin B receptor expression in advanced prostate cancer. Cancer Res 1996; 56:663–668.
35. Peters CM, Lindsay TH, Pomonis JD, et al. Endothelin and the tumorigenic component of bone cancer pain. Neuroscience 2004; 126:1043–1052.
36. Rosano L, Spinella F, Salani D, et al. Therapeutic targeting of the endothelin a receptor in human ovarian carcinoma. Cancer Res 2003; 63(10):2447–2453.
37. Yin JJ, Mohammad KS, Kakonen SM, et al. A causal role for endothelin-1 in the pathogenesis of osteoblastic bone metastases. Proc Natl Acad Sci USA 2003; 100:10954–10959.
38. Nelson JB, Carducci MA. The role of the endothelin axis in prostate cancer. Prostate J 1999; 1(3):126–130.
39. Nelson JB. Endothelin inhibition: novel therapy for prostate cancer. J Urol 2003; 170:S65–S67.
40. Petrylak DP, Tangen CM, Hussain MHA, et al. Docetaxel and estramustine compared with mitoxantrone and prednisone for advanced refractory prostate cancer. N Engl J Med 2004; 351:1513–1520.
41. Tannock IF, de Wit R, Berry WR, et al. docetaxel plus prednisone or mitoxantrone plus prednisone for advanced prostate cancer. N Engl J Med 2004; 351:1502–1512.
42. Neville-Webbe HL, Rostami-Hodjegan A, Evans CA, et al. Sequence and schedule dependent enhancement of zoledronic acid induced apoptosis by doxorubicin in breast and prostate cancer cells. Int J Cancer 2005; 113:364–371.
43. Kim S-J, Uehara H, Yazici S, et al. Modulation of bone microenvironment with zoledronate enhances the therapeutic effects of STI571 and paclitaxel against experimental bone metastasis of human prostate cancer Cancer Res 2005; 65(9):3707–3715.
44. Saitoh H, Hida M, Shimbo T, et al. Metastatic patterns of prostatic cancer. Cancer 1984; 54:3078–3084.
45. Carlin B, Andriole GL. The natural history, skeletal complications and management of bone metastases in patients with prostate carcinoma. Cancer 2000; 88:2989–2994.
46. Libouban,H, Moreau,M-F, Basle MF, et al. Increased bone remodeling due to ovariectomy dramatically increases tumoral growth in the 5T2 multiple myeloma mouse model. Bone 2003; 33:283–292.
47. Mason MD, Collaborators MP. Development of bone metastases from prostate cancer: First results from the MRC PR04 trial (ISCRTN 61384873). J Clin Oncol 2004 (suppl abstract 4511).

48. Smith MR, Kabbinavar F, Saad F, et al. Natural history of rising serum prostate-specific antigen in men with castrate nonmetastatic prostate cancer. J Clin Oncol 2005; 23: 2918–2925.
49. Hunter KW. Allelic diversity in the host genetic background may be an important determinant in tumor metastatic dissemination. Cancer Lett 2003; 200:97–103.
50. Eaton CL, Wells JM, Holen I, et al. Serum osteoprotegerin (OPG) levels are associated with disease progression and response to androgen ablation in patients with prostate cancer. Prostate 2004; 59(3):304–310.
51. Brown JM, Vessella RL, Kostenuik PJ, et al. Serum osteoprotegerin levels are increased in patients with advanced prostate cancer. Clin Cancer Res 2001; 7:2977–2983.
52. Holen I, Croucher PI, Hamdy FC, Eaton CL. Osteoprotegerin (OPG) is a survival factor for human prostate cancer cells. Cancer Res 2002; 62:1619–1623.
53. Nyambo R, Cross N, Lippitt J, et al. Human bone marrow stromal cells protect prostate cancer cells from TRAIL induced apoptosis. J Bone Miner Res 2004; 19(10):1712–1721.
54. Zhang J, Dai J, Yao Z, et al. Soluble receptor activator of nuclear factor kB Fc diminishes prostate cancer. Prog Bone Cancer Res 2003; 63:7883–7890.
55. de la Mata J, Uy HL, Guise TA, et al. IL-6 enhances hypercalcemia and bone resorption mediated by PTHrP in vivo. J Clin Invest 1995; 95:2846–2852.
56. Tsangari H, Findlay DM, Kuliwaba JS, et al. Increased expression of IL-6 and RANK mRNA in human trabecular bone from fragility fracture of the femoral neck. Bone 2004; 35(1):334–342.
57. Borsellino N, Belldegrun A, Bonavida B. Endogenous interleukin 6 is a resistance factor for cis-diamminedichloroplatinum and etoposide-mediated cytotoxicity of human prostate carcinoma cell lines. Cancer Res 1995; 55:4633–4639.
58. Okamoto M, Lee C, Oyasu R. Interleukin-6 as a paracrine and autocrine growth factor in human prostatic carcinoma cells in vitro. Cancer Res 1997; 57:141–146.
59. Ponomaryov T, Peled A, Petit I, et al. Induction of the chemokine stromal-derived factor-1 following DNA damage improves human stem cell function. J Clin Invest 2000; 106:1331–1339.
60. Taichman RS, Cooper C, Keller ET, et al. Use of the stromal cell-derived factor-1/CXCR4 pathway in prostate cancer metastasis to bone Cancer Res 2002; 62:1832–1837.
61. Sun Y-X, Schneider A, Jung Y, et al. Skeletal localization and neutralization CXCR4 axis blocks prostate cancer metastasis osseous sites in vivo. J Bone Miner Res 2005: 20:318–329.

15 Inhibiting the Proteasome in Advanced Prostate Cancer

Robert Dreicer

Department of Solid Tumor Oncology, The Glickman Urologic Institute and The Taussig Cancer Center, Cleveland Clinic Foundation, Cleveland, Ohio, U.S.A.

OVERVIEW OF THE PROTEASOME AND ITS FUNCTION

The proteasome is a large subcellular organelle present in all cells and is composed of a multisubunit protein complex that is the site for ATP-dependent degradation of ubiquitin-tagged proteins. The proteasome is responsible for the degradation of the majority of intracellular proteins in eukaryotic cells (1). The 26S proteasome is composed of a 20S proteolytic core flanked at each end by 19S regulatory complexes (Fig. 1). The 20S core consists of two alpha and two beta rings. Each beta ring consists of three active sites with trypsin, chymotrypsin, and postglutamylline hydrolytic activities. The amino terminus of the alpha subunits block access to the proteolytic chamber (2). The 26S proteasome is responsible for the degradation of the majority of regulatory proteins that control the cell cycle, transcription factor activation, apoptosis, and cell trafficking (3–5).

Ubiquitin is an essential 9-kd protein that acts as a covalent modifier of other proteins targeting them for both activation and degradation depending upon the degree of ubiquitin ligation. Chains of at least four ubiquitin adducts target proteins for proteasomal degradation. Ubiquitination is a steady-state process that can be reversed by deubiquitinating enzymes. Polyubiquitination targets proteins to the 26S proteasome and regulates proteasomal degradation, which in turn is a vital component of a range of cellular processes including cell cycle regulation, induction of the inflammatory response, and antigen presentation (1). For a detailed discussion of the ubiquitin–proteasome pathway the reader is advised to consult several excellent recently published reviews (1,6).

Recognition that a number of oncogene and suppressor gene products were found to be targets of ubiquitination led numerous investigators to propose and explore various hypotheses to explain the potential for manipulating the ubiquitin–proteasome pathway, i.e., proteasome inhibition as a target for therapeutic intervention (1).

BORTEZOMIB

Bortezomib, previously known as PS-341, is a specific and reversible inhibitor of the proteasome. It has a unique pattern of growth inhibitory and cytotoxic activity against a variety of human cancer cell lines in which cells accumulate in G2-M phase followed by apoptosis (5). An important observation that appears to be consistent across both solid and hematologic malignancies is that tumor cells appear to be more sensitive to proteasome inhibition than their normal counterparts (7,8).

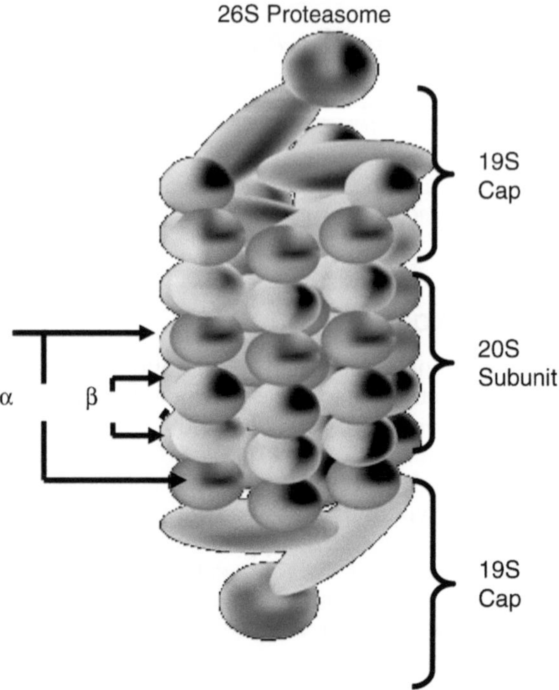

- Degrades ubiquitinated proteins.
- Proteolysis is ATP*-dependent.

FIGURE 1 (*See color insert*) 26S Proteasome. *Source*: Courtesy of Millennium Pharmaceuticals, Inc.

Phase I studies of bortezomib provided evidence of intriguing activity in heavily treated patients with multiple myeloma (9). These results provided the rationale to conduct a series of Phase II studies in relapsed and refractory myeloma patients, which formed the basis of the regulatory approval by both the Food and Drug Administration and the European Medicine Evaluation Agency (10,11). A subsequent Phase III trial in pretreated patients with myeloma demonstrated an improvement in time to disease progression and overall survival for patients treated with bortezomib compared to those patients receiving high-dose dexamethasone (12).

INHIBITING THE PROTEASOME IN PROSTATE CANCER

Notwithstanding recent important developments in the management of androgen-independent metastatic prostate cancer, there remains a pressing need for new therapeutic options. Proteasome inhibition gained early traction as a potential therapeutic strategy in prostate cancer when preclinical work demonstrated that bortezomib induced growth arrest and apoptosis in both the androgen-sensitive line LNCaP and the androgen-independent lines PC-3 and DU-145 (5,13,14). Ikezoe and colleagues working with LNCaP cells demonstrated that bortezomib induced growth arrest and apoptosis in conjunction with markedly upregulated levels of p21 (waf1) and p53. In addition, they noted that bortezomib downregulated both 5α-dihydrotestosterone (DHT)- and interleukin-6–induced expression of prostate-specific antigen (PSA) as measured by Western blot analysis. While bortezomib downregulated basal levels of the androgen receptor in the nucleus, it apparently did not affect DHT-induced nuclear translocation of the androgen receptor in these cells. Taken together, these observations led investigators to hypothesize that bortezomib induced growth arrest and apoptosis of LNCaP cells by blockade of the androgen receptor signaling pathway (15).

Whang et al. recently presented intriguing findings from a murine, prostate cancer bone model. Using a murine intratibial injection model, they examined the effects of the bortezomib on the establishment and progression of osteolytic bone lesions induced by the human prostate cancer PC-3 cell line. In this study, the intravenous administration of bortezomib (1 mg/kg) did not prevent the initial formation of osteolytic lesions but did appear to inhibit their growth in a time-dependent fashion. In contrast, bortezomib therapy effectively inhibited the establishment and progression of subcutaneous PC-3 tumors, which served as a positive control (16). Adams and colleagues, using PC-3 mouse xenograft models, have provided evidence for dose-dependent reductions in tumors with four weekly intravenous doses of bortezomib (5).

CLINICAL EXPERIENCE OF BORTEZOMIB IN PROSTATE CANCER

Several Phase I studies of bortezomib have evaluated several different administration schedules. Aghajanian and colleagues evaluated a schedule of twice-weekly therapy × two weeks with a one-week recovery period. Forty-three heavily pretreated patients typical of a Phase I population were treated (four with prostate cancer). Dose-limiting toxicities (DLT) on this schedule were diarrhea and sensory neurotoxicity, there was no hematologic DLT. One major response in a patient with nonsmall cell lung cancer was observed and the recommended Phase II dose was 1.56 mg/m^2/dose using this schedule (17). Popandreou et al. evaluated a weekly schedule of four out of five weeks of therapy in a Phase I trial conducted at MD Anderson. Of the 53 patients enrolled onto this study, 48 had androgen-independent metastatic prostate cancer. In accord with observations by Aghajanian and colleagues, a dose-dependent inhibition of 20S proteasome activity was observed. Dose-limiting toxicities of diarrhea and hypotension was observed at the 2.0 mg/m^2 dose. Of the 48 patients with androgen-independent metastatic prostate cancer, 43 (84%) had received prior chemotherapy. Two (4%) of the 47 patients with elevated PSA levels had a greater than 50% decline in PSA documented. Two (9.5%) of 21 patients with measurable disease obtained a partial response (both in nodal disease sites); one patient obtained a partial response (PR) after two cycles at the 0.4 mg/m^2 dose, the second after two cycles at the 1.6 0.4 mg/m^2 dose. The maximal tolerated dose (MTD) and recommended Phase II dose of bortezomib using this schedule was 1.6 mg/m^2.

Morris and colleagues performed a Phase II study to determine the efficacy of bortezomib and prednisone. In this Phase II design, patients with progressive, castrate, metastatic prostate cancer were divided into two patient subsets. Patients in Group 1 were heavily pretreated with both chemotherapy and secondary hormonal manipulations and received induction with bortezomib using 1.5 mg/m^2 IV twice weekly on weeks 1, 2, 4, and 5. Starting week 7, patients received 1.6 mg/m^2 weekly, four out of every six weeks, as maintenance. Prednisone at a daily dose of 10 mg was administered continuously. Group 2 was restricted to patients with one or fewer prior chemotherapeutic regimens and less than six months of prior steroid use. This group received 1.3 mg/m^2 induction and 1.6 mg/m^2 maintenance with the same schedule as for Group 1. Group 2 patients received 10 mg of prednisone daily if their PSA rose by $\geq$25% after six weeks of bortezomib alone. PSA levels were assessed at weeks 1, 4, 7, 13, and 19; scans were obtained every 12 weeks. Of 18 patients in Group 1, 13 were assessable for response. Twelve of these patients had received prior chemotherapy and 17 received prior steroids. Of the 12 patients in Group 2, nine were assessable for response, four of whom crossed over to receive prednisone. None of these patients had received prior chemotherapy and only three patients had received prior steroids. PSA declines $>$50% were not seen in either cohort. Overall, two patients had stable disease as their best response at 12 weeks, while all others progressed. Grade 4 toxicities were felt not to be attributable to drug. Grade 3 toxicities felt possibly to be drug related included anemia (13%), leukopenia (30%), neuropathy (3%), thrombocytopenia (20%), and syncope (3%). No significant differences in toxicity were seen between groups (18).

DOCETAXEL + BORTEZOMIB

The preclinical activity of bortezomib makes it a promising agent for overcoming chemotherapy resistance. Preclinical testing has demonstrated synergy between bortezomib and the topoisomerase I inhibitor irinotecan (19). Activation of the transcription factor NF-kB by irinotecan and cisplatin, among others has been shown to be protective from cell killing. Proteasome inhibition has been shown to inhibit drug-induced NF-kB, thus sensitizing cells to drug-induced apoptosis (20).

Nawrocki and colleagues examined the antitumor activity of combination therapy with bortezomib + docetaxel in two human pancreatic cancer cell lines selected for their divergent responses to bortezomib alone. Bortezomib blocked docetaxel-induced apoptosis in the MiaPaCa-2 cells and failed to enhance docetaxel-induced apoptosis in L3.6pl cells in vitro but did interact positively with docetaxel to inhibit clonogenic survival. In orthotopic xenografts, combination therapy produced significant reductions in tumor weight and volume in both the models associated with accumulation of p21, inhibition of proliferation, and increased apoptosis. Combination therapy also reduced tumor microvessel densities, effects that were associated with reductions in tumor cell production of vascular endothelial growth factor and increased levels of apoptosis in tumor-associated endothelial cells. Together, these results suggested that bortezomib enhanced the antitumoral activity of taxanes by enforcing cell growth arrest and by inhibiting angiogenesis (21).

Docetaxel has broad antitumor activity including significant activity in breast, lung, and prostate cancer. It stabilizes the β-subunit of tubulin, phosphorylates and inactivates the antiapoptotic protein Bcl-2, and stabilizes the tumor-suppressor protein p27, resulting in cell cycle arrest at M-phase and apoptosis. Proteasome inhibition can lead to inhibition of degradation of proteins such as p27 or p53, and bortezomib causes G1 and G2 cell cycle arrest. As a consequence of botezomib's inhibition of cell cycling, various investigators have raised concern that it may be antagonistic to the activity of taxanes or may limit the activity of taxanes, which show their greatest activity in M-phase (21).

Farneth et al. evaluated various sequences of docetaxel and bortezomib using both the LNCaP and the PC-3 cell lines. Flow cytometric analysis of DNA content was done to estimate the proportion of PC3 (p53 null) or LNCaP (p53 wild-type) cells in each cell cycle phase as well as sub-G1. Western blot analysis was used to evaluate protein levels. In PC3 cells, as single-agent docetaxel was more effective than bortezomib (sub-G1: 21.8% and 7.3%, respectively). In combination, the sequence of docetaxel followed by bortezomib (sub-G1: 47.4%) was more effective than either bortezomib followed by docetaxel (sub-G1: 25.7%) or coadministration of both agents (sub-G1: 6.3%). In LNCaP cells, there was little difference between docetaxel and bortezomib as single agents (sub-G1: 18.8% and 14.7%, respectively). However, docetaxel + bortezomib (sub-G1: 39.3%) given concurrently was more effective than sequential administration of either bortezomib followed by docetaxel or docetaxel followed by bortezomib (sub-G1: 14.7 and 14.4%) (22).

The principal mode of bortezomib detoxification is via deboronization involving cytochrome P4503A (CYP3A), which also metabolizes docetaxel. Messersmith et al. performed a Phase I study of bortezomib and docetaxel in a refractory group of patients with solid tumors, to define the maximal tolerated dose of this combination and to explore the potential impact of bortezomib on the pharmacokinetics of docetaxel. Patients received escalating doses of weekly docetaxel administered on days 1 and 8 with twice-weekly bortezomib (days 2, 5, 9, 12) in three-week cycles. Two patients were enrolled at each dose level, with cohort expansion to six patients for dose limiting toxicity (DLT). The first three dose levels consisted of docetaxel/bortezomib 25/0.8, 25/1.0, and 30/1.0 mg/m^2, respectively. CYP3A activity, determined using the erythromycin breath test and docetaxel PK were evaluated during weeks 1 (docetaxel alone) and 5 (docetaxel + bortezomib). Thirteen patients received a total of 31 cycles. Dose level 2 was expanded for DLT, which occurred in two of six patients (febrile neutropenia and thrombocytopenia). Dose level 1 was then expanded to six patients where no DLTs occurred, defining the maximally tolerated dose of the combination using this schedule as 25/0.8 mg/m^2. Bortezomib treatment did not alter CYP3A activity and docetaxel clearance (23).

Dreicer and colleagues explored a somewhat different docetaxel/bortezomib schedule in a multicenter Phase I/II trial. Eligible patients were required to have castrate, androgen-independent prostate cancer with clinical or biochemical progression following antiandrogen withdrawal. Patients were required to have adequate organ function and have a 60% or better Karnofsky performance status and less than a grade 2 neuropathy at study entry. Prior systemic chemotherapy was permitted. Docetaxel with standard dexamethasone premedication was given at 25, 30, 35, and 40 mg/m^2 (cohorts 1–4) IV over 30 minutes on days 1 and 8. For the first four cohorts, bortezomib was given 24 hours after docetaxel at a fixed dose of 1.3 mg/m^2 IV push on days 2 and 9; a fifth cohort evaluated bortezomib at 1.6 mg/m^2 with 40 mg/m^2 of docetaxel, with treatment in all cohorts repeated every 21 days. In Phase I portion of the study no maximally tolerated dose was determined. Two expanded Phase II cohorts were then enrolled treated with docetaxel administered at 40 mg/m^2 IV on days 1 and 8, with bortezomib 24 hours after docetaxel at doses of 1.3 and 1.6 mg/m^2 on days 2 and 9, respectively. Thirty-two patients were enrolled in the low expanded cohort (docetaxel 40 mg/m^2, bortezomib 1.3 mg/m^2). Median age was 68 (52–81), median Karnofsky performance status was 80%, and median pre-therapy PSA was 227 ng/mL. Twenty-one patients had received prior chemotherapy, 11 with a taxane-containing regimen. Six patients (24%) achieved a greater than 50% reduction of PSA maintained for at least 30 days, with four (16%) having a greater than 90% reduction. Of these six patients, four had evidenced disease progression following nontaxane chemotherapy. Three patients (23%) achieved a partial response Response Evaluation Criteria in Solid Tumors (RECIST) to therapy; all three patients had received prior chemotherapy, one taxane based. This combination therapy was well tolerated. Anemia of greater than or equal to grade 3 toxicity occurred in two of 32 patients; however, other reported adverse events of greater than or equal to grade 3 occurred in only one patient each and included fatigue, weakness, dizziness, peripheral neuropathy, hyperglycemia, congestive heart failure, hematuria, leukopenia, lymphopenia, gastrointestinal hemorrhage, kidney infection, peripheral swelling, hip fracture, discolored feces, renal vein thrombosis, hematemesis, fluid overload, and proctalgia (24).

SUMMARY

Preclinical studies and work with prostate cancer animal models suggest that proteasome inhibition is a viable, novel therapeutic strategy in the management of prostate cancer. Bortezomib as a single agent in prostate cancer appears to have limited therapeutic activity; however, there is evidence suggesting that bortezomib has both additive and potentially synergistic activity with chemotherapy. Sequence issues remain an important challenge to overcome. Early studies in combination with docetaxel have demonstrated activity, with some intriguing activity in patients with progressive disease following taxane therapy. Additional trials will be required to tease out the appropriate sequencing of therapy and its ultimate clinically utility.

REFERENCES

1. Mani A, Gelman E. The ubiquitin-proteasome pathway and its role in cancer. J Clin Oncol 2005; 23:4776–4789.
2. Groll M, Bajorek M, Kohler M, et al. A gated channel into the proteasome core particle. Nat Struct Biol 2000; 7:1062–1027.
3. Read M, Neish A, Luscinskas F, et al. The proteasome pathway is required for cytokine-induced endothelial-leukocyte adhesion molecule expression. Immunity 1995; 2: 493–506.
4. Palombella V, Rando O, Goldberg A, Maniatis T. The ubiquitin-proteasome pathway is required for processing the NF-kappa B1 precursor protein and the activation of NF-kappa B. Cell 1994; 78:773–785.
5. Adams J, Palombella V, Sausville E, et al. Proteasome inhibitors: a novel class of potent and effective antitumor agents. Cancer Res 1999; 59:2615–2622.
6. Hershko A. The ubiquitin system for protein degradation and some of its roles in the control of the cell division cycle. Cell Death Differ 2005; 12:1191–1197.
7. Hideshima T, Richardson P, Chauhan D, et al. The proteasome inhibitor PS-341 inhibits growth, induces apoptosis, and overcomes drug resistance in human multiple myeloma cells. Cancer Res 2001; 61:3071–3076.
8. Orlowski R, Eswara J, Lafond-Walker A, Grever M, Orlowski M, Dang C. Tumor growth inhibition induced in a murine model of human Burkitt's lymphoma by a proteasome inhibitor. Cancer Res 1998; 58:4342–4348.
9. Orlowski R, Stinchcombe T, Mitchell B, et al. Phase I trial of the proteasome inhibitor PS-341 in patients with refractory hematologic malignancies. J Clin Oncol 2002; 22:4420–4427.
10. Jagannath S, Barlogie B, Berenson J, et al. A phase 2 study of two doses of bortezomib in relapsed or refractory myeloma. Br J Haematol 2004; 127:165–172.

11. Richardson P, Barlogie B, Berenson J, et al. A phase 2 study of bortezomib in relapsed, refractory myeloma. N Engl J Med 2003; 348:2609–2617.
12. Richardson P, Sonneveld P, Schuster M, et al. Bortezomib or high-dose dexamethasone for relapsed multiple myeloma. N Engl J Med 2005; 352:2487–2498.
13. Pervan M, Pajonk F, Sun J, Withers H, McBride W. Molecular pathways that modify tumor radiation response. Am J Clin Oncol 2001; 24:481–485.
14. Herrmann J, Briones F, Brisbay S, Logothetis C, McDonnell T. Prostate carcinoma cell death resulting from inhibition of proteasome activity is independent of functional Bcl-2 and p53. Oncogene 1998; 17:2889–2899.
15. Ikezoe T, Yang Y, Saito T, Koeffler HP, Taguchi H. Proteasome inhibitor PS-341 down-regulates prostate-specific antigen (PSA) and induces growth arrest and apoptosis of androgen-dependent human prostate cancer LNCaP cells. Cancer Sci 2004; 95:271–275.
16. Whang P, Gamradt S, Gates J, Lieberman J. Effects of the proteasome inhibitor bortezomib on osteolytic human prostate cancer cell metastases. Prostate Cancer Prostatic Dis 2005; 8:327–334.
17. Aghajanian C, Soignet S, Dizon D, et al. A phase I trial of the novel proteasome inhibitor PS341 in advanced solid tumor malignancies. Clin Cancer Res 2002; 8:2505–2511.
18. Morris M, Beekman K, Kelly W, et al. Phase II study of bortezomib for castrate metastatic prostate cancer. Proc Am Soc Clin Oncol 2005; 23:411S; abstr 4633.
19. Cusack J, Liu R, Houston M, et al. Enhanced chemosensitivity to CPT-11 with proteasome inhibitor PS-341: implications for systemic nuclear factor-kappaB inhibition. Cancer Res 2001; 61:3535–3540.
20. Cusack J. Rationale for the treatment of solid tumors with the proteasome inhibitor bortezomib. Cancer Treat Rev 2003; 29(suppl 1):21–31.
21. Nawrocki S, Sweeney-Gotsch B, Takamori R, et al. The proteasome inhibitor bortezomib enhances the activity of docetaxel in orthotopic human pancreatic tumor xenografts. Mol Cancer Ther 2004; 3:59–70.
22. Farneth N, Holland W, Kenosi T, et al. Proteasome inhibition with bortezomib in combination with docetaxel in prostate cancer cells and xenografts. Proc Am Soc Clin Oncol 2005; 23:239s; abstr 3192.
23. Messersmith W, Baker S, Dinh K, et al. Phase I trial of bortezomib (PS-341) in combination with docetaxel in patients with advanced solid tumors. Proc Am Soc Clin Oncol 2004; 22:208s; abstr 3052.
24. Dreicer R, Roth B, Petrylak D, et al. Phase I/II trial of bortezomib plus docetaxel in patients with advanced androgen-independent prostate cancer. Proc Am Soc Clin Oncol 2004; 22:abstr 4654.

16 Hsp90: A Target for Prostate Cancer Therapy

David B. Solit

Department of Medicine and the Human Oncology and Pathogenesis Program, Memorial Sloan-Kettering Cancer Center, New York, New York, U.S.A.

Howard I. Scher

Genitourinary Oncology Service, Department of Medicine, Memorial Sloan-Kettering Cancer Center, New York, New York, U.S.A.

Neal Rosen

Department of Medicine, Pharmacology and Chemistry, Memorial Sloan-Kettering Cancer Center, New York, New York, U.S.A.

INTRODUCTION

Androgen ablation is standard initial treatment for patients with metastatic prostate cancer. Though effective, patients invariably develop resistance and progress to a so-called "androgen-independent" state (1). These patients often respond to second- and third-line hormonal therapies, suggesting that their tumors remain dependent upon steroid receptor signaling. Molecular profiling studies of androgen-independent tumors suggest that androgen receptor (AR) reactivation is a common feature of prostate cancer progression following androgen withdrawal (2,3). These findings support the contention that most castration resistant prostate cancers remain AR-dependent.

The mechanisms underlying prostate cancer progression following castration remain poorly understood. Several molecular changes have been associated with this process including mutations or amplification of the AR and ligand-independent activation of AR by growth factor signaling pathways (4,5). As the common feature of these resistance mechanisms is restoration of AR signaling, agents that induce AR degradation represent a potential treatment strategy for patients with advanced prostate cancer. 17-AAG is a selective inhibitor of the Hsp90 chaperone protein. Inhibition of Hsp90 by 17-AAG leads to the degradation of a subset of "Hsp90 clients" including the AR that require Hsp90 for either conformational maturation or stability. This chapter will focus on the role of Hsp90 in regulating AR activity and expression and the potential utility of Hsp90 inhibitors as treatments for patients with prostate cancer.

AR STABILITY AND ACTIVITY ARE REGULATED BY HSP90

AR is a member of the nuclear receptor superfamily of ligand-activated transcription factors. The AR protein is composed of four functional domains: an N-terminal transcriptional activation domain, the central DNA-binding domain, the hinge region, and a C-terminal steroid binding domain (6). The hinge region with its nuclear localization signal plays a role in AR localization, whereas the

DNA-binding domain interacts with specific DNA sequences called androgen response elements.

In the absence of ligand, AR is localized in the cytoplasm where it is associated with a stabilizing chaperone complex that includes Hsp90 and other co-chaperones (7,8). Hsp90 binds to the AR ligand-binding domain and this AR–Hsp90 interaction maintains AR in a high-affinity conformation required for efficient response to hormone. Therefore, Hsp90 regulates not only AR expression but also its activation by ligand (7). Following binding of hormone to AR, the receptor is released as an active transcription factor and transported to the nucleus. AR dimers then bind to specific androgen response elements. Recruitment of cofactors follows leading to activation of androgen-dependent genes.

Hsp90 is a protein chaperone with a role in protein folding, stability, and maturation. The Hsp90 family consists of four members: Hsp90α, Hsp90β, Grp94 whose expression is restricted to the endoplasmic reticulum, and Trap-1 which is expressed in the mitochondria (9–12). Much of our understanding of Hsp90 biology is derived from the study of geldanamycin (GM) and radicicol, natural products that bind a 15 Å deep pocket in the N-terminal domain of the protein, which is conserved across species (13–15). The physiological ligands of the pocket are ATP and ADP. Binding of GM, radicicol, or their analogues mimics the effects of ADP resulting in the degradation of proteins that require Hsp90 for maturation or stability (16,17). Hsp90 chaperone activity is also regulated in the cell through its association with co-chaperones that include Hsp70, Hop, p23, Cdc37, immunophilins, and Aha1 (8,18–20). These co-chaperones function by regulating the balance between the ATP- and ADP-bound states of Hsp90 (21). The co-chaperones also compete for binding to the C-terminal domain of Hsp90, which suggests that co-chaperones might also play a role in targeting Hsp90 to specific client substrates (21).

Exposure of cells to GM leads to ubiquitination of Hsp90 clients, which targets them for degradation in the proteasome. Which E3 ligase or ligases are responsible for ubiquitinating individual Hsp90 clients remains poorly understood. In the case of AR, one possibility is the E3 ligase CHIP (COOH terminus of the Hsp70-interacting protein), which has been shown to promote the Hsp90-associated ubiquitination and degradation of the glucocorticoid receptor and HER2 (22–24). A conserved binding motif for CHIP has been identified in the N-terminal domain of AR using two-hybrid and GST affinity matrix binding assays confirming that CHIP indeed interacts with AR (22).

A subset of steroid receptors [AR, estrogen receptor (ER), glucocorticotal receptor (GR)], kinases (Raf-1, Akt, HER2, Met, and IGF-1R), and transcription factors (Hif-1α) have been shown to be degraded by GM (16,17,25–31). In addition, some mutated oncoproteins are degraded by GM whereas their wild-type counterparts are either resistant or less sensitive to Hsp90 inhibitors. It is hypothesized that these mutations, though they promote tumorigenesis, confer a greater dependence on Hsp90 chaperone function. Examples include bcr-abl, v-src, V600E mutant B-Raf, and mutant epidermal growth factor receptor (31–34).

Hsp90 AS A TARGET FOR CANCER THERAPY: BASIS FOR A THERAPEUTIC INDEX

Inhibition of Hsp90 function and degradation of Hsp90 clients by GM and its analogues causes the retinoblastoma protein (R6)-dependent G1 arrest of most cancer cells (35). G1 arrest is followed in a cell-line–dependent manner by differentiation and/or apoptosis (36). Rb-negative cells are a notable exception. Cells with deficient Rb function progress normally through G1 and instead arrest in mitosis (35). This mitotic arrest is unstable and is followed invariably by apoptosis. G1 growth arrest in Rb wild-type cells results from downregulation of cyclin D/cdk4 activity by two mechanisms. Cdk4 is an Hsp90 client protein and is rapidly degraded following treatment with Hsp90 inhibitors (37). Cyclin D1 is not a direct target of these drugs but its expression is regulated by upstream kinase pathways via translational and post-translational mechanisms (38–41). Therefore, in cancer cells such as those with HER2 overexpression in which cyclin D1 expression is controlled by Akt activation, degradation of a sensitive upstream client such as HER2 leads to downregulation of cyclin D expression (42).

The effects of Hsp90 inhibitors on cancer cell proliferation and survival suggested that these agents may be useful clinically. However, as Hsp90 and its many client proteins play critical roles in normal cell physiology, we and others were initially concerned that these inhibitors would have an insufficient therapeutic index to be useful as drugs. Studies using xenograft models and the early clinical data outlined below suggest that this fear was unfounded. Several possible explanations for the apparent therapeutic index of these agents have been put forth.

First, in preclinical models, we find a wide variability in the sensitivity of individual Hsp90 client proteins to 17-AAG–induced degradation. For example, doses of 17-AAG can be identified that potently degrade HER2 but have no effect on Akt expression even though both proteins are Hsp90 clients (42). Therefore, although Hsp90 plays a role in the regulation of a number of kinases and transcription factors, only a limited subset of these Hsp90 clients may be degraded by 17-AAG in vivo at nontoxic doses. In our experience, the proteins observed to be most sensitive to GM-induced degradation are the HER2 tyrosine kinase, the estrogen and androgen receptors, and the Raf-1 kinase (28,43–45). We have therefore focused our preclinical studies of 17-AAG on the treatment of tumors dependent upon activation of these tyrosine kinase and steroid receptor pathways for tumor proliferation and survival.

For example, in prostate cancer patients with progression following castration, AR reactivation through amplification or mutation may account for resistance to androgen withdrawal (2). Alternatively, AR may be reactivated at castrate levels of testosterone though activation of AR by kinase signaling pathways such as HER2 (46–49). Akt, which is downstream of HER2, also phosphorylates AR and may modulate AR signaling in tumors with HER2 overexpression (50). Treatment of prostate cancer cell lines with 17-AAG causes the degradation of HER2, Akt, and both mutant and wild-type AR (44). Further, at nontoxic doses, 17-AAG causes a dose-dependent reduction in the expression of AR, HER2, and to a lesser extent Akt in androgen-dependent and androgen-independent prostate cancer xenografts. Degradation of Hsp90 clients by 17-AAG is accompanied by inhibition of xenograft tumor growth (44). These data suggest that inhibitors of Hsp90 may be particularly effective in androgen-independent prostate cancer patients whose tumors depend upon AR, HER2, or Akt activation for proliferation or survival.

A second explanation for the apparent therapeutic index of these drugs is their accumulation in tumor versus normal tissues (51,52). A mechanistic basis for this accumulation of drug in tumors is the higher affinity for 17-AAG and GM of Hsp90 derived from tumor lysates as compared to recombinant Hsp90 or

Hsp90 derived from normal control tissues (51,53,54). In tumors, most Hsp90 exists in an "activated state" in complex with co-chaperones. In contrast, Hsp90 from normal tissues exists primarily in a free, uncomplexed, latent state (54). One model is that the balance between these two states is dictated by the amount of mutated and misfolded proteins in the cell. Environmental stresses such as hypoxia, low pH or the low nutrient conditions found in many tumors may place added stress upon this regulatory system by increasing the number of denatured proteins. This situation may be exacerbated further in tumors by mutation or amplification of the genes encoding Hsp90 clients which increases further the requirement for Hsp90 chaperone function. This added requirement for Hsp90 in tumor tissues is the likely explanation of the overexpression of Hsp90 in tumor versus normal tissues (53). Despite this upregulation of Hsp90 expression, the combination of environmental stress and increased mutational load may lead to Hsp90 becoming limiting in tumor cells. Therefore, tumors cells in which free Hsp90 is limited may be more sensitive to partial inhibition of Hsp90 function than normal cells in which free, uncomplexed Hsp90 is found in great excess.

The differences in activation state between Hsp90 in tumor and normal tissues may also explain the synergy observed between Hsp90 inhibitors and chemotherapy, radiation, and inducers of hypoxic stress. In cell culture models, 17-AAG synergistically enhances the activity of cytotoxics including paclitaxel and doxorubicin, flutamide, and radiation (55–57). In the case of paclitaxel, sensitization is schedule dependent in cells with intact Rb function (56). As explained above, 17-AAG causes a G1 growth arrest in Rb wild-type cancer cells whereas paclitaxel induces mitotic arrest (35). 17-AAG synergistically enhances the antiproliferative and proapoptotic effects of paclitaxel when the two agents are administered either simultaneously or when the taxane proceeds 17-AAG (56). In contrast, pretreatment with 17-AAG is antagonistic and results in a reduction in paclitaxel-induced apoptosis. Schedule dependence is not seen in Rb-negative cell lines and with doxorubicin suggesting that induction of G1 block by 17-AAG likely prevents taxane-induced apoptosis in Rb wild-type cells (56). Sequence-dependent sensitization is also observed in mice with maximal enhancement occurring when the two agents are administered on the same day (58). A Phase I clinical trial of 17-AAG and Taxotere® (docetaxel) is now ongoing (Memorial Sloan Kettering Cancer Center protocol 03-006) to test this strategy in patients.

Inhibitors of angiogenesis may also sensitize tumor cells to Hsp90 inhibitors. Hypoxic tumor cells are under greater stress as a result of their low nutrient, low pH, and hypoxic environment and thus may have an excess of unfolded proteins. Hsp90 may play an enhanced role in such an environment by stabilizing or refolding key signaling proteins required for cell survival. HIF-1α is also an Hsp90 client protein and is required for survival under these conditions (59). As a model, we studied tumors that develop in Id-deficient mice. These mice demonstrate impaired angiogenesis. HER2-dependent breast tumors develop in these mice and resemble tumors treated with angiogenesis inhibitors with a thin rim of viable tumor cells surrounding a central necrotic core (60). 17-AAG was dramatically more effective in inhibiting the growth of these hypoxic tumors compared to those that arise in a setting of normal tumor angiogenesis (60). Hsp90 inhibitors may also possess antiangiogenic properties (61). 17-AAG and the second-generation inhibitor 17-dimethylaminoethylamino-17-demethoxygeldanamycin (17-DMAG) inhibit the proliferation and induce the apoptosis of human umbilical vascular endothelial cells. Oral administration of 17-DMAG also inhibits endothelial cell cord formation, an early step in tumor angiogenesis (61).

CLINICAL EXPERIENCE WITH 17-AAG

17-AAG was chosen for clinical development on the basis of its favorable toxicity profile as compared to the natural product geldanamcyin. In Phase I trials, 17-AAG was evaluated using weekly, twice weekly, daily ×5 (21-day cycle), and daily ×3 (14-day cycle) schedules (62–66). Toxicity was dose and schedule dependent, with hepatic toxicity dose-limiting with the daily schedules. Other common toxicities included diarrhea and fatigue. Pharmacokinetic studies indicate that serum concentrations greater than those required for inhibition of Hsp90 function in cell culture and xenograft model systems could be achieved with acceptable toxicity (62–66). No complete or partial response evaluation criteria in solid tumors (RECIST) criteria were reported in the initial Phase I studies. Several patients with melanoma and renal cancer had prolonged stable disease and declines in PSA were also seen with 17-AAG as a single agent in patients with androgen-independent prostate cancer. In one of these patients, a 50% decline in PSA was accompanied by a minor response by CT scan.

One limitation of 17-AAG is its poor solubility and oral bioavailability. To formulate 17-AAG for human use, the cancer therapy evalution program-sponsored studies used a Dimethylsulfoxide (DMSO)-egg phospholid diluent developed specifically for this agent by the National Cancer Institute (NCI). The inclusion of DMSO in this formulation proved to be a greater problem than first anticipated, as it was associated with a bad odor, nausea and anorexia that in many patients were the most prominent toxicities of the drug. To overcome this limitation, several novel Hsp90 formulations are currently in development. The first of these to enter the clinic was a cremaphor-based 17-AAG formulation (KOS-953) developed by Kosan Pharmaceuticals (Hayward, CA). The first solid tumor trial of this formulation was a Phase I/II study of 17-AAG and trastuzumab.

The Phase I portion of this study was open to patient with all solid tumor sites. Twenty-five patients were enrolled at four dose levels (225–450 mg/m^2) with both 17-AAG and trastuzumab administered using a weekly schedule (67). The most common toxicities were fatigue and gastrointestinal toxicities. Hepatotoxicity was minimal and no bone marrow suppression was seen. One patient with trastuzumab-refractory HER2-positive breast cancer had a confirmed partial response by RECIST. Three additional patients with breast cancer had tumor regressions of 25%, 22%, and 21%, respectively. Though preliminary, these data are the most convincing to date to suggest that Hsp90 represents a useful therapeutic target for human cancer. A parallel Phase I trial of the KOS-953 formulation of 17-AAG and bortezomib is ongoing in patients with myeloma. The early results of this trial presented at the 2005 Annual Meeting of the American Society of Hematology are promising with 50% of patients with bortezomib-refractory disease (6 of 12) responding to the combination of 17-AAG and bortezomib.

A Phase I trial of an oil-in-water nanoemulsion of 17-AAG was also recently reported by Conforma Therapeutics (San Diego, CA) (68). In this trial, 17-AAG was administered twice weekly, three out of four weeks. In this trial, no formulation-associated toxicities were noted. Three minor responses, all at doses at or above 83 mg/m^2, were observed in patients with melanoma and gastric and duodenal cancers.

One obstacle in the clinical development of this class of agents has been a lack of tumor-specific pharmacodynamic data. The optimal correlative assay in the Phase I trials would require pre- and post-treatment collection of tumor tissue for analysis of treatment-induced changes in relevant Hsp90 client proteins. In patients with prostate cancer, the difficulty and low yield of such biopsies and the low sensitivity of traditional immunohistochemical techniques for identifying partial but not complete reductions in protein expression limited the feasibility of such studies. Pharmacodynamic studies in mice further suggest that the optimal timeframe for obtaining the post-treatment biopsy may be short adding further logistical hurdles to such efforts (44,58). Data from the limited number of biopsies obtained suggest that Hsp90 clients can be degraded by 17-AAG with acceptable toxicity (69). However, most of the biopsies obtained have been in patients with melanoma and therefore little pharmacodynamic data have been generated for disease-specific clients such as HER2 and AR. As the sensitivity and kinetics of inhibition of these clients may differ significantly from the clients such as cdk4 and Raf-1 found in melanoma tumors, the magnitude and duration of AR and HER2 degradation/inhibition acheivable with 17-1. AAG remains unknown.

As an alternative to tumor biopsies, changes in chaperone and client protein expression in surrogate tissues such as skin or peripheral blood lymphocytes have been measured (62–66). These studies demonstrate that nontoxic doses of 17-AAG induce the co-chaperone Hsp70 and downregulate Hsp90 clients including Raf-1, ckd4, and lck in peripheral blood lymphocytes in some patients. Given the differences in affinity of Hsp90 for 17-AAG in tumor versus normal tissue, the relevance of such findings remains in question.

A novel pharmacodynamic approach may be the use of molecular imaging technology. Our group has developed a novel molecular imaging probe by labeling Herceptin $F(ab')_2$ fragments with ^{68}Ga using a DOTA conjugate (70,71). Using the DOTA-$F(ab')_2$ Herceptin tracer (HERScan) and a PET scanner, HER2 expression can be noninvasively quantitated in transplanted xenografts in mice pre and post-treatment with 17-AAG. The short half-life of ^{68}Ga and the rapid clearance of the $F(ab')_2$ fragments allow for daily imaging. The advantage of this approach over the use of direct tumor biopsy is that it will allow not only a quantitative assessment of the magnitude of client protein depletion but also a determination of the duration of the effect.

NOVEL HSP90 INHIBITORS THAT BIND THE N-TERMINAL ATP POCKET

17-AAG is poorly soluble, has limited oral bioavailablility, and is difficult to formulate. Because of these unfavorable pharmacologic properties, 17-AAG had to be formulated in DMSO and administered intravenously in the CTEP-sponsored Phase I and II studies. The DMSO-based formulation proved particularly troublesome, as it was associated with nonmechanistic toxicities (odor, nausea) that may have been dose-limiting with some dosing schedules. The need for intravenous dosing schedules also made dosing more frequently than twice weekly difficult. To overcome these limitations, several novel Hsp90 inhibitors are currently in development. These include ansamycin derivatives with greater solubility or selectivity and radicicol derivatives with greater in vivo stability (72–74). 17-DMAG (KOS-1022) was the first second-generation Hsp90 inhibitor to enter the clinic.

17-DMAG is a water-soluble derivative of GM with good oral bioavailability (75). Both intravenous and oral clinical trials of this agent are now ongoing.

Using the crystal structure of Hsp90, a completely synthetic Hsp90 inhibitor designed to bind the Hsp90 N-terminal pocket was also developed by Chiosis et al. (76). One potential advantage of these purine-based inhibitors over the natural product is that geldanamcyin and its analogues including 17-AAG and 17-DMAG are highly sensitive P-glycoprotein (P-gp) substrates (77). Upregulation of P-gp is observed in heavily pretreated patients and represents one mechanism of multidrug resistance. A new generation of small molecule inhibitors developed by Conforma Therapeutics was found to be resistant to P-gp and a lead compound from this series (CNF-2024) has entered Phase I testing (77). Small molecule inhibitors of Hsp90 developed by Serenex and Vernalis/Novartis are also being tested in the laboratory (78).

Hsp90 INHIBITORS THAT BIND THE C-TERMINAL DOMAIN

Novobiocin, an antibiotic inhibitor of DNA gyrase subunit B, also binds to and inhibits Hsp90 (79,80). In contrast to GM and radicicol, this agent binds to an ATP site located within the C-terminal portion of Hsp90 (80). Consistent with the effects of GM, Novobiocin disrupts the binding of Hsp90 with Hsc70 and p23, leading to depletion of Hsp90-dependent kinases including v-Src, Raf-1, and HER2. Binding of cisplatin to the C-terminal region of Hsp90 has also been reported (81). Though the primary mechanism of action of cisplatin in tumors is mediated through its binding to DNA, cisplatin also inhibits the transcriptional activity of steroid receptors including the AR by disrupting their binding to Hsp90 (82). In contrast to GM, other Hsp90-clients such as Raf-1, lck, and c-src were unaffected by cisplatin.

HDAC INHIBITORS

Histone deacetylase (HDAC) inhibitors have broad-spectrum antitumor activity in preclinical models and have demonstrated promising results in early-stage clinical trials (83,84). One regulator of Hsp90 chaperone activity is reversible acetylation, a process controlled by the deacetylase HDAC6 (85,86). Inhibition of HDAC6 leads to Hsp90 hyperacetylation, dissociation of Hsp90 from the cochaperone p23, and a loss of chaperone activity (86). The HDAC inhibitors depsipeptide, LAQ824, LBH589, and suberoylanilide hydroxamic acid (SAHA) all cause degradation of Hsp90 clients including HER2 and AR (85,87–90). Treatment of LNCaP cells with LAQ824, which inhibits HDAC6, causes Hsp90–AR dissociation and AR degradation that can be rescued with proteasome inhibition (85,88). In summary, these data suggest that inhibition of Hsp90 by HDAC inhibitors may contribute to the clinical activity of these agents.

CONCLUSIONS

In prostate cancer, AR reactivation contributes to castrate metastatic progression and agents that target AR expression represent a novel treatment approach. 17-AAG and other inhibitors of Hsp90 induce the degradation of mutant and wild-type AR, HER2, and Akt. As this agent targets several of the pathways implicated in the development of the androgen-independent state, it may represent a novel strategy for the treatment of patients with advanced prostate cancer.

REFERENCES

1. Scher HI, Heller G. Clinical states in prostate cancer: toward a dynamic model of disease progression. Urology 2000; 55:323–327.
2. Chen CD, Welsbie DS, Tran C, et al. Molecular determinants of resistance to antiandrogen therapy. Nat Med 2004; 10:33–39.
3. Scher HI, Sawyers CL. Biology of progressive, castration-resistant prostate cancer: directed therapies targeting the androgen-receptor signaling axis. J Clin Oncol 2005; 23:8253–8261.
4. Buchanan G, Yang M, Harris JM, et al. Mutations at the boundary of the hinge and ligand binding domain of the androgen receptor confer increased transactivation function. Mol Endocrinol 2001; 15:46–56.
5. Craft N, Shostak Y, Carey M, Sawyers CL. A mechanism for hormone-independent prostate cancer through modulation of androgen receptor signaling by the HER-2/neu tyrosine kinase. Nat Med 1999; 5:280–285.
6. MacLean HE, Warne GL, Zajac JD. Localization of functional domains in the androgen receptor. J Steroid Biochem Mol Biol 1997; 62:233–242.
7. Fang Y, Fliss AE, Robins DM, Caplan AJ. Hsp90 regulates androgen receptor hormone binding affinity in vivo. J Biol Chem 1996; 271:28697–28702.
8. Rao J, Lee P, Benzeno S, et al. Functional interaction of human Cdc37 with the androgen receptor but not with the glucocorticoid receptor. J Biol Chem 2001; 276:5814–5820.
9. Rebbe NF, Ware J, Bertina RM, Modrich P, Stafford DW. Nucleotide sequence of a cDNA for a member of the human 90-kDa heat-shock protein family. Gene 1987; 53:235–245.
10. Hickey E, Brandon SE, Smale G, Lloyd D, Weber LA. Sequence and regulation of a gene encoding a human 89-kilodalton heat shock protein. Mol Cell Biol 1989; 9:2615–2626.
11. Sorger PK, Pelham HR. The glucose-regulated protein grp94 is related to heat shock protein hsp90. J Mol Biol 1987; 194:341–344.
12. Song HY, Dunbar JD, Zhang YX, Guo D, Donner DB. Identification of a protein with homology to hsp90 that binds the type 1 tumor necrosis factor receptor. J Biol Chem 1995; 270:3574–3581.
13. Stebbins CE, Russo AA, Schneider C, Rosen N, Hartl FU, Pavletich NP. Crystal structure of an Hsp90-geldanamycin complex: targeting of a protein chaperone by an antitumor agent. Cell 1997; 89:239–250.
14. Prodromou C, Roe SM, O'Brien R, Ladbury JE, Piper PW, Pearl LH. Identification and structural characterization of the ATP/ADP-binding site in the Hsp90 molecular chaperone. Cell 1997; 90:65–75.
15. Grenert JP, Sullivan WP, Fadden P, et al. The amino-terminal domain of heat shock protein 90 (hsp90) that binds geldanamycin is an ATP/ADP switch domain that regulates hsp90 conformation. J Biol Chem 1997; 272:23843–23850.
16. Sepp-Lorenzino L, Ma Z, Lebwohl DE, Vinitsky A, Rosen N. Herbimycin A induces the 20 S proteasome- and ubiquitin-dependent degradation of receptor tyrosine kinases. J Biol Chem 1995; 270:16580–16587.
17. Mimnaugh EG, Chavany C, Neckers L. Polyubiquitination and proteasomal degradation of the p185c-erbB-2 receptor protein-tyrosine kinase induced by geldanamycin. J Biol Chem 1996; 271:22796–22801.
18. Panaretou B, Prodromou C, Roe SM, et al. ATP binding and hydrolysis are essential to the function of the Hsp90 molecular chaperone in vivo. Embo J 1998; 17:4829–4836.
19. Johnson BD, Schumacher RJ, Ross ED, Toft DO. Hop modulates Hsp70/Hsp90 interactions in protein folding. J Biol Chem 1998; 273:3679–3686.
20. Meyer P, Prodromou C, Liao C, et al. Structural basis for recruitment of the ATPase activator Aha1 to the Hsp90 chaperone machinery. Embo J 2004; 23:511–519.
21. Prodromou C, Pearl LH. Structure and functional relationships of Hsp90. Curr Cancer Drug Targets 2003; 3:301–323.

22. He B, Bai S, Hnat AT, et al. An androgen receptor NH2-terminal conserved motif interacts with the COOH terminus of the Hsp70-interacting protein (CHIP). J Biol Chem 2004; 279:30,643–30,653.
23. Connell P, Ballinger CA, Jiang J, et al. The co-chaperone CHIP regulates protein triage decisions mediated by heat-shock proteins. Nat Cell Biol 2001; 3:93–96.
24. Xu W, Marcu M, Yuan X, Mimnaugh E, Patterson C, Neckers L. Chaperone-dependent E3 ubiquitin ligase CHIP mediates a degradative pathway for c-ErbB2/Neu. Proc Natl Acad Sci USA 2002; 99:12847–12852.
25. Stancato LF, Silverstein AM, Owens-Grillo JK, Chow YH, Jove R, Pratt WB. The hsp90-binding antibiotic geldanamycin decreases Raf levels and epidermal growth factor signaling without disrupting formation of signaling complexes or reducing the specific enzymatic activity of Raf kinase. J Biol Chem 1997; 272:4013–4020.
26. Whitesell L, Cook P. Stable and specific binding of heat shock protein 90 by geldanamycin disrupts glucocorticoid receptor function in intact cells. Mol Endocrinol 1996; 10:705–712.
27. Czar MJ, Galigniana MD, Silverstein AM, Pratt WB. Geldanamycin, a heat shock protein 90-binding benzoquinone ansamycin, inhibits steroid-dependent translocation of the glucocorticoid receptor from the cytoplasm to the nucleus. Biochemistry 1997; 36:7776–7785.
28. Schulte TW, Blagosklonny MV, Romanova L, et al. Destabilization of Raf-1 by geldanamycin leads to disruption of the Raf- 1-MEK-mitogen-activated protein kinase signalling pathway. Mol Cell Biol 1996; 16:5839–5845.
29. Xu W, Mimnaugh E, Rosser MF, et al. Sensitivity of mature erbb2 to geldanamycin is conferred by its kinase domain and is mediated by the chaperone protein hsp90. J Biol Chem 2001; 276:3702–3708.
30. Webb CP, Hose CD, Koochekpour S, et al. The geldanamycins are potent inhibitors of the hepatocyte growth factor/scatter factor-met-urokinase plasminogen activator-plasmin proteolytic network. Cancer Res 2000; 60:342–349.
31. Whitesell L, Mimnaugh EG, De Costa B, Myers CE, Neckers LM. Inhibition of heat shock protein HSP90-pp60v-src heteroprotein complex formation by benzoquinone ansamycins: essential role for stress proteins in oncogenic transformation. Proc Natl Acad Sci USA 1994; 91:8324–8328.
32. Gorre ME, Ellwood-Yen K, Chiosis G, Rosen N, Sawyers CL. BCR-ABL point mutants isolated from patients with imatinib mesylate-resistant chronic myeloid leukemia remain sensitive to inhibitors of the BCR-ABL chaperone heat shock protein 90. Blood 2002; 100:3041–3044.
33. Grbovic OM, Basso AD, Sawai A, et al. V600E B-Raf requires the Hsp90 chaperone for stability and is degraded in response to Hsp90 inhibitors. Proc Natl Acad Sci USA 2006; 103:57–62.
34. Shimamura T, Lowell AM, Engelman JA, Shapiro GI. Epidermal growth factor receptors harboring kinase domain mutations associate with the heat shock protein 90 chaperone and are destabilized following exposure to geldanamycins. Cancer Res 2005; 65:6401–6408.
35. Srethapakdi M, Liu F, Tavorath R, Rosen N. Inhibition of Hsp90 function by ansamycins causes retinoblastoma gene product-dependent G1 arrest. Cancer Res 2000; 60: 3940–3946.
36. Munster PN, Srethapakdi M, Moasser MM, Rosen N. Inhibition of heat shock protein 90 function by ansamycins causes the morphological and functional differentiation of breast cancer cells. Cancer Res 2001; 61:2945–2952.
37. Stepanova L, Leng X, Parker SB, Harper JW. Mammalian p50Cdc37 is a protein kinase-targeting subunit of Hsp90 that binds and stabilizes Cdk4. Genes Dev 1996; 10: 1491–1502.
38. Cheng M, Sexl V, Sherr CJ, Roussel MF. Assembly of cyclin D-dependent kinase and titration of p27Kip1 regulated by mitogen-activated protein kinase kinase (MEK1). Proc Natl Acad Sci USA 1998; 95:1091–1096.
39. Muise-Helmericks RC, Grimes HL, Bellacosa A, Malstrom SE, Tsichlis PN, Rosen N. Cyclin D expression is controlled post-transcriptionally via a phosphatidylinositol 3-kinase/Akt-dependent pathway. J Biol Chem 1998; 273:29864–29872.

40. Diehl JA, Cheng M, Roussel MF, Sherr CJ. Glycogen synthase kinase-3beta regulates cyclin D1 proteolysis and subcellular localization. Genes Dev 1998; 12:3499–3511.
41. Brewer JW, Hendershot LM, Sherr CJ, Diehl JA. Mammalian unfolded protein response inhibits cyclin D1 translation and cell-cycle progression. Proc Natl Acad Sci USA 1999; 96:8505–8510.
42. Basso A, Solit D, Munster P, Rosen N. Ansamycin antibiotics inhibit Akt activation and tumor growth in human breast cancers that overexpress HER2. Oncogene 2002; 21:1159–1166.
43. Munster PN, Marchion DC, Basso AD, Rosen N. Degradation of HER2 by ansamycins induces growth arrest and apoptosis in cells with HER2 overexpression via a HER3, phosphatidylinositol 3′-kinase-AKT-dependent pathway. Cancer Res 2002; 62: 3132–3137.
44. Solit DB, Zheng FF, Drobnjak M, et al. 17-Allylamino-17-demethoxygeldanamycin induces the degradation of androgen receptor and HER-2/neu and inhibits the growth of prostate cancer xenografts. Clin Cancer Res 2002; 8:986–993.
45. Smith V, Hobbs S, Court W, Eccles S, Workman P, Kelland LR. ErbB2 overexpression in an ovarian cancer cell line confers sensitivity to the HSP90 inhibitor geldanamycin. Anticancer Res 2002; 22:1993–1999.
46. Yeh S, Lin HK, Kang HY, Thin TH, Lin MF, Chang C. From HER2/Neu signal cascade to androgen receptor and its coactivators: a novel pathway by induction of androgen target genes through MAP kinase in prostate cancer cells. Proc Natl Acad Sci USA 1999; 96:5458–5463.
47. Mellinghoff IK, Vivanco I, Kwon A, Tran C, Wongvipat J, Sawyers CL. HER2/neu kinase-dependent modulation of androgen receptor function through effects on DNA binding and stability. Cancer Cell 2004; 6:517–527.
48. Shi Y, Brands FH, Chatterjee S, et al. Her-2/neu expression in prostate cancer: high level of expression associated with exposure to hormone therapy and androgen independent disease. J Urol 2001; 166:1514–1519.
49. Shi Y, Chatterjee SJ, Brands FH, et al. Role of coordinated molecular alterations in the development of androgen-independent prostate cancer: an in vitro model that corroborates clinical observations. BJU Int 2006; 97:170–178.
50. Wen Y, Hu MC, Makino K, et al. HER-2/neu promotes androgen-independent survival and growth of prostate cancer cells through the Akt pathway. Cancer Res 2000; 60:6841–6845.
51. Vilenchik M, Solit D, Basso A, et al. Targeting wide-range oncogenic transformation via PU24FCl, a specific inhibitor of tumor Hsp90. Chem Biol 2004; 11:787–797.
52. Eiseman JL, Lan J, Lagattuta TF, et al. Pharmacokinetics and pharmacodynamics of 17-demethoxy 17-[[(2-dimethylamino)ethyl]amino]geldanamycin (17DMAG, NSC 707545) in C.B-17 SCID mice bearing MDA-MB-231 human breast cancer xenografts. Cancer Chemother Pharmacol 2005; 55:21–32.
53. Yano M, Naito Z, Tanaka S, Asano G. Expression and roles of heat shock proteins in human breast cancer. Jpn J Cancer Res 1996; 87:908–915.
54. Kamal A, Thao L, Sensintaffar J, et al. A high-affinity conformation of Hsp90 confers tumour selectivity on Hsp90 inhibitors. Nature 2003; 425:407–410.
55. Nguyen DM, Chen A, Mixon A, Schrump DS. Sequence-dependent enhancement of paclitaxel toxicity in non-small cell lung cancer by 17-allylamino 17-demethoxygeldanamycin. J Thorac Cardiovasc Surg 1999; 118:908–915.
56. Munster PN, Basso A, Solit D, Norton L, Rosen N. Modulation of Hsp90 function by ansamycins sensitizes breast cancer cells to chemotherapy-induced apoptosis in an RB- and schedule- dependent manner. Clin Cancer Res 2001; 7:2228–2236.
57. Enmon R, Yang W, Solit D, et al. Synergistic interaction of a geldanamycin analog (17AAG) and radiation in human prostate tumor spheroids. Proc AACR, 2002.
58. Solit DB, Basso AD, Olshen AB, Scher HI, Rosen N. Inhibition of heat shock protein 90 function down-regulates Akt kinase and sensitizes tumors to taxol. Cancer Res 2003; 63:2139–2144.
59. Mabjeesh NJ, Post DE, Willard MT, et al. Geldanamycin induces degradation of hypoxia-inducible factor 1alpha protein via the proteosome pathway in prostate cancer cells. Cancer Res 2002; 62:2478–2482.

60. de Candia P, Solit DB, Giri D, et al. Angiogenesis impairment in Id-deficient mice cooperates with an Hsp90 inhibitor to completely suppress HER2/neu-dependent breast tumors. Proc Natl Acad Sci USA 2003; 100:12337–12342.
61. Kaur G, Belotti D, Burger AM, et al. Antiangiogenic properties of 17-(dimethylaminoethylamino)-17-demethoxygeldanamycin: an orally bioavailable heat shock protein 90 modulator. Clin Cancer Res 2004; 10:4813–4821.
62. Banerji U, O'Donnell A, Scurr M, et al. Phase I pharmacokinetic and pharmacodynamic study of 17-allylamino, 17-demethoxygeldanamycin in patients with advanced malignancies. J Clin Oncol 2005; 23:4152–4161.
63. Goetz MP, Toft D, Reid J, et al. Phase I trial of 17-allylamino-17-demethoxygeldanamycin in patients with advanced cancer. J Clin Oncol 2005; 23:1078–1087.
64. Grem JL, Morrison G, Guo XD, et al. Phase I and pharmacologic study of 17-(allylamino)-17-demethoxygeldanamycin in adult patients with solid tumors. J Clin Oncol 2005; 23:1885–1893.
65. Ramanathan RK, Trump DL, Eiseman JL, et al. Phase I pharmacokinetic-pharmacodynamic study of 17-(allylamino)-17-demethoxygeldanamycin (17AAG, NSC 330507), a novel inhibitor of heat shock protein 90, in patients with refractory advanced cancers. Clin Cancer Res 2005; 11:3385–3391.
66. Solit D, Kelly W, Anana M, et al. Phase I trial of 17-AAG (17-allylamino-17-demethoxygeldanamycin) in patients (Pts) with advanced cancer. Proc Am Soc Clin Oncol 2003.
67. Modi S, Stopeck A, Gordon MS, et al. Trastuzumab (T) and KOS-953 (17-AAG) is feasible and active in patients (pts) with metastatic breast cancer: preliminary results of a Phase 1/2 study. SABCS Abst 2005; 1095.
68. Dragovich T, Gordon M, Saif W, et al. Phase 1 Study of CNF1010 (lipid formulation of 17-(allylamino)-17-demethoxygeldanamycin: 17-AAG). Clin Can Res 2005; 11:9117s.
69. Banerji U, Walton M, Raynaud F, et al. Pharmacokinetic-pharmacodynamic relationships for the heat shock protein 90 molecular chaperone inhibitor 17-allylamino, 17-demethoxygeldanamycin in human ovarian cancer xenograft models. Clin Cancer Res 2005; 11:7023–7032.
70. Smith-Jones PM, Solit DB, Akhurst T, et al. Imaging the pharmacodynamics of HER2 degradation in response to Hsp90 inhibitors. Nat Biotechnol 2004; 22:701–706.
71. Smith-Jones PM, Solit DB. Generation of DOTA-conjugated antibody fragments for radioimmunoimaging. Methods Enzymol 2004; 386:262–275.
72. Zheng FF, Kuduk SD, Chiosis G, et al. Identification of a geldanamycin dimer that induces the selective degradation of HER-family tyrosine kinases. Cancer Res 2000; 60:2090–2094.
73. Soga S, Sharma SV, Shiotsu Y, et al. Stereospecific antitumor activity of radicicol oxime derivatives. Cancer Chemother Pharmacol 2001; 48:435–445.
74. Yamamoto K, Garbaccio RM, Stachel SJ, et al. Total synthesis as a resource in the discovery of potentially valuable antitumor agents: cycloproparadicicol. Angew Chem Int Ed Engl 2003; 42:1280–1284.
75. Hollingshead M, Alley M, Burger AM, et al. In vivo antitumor efficacy of 17-DMAG (17-dimethylaminoethylamino-17-demethoxygeldanamycin hydrochloride), a water-soluble geldanamycin derivative. Cancer Chemother Pharmacol 2005; 56:1152s.
76. Chiosis G, Timaul MN, Lucas B, et al. A small molecule designed to bind to the adenine nucleotide pocket of Hsp90 causes Her2 degradation and the growth arrest and differentiation of breast cancer cells. Chem Biol 2001; 8:289–299.
77. Zhang H, Neely L, Yang Y-C, Burrows F. Influence of multidrug resistance proteins on the antitumor activity of natural and synthetic Hsp90 inhibitors. Clin Can Res 2005; 11:9108s–9109s.
78. Wright L, Barril X, Dymock B, et al. Structure-activity relationships in purine-based inhibitor binding to HSP90 isoforms. Chem Biol 2004; 11:775–785.
79. Marcu MG, Schulte TW, Neckers L. Novobiocin and related coumarins and depletion of heat shock protein 90-dependent signaling proteins. J Natl Cancer Inst 2000; 92:242–248.
80. Marcu MG, Chadli A, Bouhouche I, Catelli M, Neckers LM. The heat shock protein 90 antagonist novobiocin interacts with a previously unrecognized ATP-binding domain in the carboxyl terminus of the chaperone. J Biol Chem 2000; 275:37181–37186.

81. Soti C, Racz A, Csermely P. A nucleotide-dependent molecular switch controls ATP binding at the C-terminal domain of Hsp90. N-terminal nucleotide binding unmasks a C-terminal binding pocket. J Biol Chem 2002; 277:7066–7075.
82. Rosenhagen MC, Soti C, Schmidt U, et al. The heat shock protein 90-targeting drug cisplatin selectively inhibits steroid receptor activation. Mol Endocrinol 2003; 17: 1991–2001.
83. Butler LM, Agus DB, Scher HI, et al. Suberoylanilide hydroxamic acid, an inhibitor of histone deacetylase, suppresses the growth of prostate cancer cells in vitro and in vivo. Cancer Res 2000; 60:5165–5170.
84. Kelly WK, O'Connor OA, Krug LM, et al. Phase I study of an oral histone deacetylase inhibitor, suberoylanilide hydroxamic acid, in patients with advanced cancer. J Clin Oncol 2005; 23:3923–3931.
85. Bali P, Pranpat M, Bradner J, et al. Inhibition of histone deacetylase 6 acetylates and disrupts the chaperone function of heat shock protein 90: a novel basis for antileukemia activity of histone deacetylase inhibitors. J Biol Chem 2005; 280:26729–26734.
86. Kovacs JJ, Murphy PJ, Gaillard S, et al. HDAC6 regulates Hsp90 acetylation and chaperone-dependent activation of glucocorticoid receptor. Mol Cell 2005; 18:601–607.
87. Yu X, Guo ZS, Marcu MG, et al. Modulation of p53, ErbB1, ErbB2, and Raf-1 expression in lung cancer cells by depsipeptide FR901228. J Natl Cancer Inst 2002; 94:504–513.
88. Chen L, Meng S, Wang H, et al. Chemical ablation of androgen receptor in prostate cancer cells by the histone deacetylase inhibitor LAQ824. Mol Cancer Ther 2005; 4:1311–1319.
89. Bali P, Pranpat M, Swaby R, et al. Activity of suberoylanilide hydroxamic Acid against human breast cancer cells with amplification of her-2. Clin Cancer Res 2005; 11: 6382–6389.
90. George P, Bali P, Annavarapu S, et al. Combination of the histone deacetylase inhibitor LBH589 and the hsp90 inhibitor 17-AAG is highly active against human CML-BC cells and AML cells with activating mutation of FLT-3. Blood 2005; 105:1768–1776.

17 Vitamin D Analogs and Their Role in Prostate Cancer

Tomasz M. Beer[†] **and Anne Myrthue**

Division of Hematology & Medical Oncology and the OHSU Cancer Insitute, Oregon Health & Science University, Portland, Oregon, U.S.A.

INTRODUCTION

Based on both suggestive epidemiological data of a possible link between vitamin D and prostate cancer and on compelling preclinical evidence for antineoplastic activity of vitamin D receptor (VDR) ligands, considerable effort has been devoted to the development of VDR ligand-based therapy for prostate cancer. The combination of high-dose calcitriol, the naturally occurring ligand for the VDR, with docetaxel, a microtubule stabilizing cytotoxic agent, for the treatment of metastatic androgen-independent prostate cancer is entering Phase III testing after encouraging results from both single institution, and large multi-institutional Phase II clinical trials. Less attention has been devoted to the potential for VDR ligands in prostate cancer prevention.

EPIDEMIOLOGY OF VITAMIN D AND PROSTATE CANCER

Prostate Cancer Risk

The evidence linking low vitamin D levels with prostate cancer has been mixed. The global pattern of greater risk in northern regions led investigators to suggest that reduced exposure to solar UV radiation and consequent reduction in endogenous vitamin D production may be associated with an increased risk of prostate cancer (1). A case-control study from the United Kingdom showed a reduced risk with greater UV exposure (2). In a U.S. study, there was only a weak link between average regional UV-B radiation and prostate cancer mortality (3).

Studies that examined 25-OH vitamin D levels in populations with a low prevalence of severe vitamin D deficiency did not reveal a relationship between vitamin D blood levels and prostate cancer risk (4–8). Studies conducted in Nordic countries, where severe vitamin D deficiency is more common (9,10), reported increased risk in men with the lowest vitamin D levels, although one of the studies (10) also suggested an increased risk at the highest levels. Two studies suggest that low 1,25-OH_2 vitamin D levels were associated with an increased risk of aggressive prostate cancer (4,5), but overall prostate cancer risk was not associated with 1,25-OH_2 vitamin D in two recent relatively small studies (7,8).

[†] Dr. Beer has a significant financial interest in Novacea, the company that has a financial interest in the results of this research and technology. This potential conflict of interest has been reviewed and managed by the OHSU and Portland VA Conflict of Interest in Research Committees.

Studies that examined dietary vitamin D intake did not reveal a protective effect from prostate cancer (11–14). Interestingly, a number of studies have linked higher milk and higher calcium consumption with risk of the disease and a recent meta-analysis of 11 case-control studies reported a combined odds ration of 1.68 for high milk consumption (15).

In a recent paper, Edward Giovanucci suggested that loss of 1-alpha hydroxylase activity in prostate cancer cells may explain these epidemiologic findings. Normal prostate epithelial cells or colon cancer cells (16,17) express 1-alpha hydroxylase and can therefore convert 25-OH vitamin D to the active 1,25-OH_2 vitamin D. This activity can be lost when the cancer develops (18,19). The loss of this activity would be expected to render prostate cancer resistant to 25-OH vitamin D and dependent on circulating 1,25-OH_2 vitamin D for VDR-mediated activity. Circulating 1,25-OH_2 vitamin D levels are tightly controlled and largely unaffected by 25-OH vitamin D levels, except for a severe deficiency state (20–23). If this hypothesis proves correct, it would not be surprising that 25-OH vitamin D levels or behaviors that influence them (sunlight, vitamin D supplements) would have little effect on prostate cancer except in the extremes. At the same time, high milk and high calcium consumption are associated with a significant reduction in circulating 1,25-OH_2 vitamin D levels (24). This reduction in circulating 1,25-OH_2 vitamin D levels could explain excess risk. Our group has recently showed that VDRs are universally expressed in human prostate cancer specimens and that preprostatectomy high-dose 1,25 h OH_2 vitamin D treatment significantly reduces VDR expression in human prostate tumors (25). This finding is consistent with the hypothesis advanced by Giovanucci.

Prostate Cancer Outcomes

Several investigators have recently reported that the season of diagnosis and treatment as well as vitamin D blood levels are important predictors of outcome in several cancer types including prostate cancer. Zhou et al. found that patients diagnosed and surgically treated for nonsmall cell lung cancer during the summer had a better relapse-free survival than patients diagnosed and treated in the winter. The greatest difference was seen when patients who had surgery in the summer and had a high intake of vitamin D were compared to patients operated on in the winter who had low vitamin D intake (HR 0.33, 95% CI 0.15–0.74). A similar association for overall survival was also noted (26). In a Norwegian study of 115,096 breast, colon, and prostate cancer patients, Robsahm found that those diagnosed in the summer or fall had significantly lower case fatality rates than similar patients diagnosed in the winter and spring (27). For prostate cancer, the season of diagnosis was associated with a statistically significant 20% to 30% reduction in risk of death. There are no prospective studies of vitamin D supplementation or treatment with surgery or radiation for prostate cancer, but the emerging retrospective data are intriguing.

MECHANISMS OF ANTINEOPLASTIC ACTIVITY IN PRECLINICAL SYSTEMS

Vitamin D Signaling

Vitamin D signaling involves both receptor-mediated genomic and nongenomic pathways. The VDR, the mediator of the classic genomic response, is a steroid hormone receptor and acts as a ligand-activated transcription factor (28). It binds to the vitamin D response element (VDRE) present in the regulatory region of many genes after forming a heterodimer with the retinoid-X receptor and in some cases the retinoid A receptor (29–31). In the presence of coactivator complexes, the VDR heterodimer interacts with the RNA polymerase complex and initiates gene transcription. The number of genes that are recognized to have a functional VDRE is rapidly growing. Examples include a number of bone-associated genes such as osteocalcin (32), osteopontin (33), bone sialoprotein (34), receptor activator of NF-kappaB ligand (35), Runx2/Cbfa1 (36), tumor necrosis factor alpha (37), parathyroid hormone (38), parathyroid hormone-related protein (39), the insulin receptor (40), insulin-induced gene-2 (41), carbonic anhydrase II (42), human growth hormone (43); the calcium-binding proteins calbindin-D28k and calbindin-D9K (44), fructose 1,6-bisphosphatase (45); the cell cycle regulators p21 (46), growth arrest and DNA-damage-inducible protein 45 (GADD45) (47), and insulin-like growth factor binding protein3 (IGFBP3) (48,49); 25(OH)D_3 24-hydroxylase (50); cytochrome P3A4 (CYP3A4) (51); mitogen-related protein 3 (MRP3) (52); epidermal growth factor receptors (53); c-fos (54); phospholipase C (55); as well as a number of genes that regulate cell adhesion and differentiation such as fibronectin (56), β3 integrin (57), and involucrin (58). Interestingly, several of these genes have been implicated in prostate cancer or prostate cancer metastases (59–61).

In addition to the classic genomic response, vitamin D also induces rapid nontranscriptional signals leading to increases in calcium and phosphate uptake in intestinal cells (62) and the opening of Ca^{2+}-dependent K^{+}- and voltage-gated calcium and chloride channels in kidney proximal tubules and skeletal muscle, respectively (63,64). Rapid vitamin D-induced nongenomic signals also include the regulation of protein kinase C (65–67), ras- and mitogen-activated protein kinase (MAPK) (67–71), protein lipase A and prostaglandins (72,73), cyclic adenosinemonophosphate (AMP) and protein kinase A (74,75), phosphatidyl inositol 3-kinase/Akt (76,77), and the ceramide pathway (78). Ultimately, these responses regulate cellular growth, differentiation, and apoptosis (69,71,79,80) and may in part be mediated by the translocation of the VDR to the plasma membrane, cytosolic VDR, or by other unknown receptors (71,81–86).

Spectrum of Activity

After Abe reported that calcitriol induced terminal differentiation in myeloid leukemia cells (87), a number of investigators reported in vitro and/or in vivo activity in models of a broad range of human neoplasms including carcinoma of the bladder (88), breast (89), colon (90), endometrium (91), kidney (92,93), lung (94), pancreas (95), prostate (96–102), sarcomas of the soft tissues (103) and bone (104,105), neuroblastoma (106,107), glioma (108), melanoma (109), squamous cell carcinoma (110,111), and others. Vitamin D signaling is likely to be important throughout organ systems as VDR appears to be expressed in nearly all human tissues (112,113).

Mechanisms of Antineoplastic Activity

Several mechanisms of activity have been demonstrated in preclinical systems, but because vitamin D targets a broad range of genes it is not surprising that the observed mechanisms differ under different experimental conditions and in different tumor models. It is likely that more than one of these mechanisms of activity is important in humans and indeed different mechanisms may be important in different human diseases or at different stages of a human disease.

Differentiation and Inhibition of Proliferation

Inhibition of proliferation, which is associated with differentiation in some tumor models, has been extensively studied. In numerous cell lines, growth arrest in response to vitamin D occurs in the G_1 phase of the cell cycle (46,114–117). In several tumor models, the G_1 growth arrest has been linked to transcriptional activation of cyclin-dependent kinase inhibitors $p27^{Kip1}$ and $p21^{Waf1}$ (46,114). These effects are not universally observed. For example, $p21^{Waf1}$ expression increases after 24 hours and is reduced at 72 hours in PC-3 prostate cancer cells, suggesting a biphasic, time-dependent response (118). Induction of p27, which in contrast to p21 lacks a VDRE, appears to be mediated by NF-Y and SP1 (119,120) and additional effects may take place at the level of protein stability (121,122). Dephosphorylation of the retinoblastoma protein in response to vitamin D has also been reported both in normal human keratinocytes (123) and in several preclinical tumor models (110,124–127).

Vitamin D has been shown to inhibit other mitogenic signals including the extracellular-signal-regulated kinase (ERK/MAPK) pathway (70,71), c-myc (128,129), epidermal growth factor receptors (130) and the insulin-like growth factor system (131–133). Vitamin D has also been shown to induce transforming growth factor-beta (134,135). These effects vary across tumor models.

While cell differentiation accompanies growth inhibition in some experimental systems, this association is not universal and differentiation can occur even in cells resistant to vitamin D-mediated growth arrest (136,137).

Vitamin D inhibits fatty acid synthase expression by stimulating the expression of long-chain fatty-acid-CoA ligase 3 (FACL3) in LNCaP cells. The upregulation of FACL3 and subsequent inhibition of fatty acid synthase are involved in the antiproliferative effects of vitamin D (138). Interestingly, the growth inhibitory effects of vitamin D on LNCaP cells are significantly attenuated by an FACL3 activity inhibitor. Further, vitamin D is unable to regulate FACL3 expression in the absence of androgens, indicating that the upregulation of FACL3 expression by vitamin D is mediated through the androgen receptor (AR) signaling pathway (139).

Relevant to prostate cancer, androgen signaling may be important for vitamin D-mediated growth inhibition in human prostate cancer cells. In LNCaP cells and CWR22R cells, vitamin D induces AR expression. Vitamin D-mediated growth inhibition is reduced when AR signaling is blocked by antiandrogens, RNA interference, or targeted disruption of AR (140).

Apoptosis

Vitamin D-induced apoptosis has been demonstrated in several prostate cancer models (141,142). Vitamin D has been reported to downregulate the antiapoptotic protein Bcl-2 in prostate cancer (141) and several other neoplastic cell types (70,142–149). In several cell lines vitamin D-mediated apoptosis is independent of p53 status (143,150,151), although data about the role of p53 in this setting are not entirely consistent (144,152). In the prostate cancer cell lines LNCaP and ALVA-31, as well as in the MCF-7 breast cancer cells, vitamin D stimulates cytochrome c release from mitochondria by a caspase-independent mechanism (141,153).

Proapoptotic effects of vitamin D may also involve downregulation of the insulin-like growth factor receptor (154), upregulation of mitogen-activated protein kinase (MEK) kinase-1 (111), activation of the sphingomyelin-ceramide-ganglioside GD3 signaling pathway (78), downregulation of Akt (155,156), stimulation of tumor necrosis factor-α activity (157), induction of transforming growth factor-β signaling (158), and cytosolic calcium mobilization (159,160). Induction of ovarian cancer cell apoptosis by vitamin D is mediated through downregulation of telomerase (161).

Although proapoptotic activity has been demonstrated in multiple experimental systems, these effects are not universal and vitamin D-induced inhibition of apoptosis has also been described. For example, vitamin D inhibits ultraviolet B-induced apoptosis, Jun kinase activation, and interleukin-6 production in primary human keratinocytes (162).

Angiogenesis and Invasiveness

Several investigators have also reported antiangiogenic and anti-invasive effects of vitamin D in preclinical tumor models. Proliferation of tumor-derived endothelial cells (156) and sprouting and elongation of endothelial cells induced by vascular endothelial growth factor (163) are inhibited in in vitro models of angiogenesis. Antiangiogenic activity has been confirmed in mouse tumor models (163,164).

Reduction of metastases with vitamin D therapy have been demonstrated in rodent models including those of prostate cancer (88,102,165) and reduced invasiveness has been shown in in vitro assays using prostate cancer (166–168) as well as a number of other tumor types (169,170). Serine proteinase and metalloproteinase inhibition (166,168,171), decreased α6 and β4 integrin expression (167), increased E-cadherin expression (172), and inhibition of tenascin-C (173) may explain the anti-invasive activity of vitamin D.

VITAMIN D IN COMBINATION WITH OTHER ANTINEOPLASTIC AGENTS IN PRECLINICAL MODELS

Experiments in preclinical models suggest that VDR ligands enhance the activity of a broad range of antineoplastic agents.

Steroids

The antineoplastic activity of vitamin D is enhanced by dexamethasone both in vitro and in vivo (155,174). In squamous cell carciroma (SCC) cells, dexamethasone increases both VDR protein levels and ligand binding (174). Dexamethasone increases both vitamin D-induced cell cycle arrest and apoptosis. Phospho-Erk1/2 and phospho-Akt levels and tumor-derived endothelial cell growth are suppressed more completely by the combination than by vitamin D alone (110,155,156,174).

Cytotoxic Chemotherapy

Combinations of VDR ligands with several classes of chemotherapy drugs show additive or supra-additive activity in preclinical models. In prostate cancer models, enhanced activity of docetaxel (175), paclitaxel (118), platinum compounds (176), and mitoxantrone (177) have been reported. Animal model confirmation is available for paclitaxel and mitoxantrone (118,177). Similar results have been reported in several other tumor types (178–181); however, the mechanisms of these interactions remain incompletely understood.

Retinoid Receptor Ligands

VDR forms heterodimers with retinoid-X receptor, thus synergistic growth inhibition by ligands for both receptors is not unexpected (182,183). Synergistic induction of apoptosis (183) and inhibition of angiogenesis for vitamin D–retinoid combinations have also been reported (183). Common effects on IGFBP-3 may explain synergistic growth inhibition for the combination of retinoid A receptor and VDR ligands (184). Recently, the combination of 9-*cis* retinoic acid with calcitriol has been shown to inhibit the human telomerase reverse transcriptase in prostate cancer cells. This effect is not seen when either agent is tested alone (185). Common activation of target genes, such as p21 may also underlie interactions between retinoids and vitamin D.

Tamoxifen

VDR ligands significantly increase the inhibition of *N*-nitroso-*N*-methylurea-induced mammary carcinogenesis by tamoxifen in Sprague–Dawley rats (186). Both in vitro and in vivo data using MCF-7 cells demonstrate enhanced apoptosis with the combination (187,188). Interestingly, recent results in MCF-7 cells suggest that sensitivity to vitamin D varies inversely with sensitivity to antiestrogens suggesting that sequential or concurrent use of these compounds would be of significant interest (189).

Nonsteroidal Anti-Inflammatory Agents

Simultaneous treatment of LNCaP cells with VDR ligands along with ibuprofen resulted in additive suppression of growth in the absence of dihydrotestosterone and synergistic growth inhibition under dihydrotestosterone-stimulated conditions. Both decreased G_1-S transition and enhanced apoptosis were reported (190). cDNA analysis of LNCaP cells treated with calcitriol showed that the expression of prostaglandin synthesizing COX-2 gene is significantly decreased by calcitriol, while the prostaglanding inactivating 15-prostaglandin dehydrogenase gene was upregulated (191). The combination of calcitriol and nonsteroidal anti-inflammatory drugs synergistically acted to inhibit LNCaP cell growth (192).

Radiation

P21 expression, known to be induced by vitamin D in a number of tumor models, has also been shown to sensitize cells to radiation therapy (193). Potentiation of radiation-induced apoptosis with VDR ligands has been shown in several tumor models (194,195) and in one analysis increased ceramide generation may explain this interaction (196).

CLINICAL TRIALS OF CALCITRIOL IN PROSTATE CANCER

Calcitriol (1,25-dihydroxycholecalciferol, 1,25-OH_2 vitamin D) is clinically available and is indicated for patients who suffer from renal failure and therefore cannot adequately activate the storage form of vitamin D. The availability of this drug made it feasible for investigators to initiate studies in cancer. Because antineoplastic effects in vitro occur at significantly supraphysiologic concentrations (typically at or above 1 nM), dose escalation of calcitriol has been the goal of the Phase I programs.

Phase I Studies

Daily Administration

The first clinical trials in prostate cancer were designed to build on standard replacement dosing of calcitriol. Using a daily administration schedule, Osborn et al. sought to dose escalate calcitriol in 11 patients with hormone-refractory prostate cancer. No prostate specific antigen (PSA) responses were seen at doses that ranged from 0.5 to 1.5 μg daily. Further dose escalation was not pursued due to hypercalcemia (197). Gross et al. took a similar approach to the study of seven patients with a rising PSA that had not been treated with hormonal therapy previously. No PSA responses were seen; however, treatment appeared to favorably impact PSA kinetics (the PSA doubling time was reduced when compared to the same prior to treatment). Hypercalciuria was cited as the reason for avoiding doses above 2.5 μg/day (198).

Every Other Day Subcutaneous Administration

Subcutaneous administration every other day was an approach designed to test two hypotheses: both the route and the schedule of administration may reduce the calcemic toxicity of calcitriol. While hypercalcemia was the dose-limiting toxicity, this approach allowed significant escalation of the dose, with 10 μg daily the highest dose tested (199). Peak blood calcitriol concentrations of approximately 0.7 nM were observed at the 8 μg dose.

Weekly Dosing

In a dose ranging study, weekly oral administration resulted in peak blood calcitriol concentration of 3.7 to 6.0 nM without dose-limiting toxicity. Doses up to 2.8 μg/kg were examined; however, peak calcitriol concentrations (C_{max}) and the area under the concentration curve (AUC) did not increase linearly at doses above 0.48 μg/kg (200). This was the first study to report nonlinear pharmacokinetics with the commercially available formulation of calcitriol, a finding later confirmed by Muindi et al. (201). This pharmacokinetic limitation, as well as the very large number of capsules required for treatment (calcitriol is commercially available as 0.25 and 0.5 μg capsules), later led to the development of a new high-dose formulation of calcitriol, DN-101 (Novacea, Inc., South San Francisco, U.S.A.). Administered as a single dose, DN-101 exhibits a dose-proportional increase in both C_{max} and AUC across a broad range of doses (15–165 μg). As a result, peak calcitriol concentrations achieved in this study were higher than any previously reported (14.9 nM at the 165 μg dose) (202). In the preliminary report of the results with weekly dosing, grade 2 self-limited hypercalcemia was seen with repeat weekly dosing at 60 μg. Consequently, 45 μg weekly was recommended as the Phase II weekly dose (203). It is likely, however, that additional dose escalation on the weekly schedule would be feasible if either more conventional criteria for dose-limiting toxicity had been applied (grade 3 rather than grade 2 hypercalcemia) or DN-101 were coadministered with an agent capable of reducing hypercalcemia.

Dosing Three of Every Seven Days

Another approach to weekly dosing was administration of calcitriol for three consecutive days repeated every seven days. In a Phase I trial that combined calcitriol on this schedule with paclitaxel, daily doses up to 38 μg on three consecutive days every seven days were administered without dose-limiting toxicity and produced calcitriol C_{max} that ranged from 1.4 to 3.5 nM at the highest doses (201). The same schedule of calcitriol was also evaluated in combination with zoledronate, with dexamethasone added upon progression (204). Daily calcitriol doses up to 30 μg for three consecutive days every seven days were administered without dose-limiting toxicity and three patients had calcitriol dose reductions due to related laboratory abnormalities. There were no responses to calcitriol and zoledronate and one of seven patients responded when dexamethasone was added upon progression on the initial regimen.

Dosing Every Three Weeks

If calcitriol is primarily used to modify tumor response to chemotherapy, even less frequent dosing may be useful, particularly when the chemotherapy regimen is dosed infrequently. With this in mind, our group tested 60 μg of calcitriol every three weeks 24 hours before chemotherapy with docetaxel and estramustine. The study used a dose de-escalation design and demonstrated that 60 μg can be safely administered on this schedule (205). The study was not designed to measure efficacy. Fifty-five percent of chemotherapy-naïve and 9% of patients previously treated with docetaxel-containing chemotherapy responded.

The Phase I efforts of a number of investigators clearly demonstrate that significant dose escalation of calcitriol with intermittent dosing is feasible (Table 1). Indeed, most studies did not identify a maximum tolerated dose, as dose escalation was limited by the number of capsules needed and by the nonlinear pharmacokinetics of the commercially available formulation of calcitriol. The recently developed new formulation (DN-101) overcomes both of these limitations.

Phase II Studies

Weekly Dosing

Weekly calcitriol has been tested as a single agent in hormone-naïve prostate cancer and in combination with docetaxel in androgen-independent prostate cancer. In a nonrandomized study carried out in patients who had a biochemical progression after prostatectomy or radiation therapy, weekly calcitriol administered at a dose of 0.5 μg/kg was administered safely for a median of 10 months (206). There were no confirmed PSA reductions in excess of 50%, but lesser PSA reductions as well as lengthening of the PSA doubling time when compared to pretreatment were observed. While these findings are suggestive of antitumor activity, a randomized trial would be needed to determine their clinical significance.

A single-institution Phase II clinical trial enrolling patients with chemotherapy-naïve metastatic androgen-independent prostate cancer tested a regiment of oral calcitriol 0.5 μg/kg on day 1, followed by docetaxel 36 mg/m^2 intravenously on day 2. This regimen was administered weekly for six consecutive weeks, repeated every eight weeks (207). Overall toxicity was quite similar to that expected with docetaxel alone and 81% of the 37 patients had a confirmed PSA response. Fifty-three percent of the 15 patients with measurable disease met response evaluation criteria in solid tumors (RECIST) criteria for response in measurable disease and median overall survival was 19.5 months. These encouraging results led to the development of ASCENT [Androgen Independent Prostate Cancer (AIPC) Study of Calcitriol Enhancing Taxotere™ (Sanofi-aventis,

TABLE 1 Dose Escalation Studies of Calcitriol in Cancer

Investigators	Dose of calcitriol	Schedule and route	Companion drugs	Dose limiting toxicity	Peak calcitriol concentrations
Osborn et al. (1995)	0.5–1.5 μg	Daily/orally	None	Hypercalcemia	NR
Gross et al. (1998)	0.5–2.5 μg	Daily/orally	None	Hypercalciuria	
Smith et al. (1999)	2.0–10 μg	Every other day/ subcutaneous	None	Hypercalcemia	0.7 nm
Beer et al. (2001)	0.06–2.8 μg/kg	Weekly/orally	None	Not determined	3.7–6.0 nM
Muindi et al. (2002)	4–38 μg	Daily for 3 day every 7 day/orally	Paclitaxel 80 mg/m^2 weekly	Not determined	1.4–3.5 nM
Morris et al. (2004)	4–30 μg	Daily for 3 day every 7 day/orally	Zoledronate 4 mg IV monthly; dexamethosone 0.75 mg BID added at progression	Not determined	0.9–2.3 nM
Tiffany et al. (2005)	60 μg	Every 21 day/orally	Estramustine 280 mg on days 1–5, and docetaxel 70 mg/m^2 on day 2	Not determined	NR

Abbreviations: NR, not reported; BID, twice a day.
Source: From Ref. 208.

Paris, France)], a placebo-controlled multi-institutional randomized study that compared DN-101 (the new calcitriol formulation) + docetaxel to placebo + docetaxel in 250 U.S. and Canadian patients. DN-101 was dosed at a fixed dose of 45 µg 24 hours before docetaxel 36 mg/m^2. This regimen was administered weekly for three consecutive weeks and repeated every four weeks. While the results of this trial have not been published yet, preliminary results were presented at both American society of clinical oncology and European Cancer Conference meetings in 2005. Recently presented preliminary results showed that when compared to placebo, treatment with DN-101 was associated with improved survival (HR 0.67, $p = 0.035$) and a trend favoring DN-101 with respect to PSA response rates (overall 63% vs. 52%, $p = 0.07$, within six months 58% vs. 49%, $p = 0.16$). Further, the addition of DN-101 to docetaxel was not associated with an increase in treatment toxicity. ASCENT's primary end point was PSA response rate and not overall survival. Consequently, a larger prospective study that will examine overall survival as the primary end point is underway (Table 2).

Less Frequent Dosing

A small Phase II study also examined calcitriol 0.5 µg/kg in combination with carboplatin at an AUC dose of seven (six in patients with prior radiation) dosed every four weeks (209). The response rate was less than 10% and toxicity was unremarkable. It is not clear if this less encouraging result is related to the infrequent dosing schedule of calcitriol, to platinum resistance of prostate cancer, or due to chance given the small sample size ($n = 17$).

CALCITRIOL ANALOGS

While much of the clinical testing of VDR ligands has been conducted with calcitriol, the naturally occurring ligand, another approach has been to develop calcitriol analogs designed to decouple antineoplastic activity from calcemic toxicity. The most common synthetic approach has been to modify the side chain of the calcitriol molecule and many such compounds have been chemically synthesized. Differences in protein binding, VDR affinity, and drug metabolism have all been cited as explanation for reduced calcemic activity (210–212). Several of these compounds have entered clinical trials, some in prostate cancer.

After Phase I evaluation (213), Seocalcitol (EB1089, Leo Pharmaceuticals, Ballerup, Denmark) 10 µg daily was evaluated in Phase II studies in pancreatic and hepatocellular carcinoma. No objective responses were seen in patients with pancreatic cancer (214), but two of 33 assessable patients with unresectable hepatocellular carcinoma achieved complete remission that had endured beyond 29 months (last point of analysis) (215). Three of the 14 patients with locally advanced or cutaneous metastatic adenocarcinoma of the breast responded to topical calcipotriol (216).

Two of 25 AIPC patients had objective partial responses in a Phase I trial of 1-alpha-hydroxyvitamin D_2 (217). This study identified 12.5 µg as the Phase II dose after encountering dose-limiting hypercalcemia and renal insufficiency. A follow-up Phase II study examined this regimen in 26 patients with androgen-independent prostate cancer. As the investigators expected this analog to act primarily as a cytostatic agent, the trial's primary end point was progression-free survival. Median time to progression was 12 weeks (mean 19 weeks) and one patient had stable disease for greater than two years.

TABLE 2 Phase II Studies of Chemotherapy in Combination with High-Dose Calcitriol

Investigators	Dose	Schedule of oral calcitriol	Companion drugs	Number of patients	Efficacy results
Beer et al. (2004)	0.5 μg/kg	24 hours prior to carboplatin	Carboplatin AUC of 7 (6 in patients with prior radiation) every 28 day	17	1 of 17 patients had a PSA response
Beer et al. (2003)	0.5 μg/kg	24 hours prior to each dose of docetaxel	Docetaxel 36 mg/m^2 weekly for 6 consecutive wk repeated every 8 wk	37	81% had PSA response. 8 of 15 responded in measurable disease. Median overall survival 19.5 mo
Beer et al. (2005)	45 μg (DN-101)	24 hours prior to each dose of docetaxel	Docetaxel 36 mg/m^2 weekly for 3 consecutive wks repeated every 4 wk	250 (125 DN-101, 125 placebo)	Improved survival with DN-101 (hazard ratio 0.67, $p = 0.035$), trend favoring DN-101 with respect to PSA response rates (overall 63% vs. 52%, $p = 0.07$, within 6 mo 58% vs. 49%, $p = 0.16$)

Abbreviations: AUC, area under curve; PSA, prostate specific antigen.
Source: From Ref. 208.

ILX23-7553 has entered Phase I clinical trials and was safe at doses up to 45 μg/m^2/day for five consecutive days repeated every 14 days. The study was discontinued before dose-limiting toxicity was identified due to the number of capsules required. The authors suggest that further dose escalation should be pursued using a reformulated higher-dose capsule (218).

CONCLUSIONS

There are intriguing epidemiological data and strong preclinical data that support targeting the VDR for cancer therapy in general and prostate cancer therapy specifically. Most of the clinical trials conducted to date have examined supplementation with calcitriol, the naturally occurring ligand of the VDR. Significant dose escalation of this compound is not feasible when it is dosed daily due to predictable hypercalcemia. Various intermittent dosing approaches have been developed and all demonstrate that intermittent dosing allows substantial escalation of the calcitriol dose and consequently of calcitriol exposure.

An alternative approach is the development of calcitriol analogs that seek to uncouple antineoplastic activity from calcemic action. Several such analogs have entered clinical trials, but in prostate cancer have been less extensively studied than calcitriol.

Single-agent studies have largely focused on safety. Confirmed responses to single-agent calcitriol or its analogs have rarely been reported. Stabilization of disease or apparent slowing of the rate of rise in serum PSA has been more often seen. While disease stabilization or PSA slowing is a finding that is consistent with the hypothesis that VDR ligands are acting as cytostatic agents, the available studies are small and uncontrolled and are not sufficient to draw firm conclusions about the clinical meaning of these observations. Progress in single-agent VDR ligand therapy will require a commitment to larger, randomized prospective clinical trials. A better understanding of the molecular determinants of response and resistance to calcitriol would also be helpful, as it could allow for better selection of patients whose tumor are vulnerable to this class of agents.

Calcitriol is the only VDR ligand that has been studied in combination with cytotoxic chemotherapy. To date, single-institution Phase II results, followed by results from a larger placebo-controlled randomized Phase II trial, provide strong encouraging evidence that the combination of calcitriol and docetaxel is safe and may prove efficacious in androgen-independent prostate cancer. A definitive international trial with the primary end point of survival will test this hypothesis starting in early 2006.

REFERENCES

1. Hanchette CL, Schwartz GG. Geographic patterns of prostate mortality. Evidence for a protective effect of ultraviolet radiation. Cancer 1992; 70:2861–2869.
2. Luscombe CJ, Fryer AA, French ME, et al. Exposure to ultraviolet radiation: association with susceptibility and age at presentation with prostate cancer. Lancet 2001; 358(9282):641–642.
3. Grant WB. An estimate of premature cancer mortality in the U.S. due to inadequate doses of solar ultraviolet-B radiation. Cancer 2002; 94(6):1867–1875.
4. Corder EH, Guess HA, Hulka BS, et al. Vitamin D and prostate cancer: a prediagnostic study with stored sera. Cancer Epidemiol Biomarkers Prev 1993; 2(5):467–472.

5. Gann PH, Ma J, Hennekens CH, et al. Circulating vitamin D metabolites in relation to subsequent development of prostate cancer. Cancer Epidemiol Biomarkers Prev 1996; 5(2):121–126.
6. Nomura AM, Stemmermann GN, Lee J, et al. Serum vitamin D metabolite levels and the subsequent development of prostate cancer (Hawaii, United States). Cancer Causes Control 1998; 9(4):425–432.
7. Jacobs ET, Giuliano AR, Martinez ME, et al. Plasma levels of 25-hydroxyvitamin D, 1,25-dihydroxyvitamin D and the risk of prostate cancer. J Steroid Biochem Mol Biol 2004; 89–90(1–5):533–537.
8. Platz EA, Leitzmann MF, Hollis BW, et al. Plasma 1,25-dihydroxy- and 25-hydroxyvitamin D and subsequent risk of prostate cancer. Cancer Causes Control 2004; 15(3):255–265.
9. Ahonen MH, Tenkanen L, Teppo L, et al. Prostate cancer risk and prediagnostic serum 25-hydroxyvitamin D levels (Finland). Cancer Causes Control 2000; 11(9):847–852.
10. Tuohimaa P, Tenkanen L, Ahonen M, et al. Both high and low levels of blood vitamin D are associated with a higher prostate cancer risk: a longitudinal, nested case-control study in the Nordic countries. Int J Cancer 2004; 108(1):104–108.
11. Chan JM, Pietinen P, Virtanen M, et al. Diet and prostate cancer risk in a cohort of smokers, with a specific focus on calcium and phosphorus (Finland). Cancer Causes Control 2000; 11(9):859–867.
12. Giovannucci E, Rimm EB, Wolk A, et al. Calcium and fructose intake in relation to risk of prostate cancer. Cancer Res 1998; 58(3):442–447.
13. Chan JM, Giovannucci E, Andersson SO, et al. Dairy products, calcium, phosphorous, vitamin D, and risk of prostate cancer (Sweden). Cancer Causes Control 1998; 9(6): 559–566.
14. Kristal AR, Cohen JH, Qu P, et al. Associations of energy, fat, calcium, and vitamin D with prostate cancer risk. Cancer Epidemiol Biomarkers Prev 2002; 11(8):719–725.
15. Qin LQ, Xu JY, Wang PY, et al. Milk consumption is a risk factor for prostate cancer: meta-analysis of case-control studies. Nutr Cancer 2004; 48(1):22–27.
16. Cross HS, Bareis P, Hofer H, et al. 25-Hydroxyvitamin D(3)-1alpha-hydroxylase and VDR gene expression in human colonic mucosa is elevated during early cancerogenesis. Steroids 2001; 66(3–5):287–292.
17. Tangpricha V, Flanagan JN, Whitlatch LW, et al. 25-Hydroxyvitamin D-1alpha-hydroxylase in normal and malignant colon tissue. Lancet 2001; 357(9269):1673–1674.
18. Chen TC, Wang L, Whitlatch LW, et al. Prostatic 25-hydroxyvitamin D-1alpha-hydroxylase and its implication in prostate cancer. J Cell Biochem 2003; 88(2): 315–322.
19. Hsu JY, Feldman D, McNeal JE, et al. Reduced 1alpha-hydroxylase activity in human prostate cancer cells correlates with decreased susceptibility to 25-hydroxyvitamin D3-induced growth inhibition. Cancer Res 2001; 61(7):2852–2856.
20. Bouillon RA, Auwerx JH, Lissens WD, et al. Vitamin D status in the elderly: seasonal substrate deficiency causes 1,25-dihydroxycholecalciferol deficiency. Am J Clin Nutr 1987; 45(4):755–763.
21. Dandona P, Menon RK, Shenoy R, et al. Low 1,25-dihydroxyvitamin D, secondary hyperparathyroidism, and normal osteocalcin in elderly subjects. J Clin Endocrinol Metab 1986; 63(2):459–462.
22. Dubbelman R, Jonxis JH, Muskiet FA, et al. Age-dependent vitamin D status and vertebral condition of white women living in Curacao (The Netherlands Antilles) as compared with their counterparts in The Netherlands. Am J Clin Nutr 1993; 58(1):106–109.
23. Lips P, Wiersinga A, van Ginkel FC, et al. The effect of vitamin D supplementation on vitamin D status and parathyroid function in elderly subjects. J Clin Endocrinol Metab 1988; 67(4):644–650.
24. Giovannucci E. Dietary influences of 1,25(OH)2 vitamin D in relation to prostate cancer: a hypothesis. Cancer Causes Control 1998; 9(6):567–582.
25. Beer TM, Myrthue A, Garzotto M, et al. Randomized study of high-dose pulse calcitriol or placebo prior to radical prostatectomy. Cancer Epidemiol Biomarkers Prev 2004; 13(12):2225–2232.

26. Zhou W, Suk R, Liu G, et al. Vitamin D is associated with improved survival in early-stage non-small cell lung cancer patients. Cancer Epidemiol Biomarkers Prev 2005; 14(10):2303–2309.
27. Robsahm TE, Tretli S, Dahlback A, et al. Vitamin D3 from sunlight may improve the prognosis of breast-, colon- and prostate cancer (Norway). Cancer Causes Control 2004; 15(2):149–158.
28. Mangelsdorf DJ, Thummel C, Beato M, et al. The nuclear receptor superfamily: the second decade. Cell 1995; 83(6):835–839.
29. Kliewer SA, Umesono K, Mangelsdorf DJ, et al. Retinoid X receptor interacts with nuclear receptors in retinoic acid, thyroid hormone and vitamin D3 signalling. Nature 1992; 355(6359):446–449.
30. Carlberg C, Saurat JH. Vitamin D-retinoid association: molecular basis and clinical applications. J Invest Dermatol Symp Proc 1996; 1(1):82–86.
31. Conde I, Paniagua R, Fraile B, et al. Expression of vitamin D3 receptor and retinoid receptors in human breast cancer: identification of potential heterodimeric receptors. Int J Oncol 2004; 25(4):1183–1191.
32. Nanes MS, Kuno H, Demay MB, et al. A single up-stream element confers responsiveness to 1,25-dihydroxyvitamin D3 and tumor necrosis factor-alpha in the rat osteocalcin gene. Endocrinology 1994; 134(3):1113–1120.
33. Koszewski NJ, Reinhardt TA, Horst RL. VDR interactions with the murine osteopontin response element. J Steroid Biochem Mol Biol 1996; 59(5–6):377–388.
34. Kim RH, Li JJ, Ogata Y, et al. Identification of a vitamin D3-response element that overlaps a unique inverted TATA box in the rat bone sialoprotein gene. Biochem J 1996; 318(Pt 1):219–226.
35. Kitazawa R, Kitazawa S. Vitamin D(3) augments osteoclastogenesis via vitamin D-responsive element of mouse RANKL gene promoter. Biochem Biophys Res Commun 2002; 290(2):650–655.
36. Drissi H, Pouliot A, Koolloos C, et al. 1,25-(OH)2-vitamin D3 suppresses the bone-related Runx2/Cbfa1 gene promoter. Exp Cell Res 2002; 274(2):323–333.
37. Hakim I, Bar-Shavit Z. Modulation of TNF-alpha expression in bone marrow macrophages: involvement of vitamin D response element. J Cell Biochem 2003; 88(5): 986–998.
38. Hawa NS, O'Riordan JL, Farrow SM. Functional analysis of vitamin D response elements in the parathyroid hormone gene and a comparison with the osteocalcin gene. Biochem Biophys Res Commun 1996; 228(2):352–357.
39. Falzon M. DNA sequences in the rat parathyroid hormone-related peptide gene responsible for 1,25-dihydroxyvitamin D3-mediated transcriptional repression. Mol Endocrinol 1996; 10(6):672–681.
40. Maestro B, Davila N, Carranza MC, et al. Identification of a vitamin D response element in the human insulin receptor gene promoter. J Steroid Biochem Mol Biol 2003; 84(2–3):223–230.
41. Lee S, Lee DK, Choi E, et al. Identification of a functional vitamin D response element in the murine Insig-2 promoter and its potential role in the differentiation of 3T3-L1 preadipocytes. Mol Endocrinol 2005; 19(2):399–408.
42. Quelo I, Machuca I, Jurdic P. Identification of a vitamin D response element in the proximal promoter of the chicken carbonic anhydrase II gene. J Biol Chem 1998; 273(17):10638–10646.
43. Seoane S, Alonso M, Segura C, et al. Localization of a negative vitamin D response sequence in the human growth hormone gene. Biochem Biophys Res Commun 2002; 292(1):250–255.
44. Gill RK, Christakos S. Identification of sequence elements in mouse calbindin-D28k gene that confer 1,25-dihydroxyvitamin D3- and butyrate-inducible responses. Proc Natl Acad Sci USA 1993; 90(7):2984–2988.
45. Fujisawa K, Umesono K, Kikawa Y, et al. Identification of a response element for vitamin D3 and retinoic acid in the promoter region of the human fructose-1,6-bisphosphatase gene. J Biochem (Tokyo) 2000; 127(3):373–382.

46. Liu M, Lee MH, Cohen M, et al. Transcriptional activation of the Cdk inhibitor p21 by vitamin D3 leads to the induced differentiation of the myelomonocytic cell line U937. Genes Dev 1996; 10(2):142–153.
47. Jiang F, Li P, Fornace AJ Jr., et al. G2/M arrest by 1,25-dihydroxyvitamin D3 in ovarian cancer cells mediated through the induction of GADD45 via an exonic enhancer. J Biol Chem 2003; 278(48):48030–48040.
48. Peng L, Malloy PJ, Feldman D. Identification of a functional vitamin D response element in the human insulin-like growth factor binding protein-3 promoter. Mol Endocrinol 2004; 18(5):1109–1119.
49. Matilainen M, Malinen M, Saavalainen K, et al. Regulation of multiple insulin-like growth factor binding protein genes by 1alpha,25-dihydroxyvitamin D3. Nucl Acids Res 2005; 33(17):5521–5532.
50. Zierold C, Darwish HM, DeLuca HF. Identification of a vitamin D-response element in the rat calcidiol (25-hydroxyvitamin D3) 24-hydroxylase gene. Proc Natl Acad Sci USA 1994; 91(3):900–902.
51. Thompson PD, Jurutka PW, Whitfield GK, et al. Liganded VDR induces CYP3A4 in small intestinal and colon cancer cells via DR3 and ER6 vitamin D responsive elements. Biochem Biophys Res Commun 2002; 299(5):730–738.
52. McCarthy TC, Li X, Sinal CJ. VDR-dependent regulation of colon multidrug resistance-associated protein 3 gene expression by bile acids. J Biol Chem 2005; 280(24): 23232–23242.
53. McGaffin KR, Chrysogelos SA. Identification and characterization of a response element in the EGFR promoter that mediates transcriptional repression by 1,25-dihydroxyvitamin D3 in breast cancer cells. J Mol Endocrinol 2005; 35(1):117–133.
54. Candeliere GA, Jurutka PW, Haussler MR, et al. A composite element binding the VDR, retinoid X receptor alpha, and a member of the CTF/NF-1 family of transcription factors mediates the vitamin D responsiveness of the c-fos promoter. Mol Cell Biol 1996; 16(2):584–592.
55. Xie Z, Bikle DD. Differential regulation of vitamin D responsive elements in normal and transformed keratinocytes. J Invest Dermatol 1998; 110(5):730–733.
56. Polly P, Carlberg C, Eisman JA, et al. Identification of a vitamin D3 response element in the fibronectin gene that is bound by a vitamin D3 receptor homodimer. J Cell Biochem 1996; 60(3):322–333.
57. Cao X, Ross FP, Zhang L, et al. Cloning of the promoter for the avian integrin beta 3 subunit gene and its regulation by 1,25-dihydroxyvitamin D3. J Biol Chem 1993; 268(36):27371–27380.
58. Bikle DD, Ng D, Oda Y, et al. The vitamin D response element of the involucrin gene mediates its regulation by 1,25-dihydroxyvitamin D3. J Invest Dermatol 2002; 119(5): 1109–1113.
59. Tenta R, Sourla A, Lembessis P, et al. Bone microenvironment-related growth factors, zoledronic acid and dexamethasone differentially modulate PTHrP expression in PC-3 prostate cancer cells. Horm Metab Res 2005; 37(10):593–601.
60. Deftos LJ, Barken I, Burton DW, et al. Direct evidence that PTHrP expression promotes prostate cancer progression in bone. Biochem Biophys Res Commun 2005; 327(2):468–472.
61. Lynch CC, Hikosaka A, Acuff HB, et al. MMP-7 promotes prostate cancer-induced osteolysis via the solubilization of RANKL. Cancer Cell 2005; 7(5):485–496.
62. Nemere I, Yoshimoto Y, Norman AW. Calcium transport in perfused duodena from normal chicks: enhancement within fourteen minutes of exposure to 1,25-dihydroxyvitamin D3. Endocrinology 1984; 115(4):1476–1483.
63. Edelman A, Garabedian M, Anagnostopoulos T. Mechanisms of 1,25(OH)2D3-induced rapid changes of membrane potential in proximal tubule: role of Ca2+-dependent K+ channels. J Membr Biol 1986; 90(2):137–143.
64. De Boland AR, Boland RL. Non-genomic signal transduction pathway of vitamin D in muscle. Cell Signal 1994; 6(7):717–724.
65. de Boland AR, Morelli S, Boland R. 1,25(OH)2-vitamin D3 signal transduction in chick myoblasts involves phosphatidylcholine hydrolysis. J Biol Chem 1994; 269(12):8675–8679.

66. de Boland AR, Facchinetti MM, Balogh G, et al. Age-associated decrease in inositol 1,4,5-trisphosphate and diacylglycerol generation by 1,25(OH)2-vitamin D3 in rat intestine. Cell Signal 1996; 8(3):153–157.
67. Beno DW, Brady LM, Bissonnette M, et al. Protein kinase C and mitogen-activated protein kinase are required for 1,25-dihydroxyvitamin D3-stimulated Egr induction. J Biol Chem 1995; 270(8):3642–3647.
68. Rossi AM, Capiati DA, Picotto G, et al. MAPK inhibition by 1alpha,25(OH)2-vitamin D3 in breast cancer cells. Evidence on the participation of the VDR and Src. J Steroid Biochem Mol Biol 2004; 89–90(1–5):287–290.
69. Gniadecki R. Activation of Raf-mitogen-activated protein kinase signaling pathway by 1,25-dihydroxyvitamin D3 in normal human keratinocytes. J Invest Dermatol 1996; 106(6):1212–1217.
70. Park WH, Seol JG, Kim ES, et al. Induction of apoptosis by vitamin D3 analogue EB1089 in NCI-H929 myeloma cells via activation of caspase 3 and p38 MAP kinase. Br J Haematol 2000; 109(3):576–583.
71. Capiati DA, Rossi AM, Picotto G, et al. Inhibition of serum-stimulated mitogen activated protein kinase by 1alpha, 25(OH)2-vitamin D3 in MCF-7 breast cancer cells. J Cell Biochem 2004; 93(2):384–397.
72. Vazquez G, Boland R, de Boland AR. Modulation by 1,25(OH)2-vitamin D3 of the adenylyl cyclase/cyclic AMP pathway in rat and chick myoblasts. Biochim Biophys Acta 1995; 1269(1):91–97.
73. Bellido T, Morelli S, Fernandez LM, et al. Evidence for the participation of protein kinase C and 3′,5′-cyclic AMP-dependent protein kinase in the stimulation of muscle cell proliferation by 1,25-dihydroxy-vitamin D3. Mol Cell Endocrinol 1993; 90(2): 231–238.
74. Massheimer V, Boland R, de Boland AR. Rapid 1,25(OH)2-vitamin D3 stimulation of calcium uptake by rat intestinal cells involves a dihydropyridine-sensitive cAMP-dependent pathway. Cell Signal 1994; 6(3):299–304.
75. Santillan GE, Boland RL. Studies suggesting the participation of protein kinase A in 1, 25(OH)2-vitamin D3-dependent protein phosphorylation in cardiac muscle. J Mol Cell Cardiol 1998; 30(2):225–233.
76. Hmama Z, Nandan D, Sly L, et al. 1alpha,25-Dihydroxyvitamin D(3)-induced myeloid cell differentiation is regulated by a VDR-phosphatidylinositol 3-kinase signaling complex. J Exp Med 1999; 190(11):1583–1594.
77. Lee JS, Hmama Z, Mui A, et al. Stable gene silencing in human monocytic cell lines using lentiviral-delivered small interference RNA. Silencing of the p110alpha isoform of phosphoinositide 3-kinase reveals differential regulation of adherence induced by 1alpha,25-dihydroxycholecalciferol and bacterial lipopolysaccharide. J Biol Chem 2004; 279(10):9379–9388.
78. Bektas M, Orfanos CE, Geilen CC. Different vitamin D analogues induce sphingomyelin hydrolysis and apoptosis in the human keratinocyte cell line HaCaT. Cell Mol Biol (Noisy-le-grand) 2000; 46(1):111–119.
79. Rebsamen MC, Sun J, Norman AW, et al. 1alpha,25-Dihydroxyvitamin D3 induces vascular smooth muscle cell migration via activation of phosphatidylinositol 3-kinase. Circ Res 2002; 91(1):17–24.
80. Schwartz Z, Ehland H, Sylvia VL, et al. 1alpha,25-Dihydroxyvitamin D(3) and 24R,25-dihydroxyvitamin D(3) modulate growth plate chondrocyte physiology via protein kinase C-dependent phosphorylation of extracellular signal-regulated kinase 1/2 mitogen-activated protein kinase. Endocrinology 2002; 143(7):2775–2786.
81. Rohe B, Safford SE, Nemere I, et al. Identification and characterization of 1,25D3-membrane-associated rapid response, steroid (1,25D3-MARRS)-binding protein in rat IEC-6 cells. Steroids 2005; 70(5–7):458–463.
82. Norman AW, Okamura WH, Bishop JE, et al. Update on biological actions of 1alpha,25(OH)2-vitamin D3 (rapid effects) and 24R,25(OH)2-vitamin D3. Mol Cell Endocrinol 2002; 197(1–2):1–13.
83. Norman AW, Okamura WH, Hammond MW, et al. Comparison of 6-s-cis- and 6-s-trans-locked analogs of 1alpha,25-dihydroxyvitamin D3 indicates that the 6-s-cis

conformation is preferred for rapid nongenomic biological responses and that neither 6-s-cis- nor 6-s-trans-locked analogs are preferred for genomic biological responses. Mol Endocrinol 1997; 11(10):1518–1531.

84. Erben RG, Soegiarto DW, Weber K, et al. Deletion of deoxyribonucleic acid binding domain of the VDR abrogates genomic and nongenomic functions of vitamin D. Mol Endocrinol 2002; 16(7):1524–1537.
85. Huhtakangas JA, Olivera CJ, Bishop JE, et al. The VDR is present in caveolae-enriched plasma membranes and binds 1 alpha,25(OH)2-vitamin D3 in vivo and in vitro. Mol Endocrinol 2004; 18(11):2660–2671.
86. Mizwicki MT, Bishop JE, Olivera CJ, et al. Evidence that annexin II is not a putative membrane receptor for 1alpha,25(OH)2-vitamin D3. J Cell Biochem 2004; 91(4): 852–863.
87. Abe E, Miyaura C, Sakagami H, et al. Differentiation of mouse myeloid leukemia cells induced by 1 alpha,25-dihydroxyvitamin D3. Proc Natl Acad Sci USA 1981; 78(8): 4990–4994.
88. Konety BR, Lavelle JP, Pirtskalaishvili G, et al. Effects of vitamin D (calcitriol) on transitional cell carcinoma of the bladder in vitro and in vivo. J Urol 2001; 165(1):253–258.
89. Colston KW, Chander SK, Mackay AG, et al. Effects of synthetic vitamin D analogues on breast cancer cell proliferation in vivo and in vitro. Biochem Pharmacol 1992; 44(4):693–702.
90. Cross HS, Huber C, Peterlik M. Antiproliferative effect of 1,25-dihydroxyvitamin D3 and its analogs on human colon adenocarcinoma cells (CaCo-2): influence of extracellular calcium. Biochem Biophys Res Commun 1991; 179(1):57–62.
91. Yabushita H, Hirata M, Noguchi M, et al. VDR in endometrial carcinoma and the differentiation-inducing effect of 1,25-dihydroxyvitamin D3 on endometrial carcinoma cell lines. J Obstet Gynaecol Res 1996; 22(6):529–539.
92. Nagakura K, Abe E, Suda T, Hayakawa M, Nakamura H, Tazaki H. Inhibitory effect of 1alpha,25-dihydroxyvitamin D3 on the growth of the renal carcinoma cell line. Kidney Int 1986; 29(4):834–840.
93. Fujioka T, Hasegawa M, Ishikura K, Matsushita Y, Sato M, Tanji S. Inhibition of tumor growth and angiogenesis by vitamin D3 agent in murine renal cell carcinoma. J Urol 1998; 160(1):247–251.
94. Higashimoto Y, Ohata M, Nishio K, et al. 1 alpha, 25-Dihydroxyvitamin D3 and all-trans-retinoic acid inhibit the growth of a lung cancer cell line. Anticancer Res 1996; 16(5A):2653–2659.
95. Zugmaier G, Jager R, Grage B, et al. Growth-inhibitory effects of vitamin D analogues and retinoids on human pancreatic cancer cells. Br J Cancer 1996; 73(11):1341–1346.
96. Skowronski RJ, Peehl DM, Feldman D. Vitamin D and prostate cancer: 1,25 dihydroxyvitamin D3 receptors and actions in human prostate cancer cell lines. Endocrinology 1993; 132(5):1952–1960.
97. Peehl DM, Skowronski RJ, Leung GK, et al. Antiproliferative effects of 1,25-dihydroxyvitamin D3 on primary cultures of human prostatic cells. Cancer Res 1994; 54(3):805–810.
98. Schwartz GG, Oeler TA, Uskokovic MR, et al. Human prostate cancer cells: inhibition of proliferation by vitamin D analogs. Anticancer Res 1994; 14(3A):1077–1081.
99. Skowronski RJ, Peehl DM, Feldman D. Actions of vitamin D3, analogs on human prostate cancer cell lines: comparison with 1,25-dihydroxyvitamin D3. Endocrinology 1995; 136(1):20–26.
100. Hedlund TE, Moffatt KA, Miller GJ. VDR expression is required for growth modulation by 1 alpha, 25-dihydroxyvitamin D3 in the human prostatic carcinoma cell line ALVA-31. J Steroid Biochem Mol Biol 1996; 58(3):277–288.
101. Zhuang SH, Schwartz GG, Cameron D, et al. VDR content and transcriptional activity do not fully predict antiproliferative effects of vitamin D in human prostate cancer cell lines. Mol Cell Endocrinol 1997; 126(1):83–90.
102. Getzenberg RH, Light BW, Lapco PE, et al. Vitamin D inhibition of prostate adenocarcinoma growth and metastasis in the Dunning rat prostate model system. Urology 1997; 50(6):999–1006.

103. Shabahang M, Buffan AE, Nolla JM, et al. The effect of 1, 25-dihydroxyvitamin D3 on the growth of soft-tissue sarcoma cells as mediated by the VDR. Ann Surg Oncol 1996; 3(2):144–149.
104. Tokuumi Y. Correlation between the concentration of 1,25 alpha dihydroxyvitamin D3 receptors and growth inhibition, and differentiation of human osteosarcoma cells induced by vitamin D3. Nippon Seikeigeka Gakkai Zasshi 1995; 69(4):181–190.
105. Hara K, Kusuzaki K, Takeshita H, et al. Oral administration of 1 alpha hydroxyvitamin D3 inhibits tumor growth and metastasis of a murine osteosarcoma model. Anticancer Res 2001; 21(1A):321–324.
106. Veenstra T, Londowski JM, Windebank AJ, Brimijoin S, Kumar R. Effects of 1,25-dihydroxyvitamin D3 on growth of mouse neuroblastoma cells. Brain Res Dev Brain Res 1997; 99(1):53–60.
107. Celli A, Treves C, Stio M. VDR in SH-SY5Y human neuroblastoma cells and effect of 1,25-dihydroxyvitamin D3 on cellular proliferation. Neurochem Int 1999; 34(2): 117–124.
108. Naveilhan P, Berger F, Haddad K, et al. Induction of glioma cell death by 1,25(OH)2 vitamin D3: toward an endocrine therapy of brain tumors? J Neurosci Res 1994; 37(2):271–277.
109. Colston K, Colston MJ, Feldman D. 1,25-dihydroxyvitamin D3 and malignant melanoma: the presence of receptors and inhibition of cell growth in culture. Endocrinology 1981; 108(3):1083–1086.
110. Hershberger PA, Modzelewski RA, Shurin ZR, et al. 1,25-Dihydroxycholecalciferol (1,25-D3) inhibits the growth of squamous cell carcinoma and down-modulates p21(Waf1/Cip1) in vitro and in vivo. Cancer Res 1999; 59(11):2644–2649.
111. McGuire TF, Trump DL, Johnson CS. Vitamin D(3)-induced apoptosis of murine squamous cell carcinoma cells. Selective induction of caspase-dependent mitoger-activated protein kinase (MEK) cleavage and up-regulation of MEKK-1. J Biol Chem 2001; 276(28):26365–26373.
112. Berger U, Wilson P, McClelland RA, et al. Immunocytochemical detection of 1,25-dihydroxyVDRs in normal human tissues. J Clin Endocrinol Metab 1988; 67(3):607–613.
113. Holick MF. Vitamin D: a millenium perspective. J Cell Biochem 2003; 88(2):296–307.
114. Wang QM, Jones JB, Studzinski GP. Cyclin-dependent kinase inhibitor p27 as a mediator of the G1-S phase block induced by 1,25-dihydroxyvitamin D3 in HL60 cells. Cancer Res 1996; 56(2):264–267.
115. Sheikh MS, Rochefort H, Garcia M. Overexpression of p21WAF1/CIP1 induces growth arrest, giant cell formation and apoptosis in human breast carcinoma cell lines. Oncogene 1995; 11(9):1899–1905.
116. Zhuang SH, Burnstein KL. Antiproliferative effect of 1alpha,25-dihydroxyvitamin D3 in human prostate cancer cell line LNCaP involves reduction of cyclin-dependent kinase 2 activity and persistent G1 accumulation. Endocrinology 1998; 139(3): 1197–1207.
117. Campbell MJ, Koeffler HP. Toward therapeutic intervention of cancer by vitamin D compounds. J Natl Cancer Inst 1997; 89(3):182–185.
118. Hershberger PA, Yu WD, Modzelewski RA, et al. Calcitriol (1,25-dihydroxycholecalciferol) enhances paclitaxel antitumor activity in vitro and in vivo and accelerates paclitaxel-induced apoptosis. Clin Cancer Res 2001; 7(4):1043–1051.
119. Inoue T, Kamiyama J, Sakai T. Sp1 and NF-Y synergistically mediate the effect of vitamin D(3) in the p27(Kip1) gene promoter that lacks vitamin D response elements. J Biol Chem 1999; 274(45):32309–32317.
120. Huang YC, Chen JY, Hung WC. Vitamin D3 receptor/Sp1 complex is required for the induction of p27Kip1 expression by vitamin D3. Oncogene 2004; 23(28):4856–4861.
121. Lin R, Wang TT, Miller WH Jr., et al. Inhibition of F-Box protein p45(SKP2) expression and stabilization of cyclin-dependent kinase inhibitor p27(KIP1) in vitamin D analog-treated cancer cells. Endocrinology 2003; 144(3):749–753.
122. Yang ES, Burnstein KL. Vitamin D inhibits G1 to S progression in LNCaP prostate cancer cells through p27Kip1 stabilization and Cdk2 mislocalization to the cytoplasm. J Biol Chem 2003; 278(47):46862–46868.

123. Kobayashi T, Hashimoto K, Yoshikawa K. Growth inhibition of human keratinocytes by 1,25-dihydroxyvitamin D3 is linked to dephosphorylation of retinoblastoma gene product. Biochem Biophys Res Commun 1993; 196(1):487–493.
124. Fan FS, Yu WC. 1,25-Dihydroxyvitamin D3 suppresses cell growth, DNA synthesis, and phosphorylation of retinoblastoma protein in a breast cancer cell line. Cancer Invest 1995; 13(3):280–286.
125. Jensen SS, Madsen MW, Lukas J, et al. Inhibitory effects of 1alpha,25-dihydroxyvitamin D(3) on the G(1)-S phase-controlling machinery. Mol Endocrinol 2001; 15(8):1370–1380.
126. Hager G, Formanek M, Gedlicka C, et al. 1,25(OH)2 vitamin D3 induces elevated expression of the cell cycle-regulating genes P21 and P27 in squamous carcinoma cell lines of the head and neck. Acta Otolaryngol 2001; 121(1):103–109.
127. Yen A, Varvayanis S. Late dephosphorylation of the RB protein in G2 during the process of induced cell differentiation. Exp Cell Res 1994; 214(1):250–257.
128. Reitsma PH, Rothberg PG, Astrin SM, et al. Regulation of myc gene expression in HL-60 leukaemia cells by a vitamin D metabolite. Nature 1983; 306(5942):492–494.
129. Matsumoto K, Hashimoto K, Nishida Y, et al. Growth-inhibitory effects of 1,25-dihydroxyvitamin D3 on normal human keratinocytes cultured in serum-free medium. Biochem Biophys Res Commun 1990; 166(2):916–923.
130. Tong WM, Kallay E, Hofer H, et al. Growth regulation of human colon cancer cells by epidermal growth factor and 1,25-dihydroxyvitamin D3 is mediated by mutual modulation of receptor expression. Eur J Cancer 1998; 34(13):2119–2125.
131. Vink-van Wijngaarden T, Pols HA, Buurman CJ, et al. Inhibition of insulin- and insulin-like growth factor-I-stimulated growth of human breast cancer cells by 1,25-dihydroxyvitamin D3 and the vitamin D3 analogue EB1089. Eur J Cancer 1996; 32A(5):842–848.
132. Drivdahl RH, Loop SM, Andress DL, et al. IGF-binding proteins in human prostate tumor cells: expression and regulation by 1,25-dihydroxyvitamin D3. Prostate 1995; 26(2):72–79.
133. Scharla SH, Strong DD, Subburaman M, et al. 1,25-Dihydroxyvitamin D3 differentially regulates the production of insulin-like growth factor I (IGF-I) and IGF-binding protein-4 in mouse osteoblasts. Endocrinology 1991; 129(6):3139–3146.
134. Haugen JD, Pittelkow MR, Zinsmeister AR, et al. 1alpha,25-Dihydroxyvitamin D3 inhibits normal human keratinocyte growth by increasing transforming growth factor b2 release. Biochem Biophys Res Commun 1996; 229:618–623.
135. Wu Y, Haugen JD, Zinsmeister AR, et al. 1 alpha,25-Dihydroxyvitamin D3 increases transforming growth factor and transforming growth factor receptor type I and II synthesis in human bone cells. Biochem Biophys Res Commun 1997; 239(3):734–739.
136. Elstner E, Linker-Israeli M, Said J, et al. 20-epi-Vitamin D3 analogues: a novel class of potent inhibitors of proliferation and inducers of differentiation of human breast cancer cell lines. Cancer Res 1995; 55(13):2822–2830.
137. Studzinski GP, Rathod B, Wang QM, et al. Uncoupling of cell cycle arrest from the expression of monocytic differentiation markers in HL60 cell variants. Exp Cell Res 1997; 232(2):376–387.
138. Qiao S, Tuohimaa P. Vitamin D3 inhibits fatty acid synthase expression by stimulating the expression of long-chain fatty-acid-CoA ligase 3 in prostate cancer cells. FEBS Lett 2004; 577(3):451–454.
139. Qiao S, Tuohimaa P. The role of long-chain fatty-acid-CoA ligase 3 in vitamin D3 and androgen control of prostate cancer LNCaP cell growth. Biochem Biophys Res Commun 2004; 319(2):358–368.
140. Bao BY, Hu YC, Ting HJ, et al. Androgen signaling is required for the vitamin D-mediated growth inhibition in human prostate cancer cells. Oncogene 2004; 23(19): 3350–3360.
141. Guzey M, Kitada S, Reed JC. Apoptosis induction by 1alpha, 25-dihydroxyvitamin D3 in prostate cancer. Mol Cancer Ther 2002; 1(9):667–677.
142. Modzelewski RA, Hershberger PA, Johnson CS, et al. Apoptotic effects of paclitaxel and calcitriol in rat dunning MLL and human PC-3 prostate tumors in vitro. Proc AACR 1999; 40:580.

143. Pepper C, Thomas A, Hoy T, et al. The vitamin D3 analog EB1089 induces apoptosis via a p53-independent mechanism involving p38 MAP kinase activation and suppression of ERK activity in B-cell chronic lymphocytic leukemia cells in vitro. Blood 2003; 101(7):2454–2460.
144. James SY, Mackay AG, Colston KW. Effects of 1,25 dihydroxyvitamin D3 and its analogues on induction of apoptosis in breast cancer cells. J Steroid Biochem Mol Biol 1996; 58(4):395–401.
145. Wagner N, Wagner KD, Schley G, et al. 1,25-Dihydroxyvitamin D3-induced apoptosis of retinoblastoma cells is associated with reciprocal changes of Bcl-2 and bax. Exp Eye Res 2003; 77(1):1–9.
146. Simboli-Campbell M, Narvaez CJ, Tenniswood M, et al. 1,25-Dihydroxyvitamin D3 induces morphological and biochemical markers of apoptosis in MCF-7 breast cancer cells. J Steroid Biochem Mol Biol 1996; 58(4):367–376.
147. Sergeev IN RW, Norman AW. 1,25-Dihydroxyvitamin D3, intracellular Ca2+ and apoptosis in breast cancer cell lines. In: Norman AW BR, Thomasset M, eds. Vitamin D Chemistry, Biology and Clinical Applications of the Steroid Hormone. Riverside, CA: University of California, 1997:473–474.
148. Vandewalle B, Wattez N, Lefebvre J. Effects of vitamin D3 derivatives on growth, differentiation and apoptosis in tumoral colonic HT 29 cells: possible implication of intracellular calcium. Cancer Lett 1995; 97(1):99–106.
149. Elstner E, Linker-Israeli M, Umiel T, et al. Combination of potent 20-epi-vitamin D3 analogue (KH 1060) with 9-cis-retinoic acid irreversibly inhibits clonal growth, decreases bcl-2 expression, and induces apoptosis in HL-60 leukemic cells. Cancer Res 1996; 56(15):3570–3576.
150. Mathiasen IS, Lademann U, Jaattela M. Apoptosis induced by vitamin D compounds in breast cancer cells is inhibited by Bcl-2 but does not involve known caspases or p53. Cancer Res 1999; 59(19):4848–4856.
151. Polek TC, Stewart LV, Ryu EJ, et al. p53 is required for 1,25-dihydroxyvitamin D3-induced G0 arrest but is not required for G1 accumulation or apoptosis of LNCaP prostate cancer cells. Endocrinology 2003; 144(1):50–60.
152. Galbiati F, Polastri L, Thorens B, et al. Molecular pathways involved in the antineoplastic effects of calcitriol on insulinoma cells. Endocrinology 2003; 144(5):1832–1841.
153. Narvaez CJ, Welsh J. Role of mitochondria and caspases in vitamin D-mediated apoptosis of MCF-7 breast cancer cells. J Biol Chem 2001; 276(12):9101–9107.
154. Xie SP, James SY, Colston KW. Vitamin D derivatives inhibit the mitogenic effects of IGF-I on MCF-7 human breast cancer cells. J Endocrinol 1997; 154(3):495–504.
155. Bernardi RJ, Trump DL, Yu WD, et al. Combination of 1alpha,25-dihydroxyvitamin D(3) with dexamethasone enhances cell cycle arrest and apoptosis: role of nuclear receptor cross-talk and Erk/Akt signaling. Clin Cancer Res 2001; 7(12):4164–4173.
156. Bernardi RJ, Johnson CS, Modzelewski RA, et al. Antiproliferative effects of 1alpha,25-dihydroxyvitamin D(3) and vitamin D analogs on tumor-derived endothelial cells. Endocrinology 2002; 143(7):2508–2514.
157. Rocker D, Ravid A, Liberman UA, et al. 1,25-Dihydroxyvitamin D3 potentiates the cytotoxic effect of TNF on human breast cancer cells. Mol Cell Endocrinol 1994; 106(1–2):157–162.
158. Murthy S, Weigel NL. 1alpha,25-Dihydroxyvitamin D3 induced growth inhibition of PC-3 prostate cancer cells requires an active transforming growth factor beta signaling pathway. Prostate 2004; 59(3):282–291.
159. Sergeev IN, Rhoten WB. Regulation of intracellular calcium in human breast cancer cells. Endocrine 1998; 9(3):321–327.
160. Sergeev IN. Calcium as a mediator of 1,25-dihydroxyvitamin D3-induced apoptosis. J Steroid Biochem Mol Biol 2004; 89–90(1–5):419–425.
161. Jiang F, Bao J, Li P, et al. Induction of ovarian cancer cell apoptosis by 1,25-dihydroxyvitamin D3 through the down-regulation of telomerase. J Biol Chem 2004; 279(51):53213–53221.

162. De Haes P, Garmyn M, Degreef H, et al. 1,25-Dihydroxyvitamin D3 inhibits ultraviolet B-induced apoptosis, Jun kinase activation, and interleukin-6 production in primary human keratinocytes. J Cell Biochem 2003; 89(4):663–673.
163. Mantell DJ, Owens PE, Bundred NJ, et al. 1 alpha,25-Dihydroxyvitamin D(3) inhibits angiogenesis in vitro and in vivo. Circ Res 2000; 87(3):214–220.
164. Majewski S, Skopinska M, Marczak M, et al. Vitamin D3 is a potent inhibitor of tumor cell-induced angiogenesis. J Invest Dermatol Symp Proc 1996; 1(1):97–101.
165. Yudoh K, Matsuno H, Kimura T. 1alpha,25-Dihydroxyvitamin D3 inhibits in vitro invasiveness through the extracellular matrix and in vivo pulmonary metastasis of B16 mouse melanoma. J Lab Clin Med 1999; 133(2):120–128.
166. Schwartz GG, Wang MH, Zang M, et al. 1 alpha,25-Dihydroxyvitamin D (calcitriol) inhibits the invasiveness of human prostate cancer cells. Cancer Epidemiol Biomarkers Prev 1997; 6(9):727–732.
167. Sung V, Feldman D. 1,25-Dihydroxyvitamin D3 decreases human prostate cancer cell adhesion and migration. Mol Cell Endocrinol 2000; 164(1–2):133–143.
168. Bao BY, Yeh SD, Lee YF. 1{alpha},25-Dihydroxyvitamin D3 inhibits prostate cancer cell invasion via modulation of selective proteases. Carcinogenesis 2006; 27(1):32–42.
169. Hansen CM, Frandsen TL, Brunner N, et al. 1 alpha,25-Dihydroxyvitamin D3 inhibits the invasive potential of human breast cancer cells in vitro. Clin Exp Metastasis 1994; 12(3):195–202.
170. Young MR, Ihm J, Lozano Y, et al. Treating tumor-bearing mice with vitamin D3 diminishes tumor-induced myelopoiesis and associated immunosuppression, and reduces tumor metastasis and recurrence. Cancer Immunol Immunother 1995; 41(1):37–45.
171. Koli K, Keski-Oja J. 1alpha,25-Dihydroxyvitamin D3 and its analogues down-regulate cell invasion-associated proteases in cultured malignant cells. Cell Growth Differ 2000; 11(4):221–229.
172. Campbell MJ, Elstner E, Holden S, et al. Inhibition of proliferation of prostate cancer cells by a 19-nor-hexafluoride vitamin D3 analogue involves the induction of p21waf1, p27kip1 and E-cadherin. J Mol Endocrinol 1997; 19(1):15–27.
173. Gonzalez-Sancho JM, Alvarez-Dolado M, Munoz A. 1,25-Dihydroxyvitamin D3 inhibits tenascin-C expression in mammary epithelial cells. FEBS Lett 1998; 426(2):225–228.
174. Yu WD, McElwain MC, Modzelewski RA, et al. Enhancement of 1,25-dihydroxyvitamin D3-mediated antitumor activity with dexamethasone. J Natl Cancer Inst 1998; 90(2):134–141.
175. Beer TM, Hough KM, Garzotto M, et al. Weekly high-dose calcitriol and docetaxel in advanced prostate cancer. Semin Oncol 2001; 28(4 suppl 15):49–55.
176. Moffatt KA, Johannes WU, Miller GJ. 1alpha,25Dihydroxyvitamin D3 and platinum drugs act synergistically to inhibit the growth of prostate cancer cell lines. Clin Cancer Res 1999; 5(3):695–703.
177. Ahmed S, Johnson CS, Rueger RM, et al. Calcitriol (1,25-dihydroxycholecalciferol) potentiates activity of mitoxantrone/dexamethasone in an androgen independent prostate cancer model. J Urol 2002; 168(2):756–761.
178. Light BW, Yu WD, McElwain MC, et al. Potentiation of cisplatin antitumor activity using a vitamin D analogue in a murine squamous cell carcinoma model system. Cancer Res 1997; 57(17):3759–3764.
179. Wieder R, Wang Q, Uytingco M, et al. 1,25-Dihydroxyvitamin D3 and all-trans retinoic acid promote apoptosis and sensitize breast cancer cells to the effects of chemotherapeutic agents. Proc Am Soc Clin Onc 1998; 17:107a.
180. Sundaram S, Chaudhry M, Reardon D, et al. The vitamin D3 analog EB 1089 enhances the antiproliferative and apoptotic effects of adriamycin in MCF-7 breast tumor cells. Breast Cancer Res Treat 2000; 63(1):1–10.
181. Torres R, Calle C, Aller P, et al. Etoposide stimulates 1,25-dihydroxyvitamin D3 differentiation activity, hormone binding and hormone receptor expression in HL-60 human promyelocytic cells. Mol Cell Biochem 2000; 208(1–2):157–162.

182. Koga M, Sutherland RL. Retinoic acid acts synergistically with 1,25-dihydroxyvitamin D3 or antioestrogen to inhibit T-47D human breast cancer cell proliferation. J Steroid Biochem Mol Biol 1991; 39(4A):455–460.
183. Guzey M, Sattler C, DeLuca HF. Combinational effects of vitamin D3 and retinoic acid (all trans and 9 cis) on proliferation, differentiation, and programmed cell death in two small cell lung carcinoma cell lines. Biochem Biophys Res Commun 1998; 249(3): 735–744.
184. Peehl DM, Feldman D. Interaction of nuclear receptor ligands with the vitamin D signaling pathway in prostate cancer. J Steroid Biochem Mol Biol 2004; 92(4):307–315.
185. Ikeda N, Uemura H, Ishiguro H, et al. Combination treatment with 1alpha, 25-dihydroxyvitamin D3 and 9-cis-retinoic acid directly inhibits human telomerase reverse transcriptase transcription in prostate cancer cells. Mol Cancer Ther 2003; 2(8):739–746.
186. Anzano MA, Smith JM, Uskokovic MR, et al. 1 alpha,25-Dihydroxy-16-ene-23-yne-26,27-hexafluorocholecalciferol (Ro24–5531), a new deltanoid (vitamin D analogue) for prevention of breast cancer in the rat. Cancer Res 1994; 54(7):1653–1656.
187. Welsh J. Induction of apoptosis in breast cancer cells in response to vitamin D and antiestrogens. Biochem Cell Biol 1994; 72(11–12):537–545.
188. Abe-Hashimoto J, Kikuchi T, Matsumoto T, et al. Antitumor effect of 22-oxa-calcitriol, a noncalcemic analogue of calcitriol, in athymic mice implanted with human breast carcinoma and its synergism with tamoxifen. Cancer Res 1993; 53(11):2534–2537.
189. Christensen GL, Jepsen JS, Fog CK, et al. Sequential versus combined treatment of human breast cancer cells with antiestrogens and the vitamin D analogue EB1089 and evaluation of predictive markers for vitamin D treatment. Breast Cancer Res Treat 2004; 85(1):53–63.
190. Gavrilov V, Steiner M, Shany S. The combined treatment of 1,25-dihydroxyvitamin D3 and a non-steroid anti-inflammatory drug is highly effective in suppressing prostate cancer cell line (LNCaP) growth. Anticancer Res 2005; 25(5):3425–3429.
191. Moreno J, Krishnan AV, Feldman D. Molecular mechanisms mediating the anti-proliferative effects of vitamin D in prostate cancer. J Steroid Biochem Mol Biol 2005; 97(1–2):31–36.
192. Moreno J, Krishnan AV, Swami S, et al. Regulation of prostaglandin metabolism by calcitriol attenuates growth stimulation in prostate cancer cells. Cancer Res 2005; 65(17):7917–7925.
193. Hsiao M, Tse V, Carmel J, et al. Functional expression of human p21(WAF1/CIP1) gene in rat glioma cells suppresses tumor growth in vivo and induces radiosensitivity. Biochem Biophys Res Commun 1997; 233(2):329–335.
194. Dunlap N, Schwartz GG, Eads D, et al. 1alpha,25-Dihydroxyvitamin D(3) (calcitriol) and its analogue, 19-nor-1alpha,25(OH)(2)D(2), potentiate the effects of ionising radiation on human prostate cancer cells. Br J Cancer 2003; 89(4):746–753.
195. Polar MK, Gennings C, Park M, et al. Effect of the vitamin D3 analog ILX 23-7553 on apoptosis and sensitivity to fractionated radiation in breast tumor cells and normal human fibroblasts. Cancer Chemother Pharmacol 2003; 51(5):415–421.
196. DeMasters GA, Gupta MS, Jones KR, et al. Potentiation of cell killing by fractionated radiation and suppression of proliferative recovery in MCF-7 breast tumor cells by the vitamin D3 analog EB 1089. J Steroid Biochem Mol Biol 2004; 92(5):365–374.
197. Osborn JL, Schwartz GG, Smith DC, et al. Phase II trial of oral 1,25-dihydroxyvitamin D (calcitriol) in hormone refractory prostate cancer. Urol Oncol 1995; 1(5):195–198.
198. Gross C, Stamey T, Hancock S, et al. Treatment of early recurrent prostate cancer with 1,25-dihydroxyvitamin D3 (calcitriol). J Urol 1998; 159(6):2035–2039; discussion 2039–2040.
199. Smith DC, Johnson CS, Freeman CC, et al. A phase I trial of calcitriol (1,25-dihydroxycholecalciferol) in patients with advanced malignancy. Clin Cancer Res 1999; 5(6): 1339–1345.
200. Beer TM, Munar M, Henner WD. A Phase I trial of pulse calcitriol in patients with refractory malignancies: pulse dosing permits substantial dose escalation. Cancer 2001; 91(12):2431–2439.

201. Muindi JR, Peng Y, Potter DM, et al. Pharmacokinetics of high-dose oral calcitriol: results from a phase 1 trial of calcitriol and paclitaxel. Clin Pharmacol Ther 2002; 72(6):648–659.
202. Beer TM, Javle M, Lam GN, et al. Pharmacokinetics and tolerability of a single dose of DN-101, a new formulation of calcitriol, in patients with cancer. Clin Cancer Res 2005; 11(21):7794–7799.
203. Beer TM, Javle M, Henner WD, et al. Pharmacokinetics (PK) and tolerability of DN-101, a new formulation of calcitriol, in patients with cancer. Proc Am Assoc Cancer Res 2004; 45.
204. Morris MJ, Smaletz O, Solit D, et al. High-dose calcitriol, zoledronate, and dexamethasone for the treatment of progressive prostate carcinoma. Cancer 2004; 100(9): 1868–1875.
205. Tiffany NM, Ryan CW, Garzotto M, et al. High dose pulse calcitriol, docetaxel and estramustine for androgen independent prostate cancer: a phase I/II study. J Urol 2005; 174(3):888–892.
206. Beer TM, Lemmon D, Lowe BA, et al. High-dose weekly oral calcitriol in patients with a rising PSA after prostatectomy or radiation for prostate carcinoma. Cancer 2003; 97(5):1217–1224.
207. Beer TM, Eilers KM, Garzotto M, et al. Weekly high-dose calcitriol and docetaxel in metastatic androgen-independent prostate cancer. J Clin Oncol 2003; 21(1):123–128.
208. Beer T, Ryan C, Venner P, et al. ASCENT: A double-blinded randomized study of DN-101 vs. placebo plus docetaxel is androgen-independent prostate cancer. European J Cancer 2005; 3(2): 232.
209. Beer TM, Garzotto M, Katovic NM. High-dose calcitriol and carboplatin in metastatic androgen-independent prostate cancer. Am J Clin Oncol 2004; 27(5):535–541.
210. Kissmeyer AM, Binderup E, Binderup L, et al. Metabolism of the vitamin D analog EB 1089: identification of in vivo and in vitro liver metabolites and their biological activities. Biochem Pharmacol 1997; 53(8):1087–1097.
211. Bouillon R, Verstuyf A, Verlinden L, et al. Non-hypercalcemic pharmacological aspects of vitamin D analogs. Biochem Pharmacol 1995; 50(5):577–583.
212. Bouiloon R, Okamura WH, Norman AW. Structure-function relationships in the vitamin D endocrine system. Endocrine Rev 1995; 16(2):200–257.
213. Gulliford T, English J, Colston KW, et al. A phase I study of the vitamin D analogue EB 1089 in patients with advanced breast and colorectal cancer. Br J Cancer 1998; 78(1): 6–13.
214. Evans TR, Colston KW, Lofts FJ, et al. A phase II trial of the vitamin D analogue Seocalcitol (EB1089) in patients with inoperable pancreatic cancer. Br J Cancer 2002; 86(5):680–685.
215. Dalhoff K, Dancey J, Astrup L, et al. A phase II study of the vitamin D analogue Seocalcitol in patients with inoperable hepatocellular carcinoma. Br J Cancer 2003; 89(2):252–257.
216. Bower M, Colston KW, Stein RC, et al. Topical calcipotriol treatment in advanced breast cancer. Lancet 1991; 337(8743):701–702.
217. Liu G, Oettel K, Ripple G, et al. Phase I trial of 1alpha-hydroxyvitamin d(2) in patients with hormone refractory prostate cancer. Clin Cancer Res 2002; 8(9):2820–2827.
218. Wieder R, Novick SC, Hollis BW, et al. Pharmacokinetics and safety of ILX23-7553, a non-calcemic-vitamin D3 analogue, in a phase I study of patients with advanced malignancies. Invest New Drugs 2003; 21(4):445–452.

18 Other Novel Therapies

Arif Hussain and Richard Schraeder
University of Maryland Greenebaum Cancer Center, Baltimore, Maryland, U.S.A.

INTRODUCTION

Advanced hormone-resistant prostate cancer (HRPC) remains a major cause of morbidity and mortality, and its treatment has proven to be particularly challenging. Although mitoxantrone in combination with steroids was shown to provide palliation in metastatic HRPC without affecting survival, recently two large randomized trials have demonstrated that taxane-based chemotherapy improves survival when compared to mitoxantrone (1–4). However, progress has been incremental, with overall survival remaining less than two years in this group of patients. For patients not responding to taxanes, or those failing initial chemotherapy, the prognosis is even more dismal. Thus, there is an urgent need to identify new agents and treatment strategies in metastatic HRPC. Among the novel treatments for HRPC that are currently being investigated are the cytotoxic agents epothilones and satraplatin, which are the subject of this chapter.

EPOTHILONES

Background

The epothilones are 16-membered macrolides produced by the myxobacteria *Sorangium cellulosum*; this myxobacteria was isolated from the banks of the Zambesi River in the Republic of South Africa (5). The genes involved in the biosynthesis of epothilones have been identified (6). In *S. cellulosum*, Epothilones A and B are derived from Epothilones C and D, respectively, by the action of epoxidases (6,7). Although naturally occurring, synthesis of these molecules has been achieved in the laboratory (8). Moreover, several hundred semisynthetic analogs have been developed, some of which are entering clinical trials (8,9).

Epothilones bind to the β-tubulins and stabilize the microtubular network, thereby disrupting the cell cycle which ultimately leads to cell death (10–12). In this regard, the overall mechanism of action of the epothilones is similar to the taxanes, although these two classes of drugs are structurally quite different. Epothilones and paclitaxel can compete for the same binding site within the β-tubulins (10). However, recent crystallographic studies show that each compound engages the tubulin-binding pocket in a unique manner (13). This is also consistent with the observation that different amino-acid residues in and around the tubulin-binding pocket undergo point mutations when cell lines are selected for resistance to epothilones or paclitaxel (14–17). Furthermore, certain β-tubulin mutants that are resistant to paclitaxel are not so to the epothilones, while other mutants may show differing degrees of resistance and crossresistance to these compounds (14–17).

The mechanisms by which stabilization of the microtubules leads to cell death are complex and not completely understood; the intrinsic mitochondrial pathway plays an important role in the process. Among the various molecular mediators, p53 status of the cells can dictate relative sensitivity to taxanes and epothilones. For instance, cells with mutant p53/loss of p53 function show increased sensitivity to these drugs (18,19). The role of p53 in the process depends upon both the cellular context and the specific mutations within p53. As an example, certain point mutations within the transactivation domain of p53 can trigger apoptosis in a transcription-independent manner in response to epothilones (20). By contrast, p53-negative cells transfected with a proline-rich domain deletion mutant of p53 are relatively resistant to microtubule-damaging agents (20). Interestingly, in other cells, wild-type p53 is involved in mediating epothilone-induced cell death. In particular, epothilone-mediated increase in wild-type p53 in HCT116 human cancer cells results in an increase in the BH3-only proapoptotic protein PUMA, which in turn induces a conformational change in Bax, resulting in translocation of the latter to the mitochondria and the induction of apoptosis (20). In human breast cancer cells, the BH3-only protein Bim is involved in mediating Bax conformational change and apoptosis in response to paclitaxel-mediated microtubule stabilization (21). In addition, these agents can also potentially affect angiogenesis (22). Despite the complexities underlying the integration of various signals leading to apoptosis, the differential sensitivity of cancer cells and normal cells to microtubule stabilization has been exploited for therapeutic purposes, as demonstrated by the remarkable clinical success of the taxanes (paclitaxel and docetaxel).

Given that the microtubules represent an important cellular target in the treatment of cancer, epothilones potentially offer certain advantages over the taxanes. These compounds have a simpler overall structure that is more amenable to synthesis and manipulation (8). In general, these compounds tend to be more water soluble than the taxanes. Further, they are not substrates for p-glycoprotein, a drug efflux pump that can confer resistance to taxanes (10). Several in vitro, cell culture and human cancer xenograft studies suggest that epothilones may possess greater activity than paclitaxel, although the extent of tubulin polymerization does not necessarily correlate with their cytotoxicity (10,17,23–27).

Clinical Studies

Of the numerous epothilone derivatives, four have undergone various degrees of clinical evaluation in the Phase I and II settings (9). These include the naturally occurring Epothilone B (patupilone, EPO906), two semisynthetic analogs, i.e., aza-Epothilone B (ixabepilone and BMS-247550) and BMS-310705 (a water-soluble Epothilone B derivative), and Epothilone D (KOS-862). Various treatment schedules have been evaluated in patients; these include every three week, weekly, and daily × 3 or daily × 5 (repeated every 21 days) dosing schedules (9). The major dose-limiting toxicities (DLT) observed with this group of drugs include myelosuppression, neuropathies, and diarrhea, with a proportion of patients also experiencing grade 3/4 fatigue, nausea, and vomiting (9,28–30). The toxicity profiles depend not only on the specific epothilone, but also on the drug formulation used and the schedule of drug delivery (9,28–30). For instance, myelosuppression and neuropathy are commonly observed with every three-week ixabepilone, while diarrhea has been a major issue with weekly patupilone. Neurologic symptoms are also more common with BMS-310705 and Epothilone D.

In the treatment of prostate cancer, ixabepilone has been most extensively studied (31–33). A Phase I trial investigated the maximum tolerated dose (MTD) of ixabepilone administered in combination with estramustine (EMP) in patients with HRPC (31). This trial was part of a two-step program to rapidly investigate ixabepilone in this disease, and results of the Phase II component have also been recently published (32). Thirteen patients were accrued to the Phase I trial; one patient was taken off study because of hypersensitivity reaction to ixabepilone (31). All patients enrolled had castrate levels of serum testosterone and were chemotherapy naïve. EMP was administered 280 mg orally (po) t.i.d. on days 1 to 5, and ixabepilone was administered IV over three hours on day 2 every 21 days. Patients received thromboembolic prophylaxis with warfarin 2 mg po daily as well as hypersensitivity reaction prophylaxis. Two dose levels of ixabepilone were evaluated, i.e., 35 and 40 mg/m^2. Grade 4 neutropenia was observed in three of six patients at the 40 mg/m^2 dose, and thus the MTD for ixabepilone given in combination with EMP on the above dosing schedule was determined to be 35 mg/m^2. As in other trials investigating ixabepilone, neutropenia was the DLT. Other toxicities included grade I thrombocytopenia (9/12 patients), ≤grade 2 diarrhea (5/12 patients), grade 3 nausea (2/12 patients), and thromboembolic events (2/12 patients). Of note, eight patients developed neurotoxicity; six of these eight patients had significant neuropathy (>grade 2). Eleven of 12 assessable patients (92%) had a posttreatment prostate-specific antigen (PSA) decline greater than 50%. The median time to PSA nadir was reported as 13 weeks and median time to PSA progression was 19 weeks. The authors noted that median time to PSA progression was similar to that of EMP/taxane-based regimens.

The second phase of the two-stage study was a randomized Phase II trial of ixabepilone with or without EMP in patients with progressive HRPC (32). Ninety-two patients were accrued, and were randomly assigned to receive ixabepilone 35 mg/m^2 every three weeks (45 patients), or ixabepilone 35 mg/m^2 on day 2 with EMP 280 mg po t.i.d. daily on days 1 to 5 (47 patients). As in the first step Phase I trial, all patients were chemotherapy naïve and had castrate, progressive metastatic prostate cancer. All patients had hypersensitivity prophylaxis, and those on the combination arm also received warfarin 2 mg daily. The primary end point was the proportion of patients achieving a 50% or greater post-therapy decline in PSA. Dose reduction was required in 12 of the 264 total cycles administered in the combination arm (nine dose reductions of ixabepilone and three dose reductions of EMP), and in eight of the 268 total cycles administered on the ixabepilone alone arm.

Twelve-month follow-up revealed 44 of 45 patients on the combination arm and 46 of 47 patients on the ixabepilone alone arm stopped therapy. Patients received a median of five cycles on the ixabepilone plus EMP arm, and a median of four cycles on the ixabepilone alone arm. The most common reasons for termination of treatment in both arms were progression of disease (34% in the combination arm and 50% in the ixabepilone alone arm) and toxicity (36% and 35%, respectively). Neuropathy was the most common toxicity leading to discontinuation of treatment (18% combination arm and 28% single arm). Grade 3 or 4 toxicities included neutropenia (29%), febrile neutropenia (9%), fatigue (9%), neuropathy (7%), and thrombosis (6%) on the combination arm, and neutropenia (22%), fatigue (9%), and neuropathy (13%) on the single-agent arm. Nausea and vomiting were not significant adverse events. Peripheral neuropathy occurred commonly, and was observed in 73% of patients on the combination arm and 67% on the single arm; this neuropathy appeared to improve with time post discontinuation of therapy (median time to improvement was 46 days). A decline in PSA of 50% or greater occurred in 69% of patients on the combination arm and 48% on the ixabepilone alone arm, with time to PSA progression being 5.2 and 4.4 months, respectively, on the combination and single-agent arms. It was concluded that ixabepilone, with or without EMP, is active in patients with HRPC.

The Southwest Oncology Group also recently published a Phase II trial which evaluated single-agent ixabepilone in patients with HRPC (33). Forty-eight patients were enrolled (42 were eligible) in this trial and received ixabepilone 40 mg/m^2 IV over three hours every 21 days. Enrolled patients had progressive, metastatic HRPC and were chemotherapy naïve. The primary end point of the trial was proportion of patients with $\geq$50% decline in serum PSA; secondary end points included overall survival and progression-free survival. One-level dose reduction was required in 11 patients, and one patient required a two-level dose reduction. Treatment was discontinued after progression of disease, unacceptable toxicity, or treatment delay of more than three weeks. Grade 4 toxicities included neuropenia (7%) and leukopenia (2%). The most common grade 3 adverse events were neurologic toxicity (19%), hematologic toxicity (7%), flu-like symptoms (12%), and infection (12%). Thirteen patients were removed from treatment because of toxicity, 10 because of peripheral neuropathy, and three due to fatigue. Overall, 60% of the treated patients experienced some form of neurotoxicity. Fourteen (33%) patients had a confirmed PSA response, with median progression-free survival and median survival being 6 and 18 months, respectively. This trial confirmed the results of the other previous Phase II trial, demonstrating activity of ixabepilone in chemotherapy-naïve metastatic HRPC.

Patupilone is the other epothilone that has been evaluated in a Phase II, multicenter trial in patients with HRPC, and preliminary results reported in abstract form (34). In contrast to the two Phase II ixabepilone trials, 29 (64%) of the 45 patients treated with patupilone had received prior chemotherapy. Patupilone was given at 2.5 mg/m^2 IV over five minutes three out of every four weeks. No significant myelosuppression or neuropathy was reported but grade 3 diarrhea occurred in 22% of the treated patients. Of note is that three of six PSA-responding patients had received prior taxanes.

Although experience with epothilone is still limited in advanced prostate cancer, it is apparent that they do have activity in this disease. Whether they will provide any advantage over the taxanes either in the first- or second-line setting in metastatic HRPC, however, remains to be determined. Further, their toxicity profile has to be put in proper context with that observed with the taxanes, and relative benefit–toxicity ratios clarified.

SATRAPLATIN

Background

Bis-Aceto-ammine-dichloro-cyclohexylamine-platinum (IV) [also known as satraplatin, BMS-182751, or JM216 (Johnson Mathey Technology Center, Reading, United Kingdom)] is a third-generation, oral platinum complex currently being evaluated in several malignancies, including HRPC. Like tetraplatin and the new platinum drug (OC-6-43)-bis (acatato) (1-adamantylamine) amminedichloroplatinum (IV) (coded LA-12), satraplatin is a platinum (IV) compound, whereas cisplatin, carboplatin, and oxaliplatin are platinum (II) compounds (35–37). Satraplatin is essentially a prodrug that undergoes rapid biotransformation in blood, generating several platinum (II) and platinum (IV) metabolites that retain activity (38,39). As with other platinum analogs, satraplatin forms intrastrand and interstrand DNA adducts, resulting in cellular toxicity. Several mechanisms can lead to resistance to the platinum class of drugs, including alterations in cellular drug uptake, enhanced detoxification (e.g., via glutathiones and metallothioneins), and repair of the platinum-induced DNA lesions by nucleotide excision repair pathways, and in some cases also by DNA mismatch repair (40,41). Studies suggest that, compared to cisplatin, resistance to satraplatin may be less likely to occur due to decreased drug accumulation (42). Further, in some tumor models satraplatin also demonstrates greater activity than other platinum compounds (43). Whether such properties translate into a more effective platinum drug has yet to be clearly established. Nevertheless, satraplatin offers several potential advantages, including the fact that it is orally bioavailable; the other oral platinum currently undergoing evaluation is the platinum (IV) drug LA-12 (44). In addition, satraplatin has not been associated with significant neurotoxicity or nephrotoxicity, although myelosuppression and gastrointestinal side effects can be prominent (45,46). In terms of schedule of administration, preclinical in vivo studies demonstrate that, compared to single dose or chronic daily dosing, daily × 5 oral administration produces better antitumor activity as well as tolerability; as a result, this schedule has been adopted in many satraplatin clinical trials (47).

Clinical Studies

Data with satraplatin in advanced HRPC are limited. Results of a completed small Phase II trial have been reported recently (48). In this trial, satraplatin was administered orally daily × 5 days in patients with HRPC. Thirty-nine patients were enrolled, and a total of 155 courses of drug were administered. Patients received satraplatin 120 mg/m^2/day for 5 consecutive days every 28 days (the dose interval was initially every 21 days but was amended after the first five patients experienced delayed hematologic recovery). All enrolled patients had received no prior cytotoxic agents or large field (>30% of marrow-bearing area) radiotherapy. The median age of the enrolled patients was 69 years, and overall they had good performance status and no significant medical comorbidities. The most common serious adverse events (grade 3 or higher) included thrombocytopenia (54%), neutropenia (52%), diarrhea (28%), anemia (24%), vomiting (16%), and nausea (13). Approximately a third of the patients experienced an elevation in liver function tests, with three requiring discontinuation of therapy due to this. Except for gastrointestinal toxicities, nonhematologic toxicities were generally grade 1 and 2. Of note, one patient developed a myelodysplastic syndrome approximately 11 months after treatment. Nineteen (49%), 13 (33%), and 5 (13%) patients had treatment discontinued due to progressive disease, treatment-related toxicity, or upon patient request, respectively (48). PSA response was evaluated in 32 patients; 10 (26%) had partial response, 14 (36%) stable disease, and 8 (21%) PSA progression. Of the 20 patients with measurable disease, two had an objective partial response. The median overall survival was 16.7 months, median PSA response duration was 3.8 months, and median progression-free survival was 7.7 months in the 32 assessable patients. An unexpected finding of prolonged myelosuppression was noted (the median cycle interval was prolonged at 38 days). It was concluded that while satraplatin demonstrated moderate activity in patients with chemotherapy-naïve HRPC, the toxicities (particularly late recovery of neutropenia and thrombocytopenia and gastrointestinal toxicities) encountered in this group of patients was significant and complicated management. The authors suggested that future clinical studies utilizing satraplatin in the treatment of HRPC should evaluate lower starting doses with longer cycle duration (48).

A Phase III randomized trial of satraplatin plus prednisone versus prednisone alone was also launched in patients with HRPC. The primary end points were to determine overall survival and time to pain progression. The initial study design planned for a sample size of 380 patients. However, after 50 patients were enrolled, the trial was closed prematurely by the sponsoring company. Hence, the statistical power of a Phase III trial was not achieved and no definitive conclusions on the study's primary end points can be made. Although the trial was far from meeting its target accrual, an ad hoc analysis on the 50 randomized patients has been performed (49).

Patients with metastatic chemotherapy-naïve HRPC were randomized either to satraplatin 100 mg/m^2/day orally on days 1 to 5 every 35 days plus prednisone 10 mg orally b.i.d. continuously or prednisone 10 mg orally b.i.d. alone (49). Twenty-seven patients were randomized to the combination arm and 23 to the prednisone alone arm. Overall, patients characteristics were not significantly different on the two treatment arms. Patients on the combination arm received antiemetic prophylaxis on the days of satraplatin therapy. Dose reductions due to toxicities were rare. A median of four cycles were administered on the combination arm, and a median of three cycles on the prednisone alone arm. Treatment was discontinued in all but three patients due to disease progression (two patients on the combination arm were taken off study due to toxicity). None of the patients on the prednisone arm experienced grade 3 or 4 hematologic toxicities, while on the combination arm 30% had grade 3 thrombocytopenia, 26% grade 3 leukopenia, and 15% grade 3 or 4 neutropenia. Grade 3 vomiting or diarrhea were noted in 7% of the patients receiving combined therapy and in none in the control arm. One patient in each treatment arm was suspected to have died from presumed steroid-related stomach perforation. At the time of study submission for publication, 48 of the 50 patients had progressed and 42 died, mostly due to prostate cancer. Overall survival was 14.9 months on the combination arm and 11.9 months on the prednisone alone arm ($p = 0.579$). A greater than 50% decline in PSA was seen in 33% of patients on the combination arm and 8.7% on the prednisone arm ($p = 0.046$), while progression-free survival was 5.2 and 2.5 months ($p = 0.023$), respectively (49,50). Due to the small number of patients, although the analysis lacked significant power and no definitive conclusions on the impact of satraplatin plus prednisone on pain or overall survival could be made, a trend towards better PSA response and longer time to progression were noted with the combination therapy.

The potential role of satraplatin is also being evaluated in patients with metastatic HRPC who have failed one (but not more than one) prior chemotherapy regimen in the satraplatin and prednisone against refractory cancer (SPARC) trial (50). This is a multicenter, placebo-controlled, double-blind study with a target accrual of over 900 patients and a 2:1 randomization favoring the satraplatin arm. The satraplatin dose has been reduced by 20% in this study, i.e., patients receive satraplatin at 80 mg/m^2/day on days 1 to 5 every five weeks plus prednisolone 5 mg b.i.d. continuously along with prophylactic antiemetics; in the control arm patients receive placebo (including antiemetic placebo) plus prednisolone. The primary end point of the study is time to progression, defined as first occurrence of tumor progression. Overall survival is a secondary end point. Accrual to the study was recently completed, and results are awaited.

CONCLUSION

Over the last few years it has become apparent that metastatic HRPC is a relatively chemotherapy-responsive disease. However, chemotherapy is largely palliative, and the majority of men with metastatic prostate cancer eventually succumb to their disease. Identification of more effective treatments, including for patients failing first-line chemotherapies, remains a significant challenge (51,52). To meet this challenge, new cytotoxics and new targets are being identified and studied. Epothilones and satraplatin are examples of some of the newer agents being evaluated in advanced prostate cancer. Although a concerted effort has been made to study these drugs, their role in the treatment of metastatic HRPC has yet to be clearly defined.

ACKNOWLEDGMENTS

This work was supported in part by a Merit Review Award from the Medical Research Service, Department of Veterans Affairs (A.H.). The authors thank Christine Webb for typing the manuscript.

REFERENCES

1. Tannock IF, Osoba D, Stockler MR, et al. Chemotherapy with mitoxantrone plus prednisone or prednisone alone for symptomatic hormone-resistant prostate cancer: a Canadian randomized trial with palliative end points. J Clin Oncol 1996; 14(6):1756–1764.
2. Kantoff PW, Halabi S, Conaway M, et al. Hydrocortisone with or without mitoxantrone in men with hormone-refractory prostate cancer: results of the Cancer and Leukemia Group B 9182 Study. J Clin Oncol 1999; 17(8):2506.
3. Tannock IF, de Wit R, Berry WR, et al. Docetaxel plus prednisone or mitoxantrone plus prednisone for advanced prostate cancer. N Engl J Med 2004; 351(15):1502–1512.
4. Petrylak DP, Tangen CM, Hussain MH, et al. Docetaxel and estramustine compared with mitoxantrone and prednisone for advanced refractory prostate cancer. N Engl J Med 2004; 351(15):1513–1520.
5. Gerth K, Bedorf N, Hofle G, et al. Epothilone A and B: antifungal and cytotoxic compounds from *Sorangium cellulosum* (Myxobacteria): production, physicochemical, and biological properties. J Antibiot 1996; 49(6):560–563.
6. Tang L, Shah S, Chung L, et al. Cloning and heterologous expression of the epothilone gene cluster. Science 2000; 287(5453):640–642.
7. Gerth K, Steinmetz H, Hofle G, et al. Studies on the biosynthesis of epothilones: The PKS and epothilone C/D monooxygenase. J Antibiot 2001; 54(2):144–148.
8. Watkins EB, Chittiboyina AG, Jung J-C, Avery MA. The epothilones and related analogues—a review of their syntheses and anti-cancer activities. Curr Pharm Des 2005; 11(13):1615–1653.
9. Goodin S, Kane MP, Rubin EH. Epothilones: mechanism of action and biologic activity. J Clin Oncol 2004; 22(10):2015–2025.
10. Bollag DM, McQueney PA, Zhu J, et al. Epothilones, a new class of microtubule-stabilizing agents with taxol-like mechanism of action. Cancer Res 1995; 55(11):2325–2333.
11. Kamath K, Jordan MA. Suppression of microtubule dynamics by epothilone B is associated with mitotic arrest. Cancer Res 2003; 63(18):6026–6031.
12. Chen J-G, Yang C-P, Cammer M, Horwitz SB. Gene expression and mitotic exit by microtubule-stabilizing drugs. Cancer Res 2003; 63(22):7891–7899.
13. Nettles JH, Li H, Cornett B, et al. The binding mode of epothilone A on α, β-tubulin by electron crystallography. Science 2004; 305(5685):866–869.
14. He L, Yang CP, Horwitz SB. Mutations in β-tubulin map to domains involved in regulation of microtubule stability in epothilone-resistant cell lines. Mol Cancer Ther 2001; 1(1):3–10.
15. Giannakakou P, Gussio R, Nogales E, et al. A common pharmacophore for epothilone and taxanes: molecular basis for drug resistance conferred by tubulin mutations in human cancer cells. Proc Natl Acad Sci USA 2000; 97(6):2904–2909.

16. Verrills NM, Flemming CL, Liu M, et al. Microtubule alterations and mutations induced by desoxyepothilone B: implications for drug-target interactions. Chem Biol 2003; 10(7):597–607.
17. Kowalski RJ, Giannakakou P, Hamel E. Activities of the microtubule-stabilizing agents epothilones A and B with purified tubulin and in cells resistant to paclitaxel (Taxol®). J Biol Chem 1997; 272(4):2534–2541.
18. Ioffe ML, White E, Nelson DA, et al. Epothilone induced cytotoxicity is dependent on p53 status in prostate cells. Prostate 2004; 61(3):243—247.
19. Wahl AF, Donaldson KL, Fairchild C, et al. Loss of normal p53 function confers sensitization to Taxol by increasing G2/M arrest and apoptosis. Nat Med 1996; 2(1):72–79.
20. Yamaguchi H, Chen J, Bhalla K, Wang H-G. Regulation of Bax activation and apoptotic response to microtubule-damaging agents by p53 transcription-dependent and -independent pathways. J Biol Chem 2004; 279(38):39,431–39,437.
21. Sunters A, Fernandez de Mattos S, Stahl M, et al. FoxO3a transcriptional regulation of Bim controls apoptosis in paclitaxel-treated breast cancer cell lines. J Biol Chem 2003; 278(50):49,795–49,805.
22. Belotti D, Vergani V, Drudis T, et al. The microtubule-affecting drug paclitaxel has antiangiogenic activity. Clin Cancer Res 1996; 2(11):1843–1849.
23. Lee FY; Borzilleri R, Fairchild CR, et al. BMS-247550: a novel epothilone analog with a mode of action similar to paclitaxel but possessing superior antitumor efficacy. Clin Cancer Res 2001; 7(5):1429–1437.
24. Sepp-Lorenzino L, Balog A, Su D-S, et al. The microtubule-stabilizing agents epothilones A and B and their desoxy-derivatives induce mitotic arrest and apoptosis in human prostate cells. Prostate Cancer Prostatic Dis 1999; 2(1):41–52.
25. Newman RA, Yang J, Finlay MR, et al. Antitumor efficacy of 26-fluoroepothilone B against human prostate cancer xenografts. Cancer Chemother Pharmacol 2001; 48(4):319–326.
26. Kolman A. Activity of epothilones. Curr Opin Invest Drugs 2005; 6(6):616–622.
27. Altmann KH, Bold G, Caravatti G, et al. Synthesis and biological evaluation of highly potent analogues of epothilones B and D. Bioorg Med Chem Lett 2000; 10(24):2765–2768.
28. Rubin EH, Rothermel J, Tesfaye F, et al. Phase I dose-finding study of weekly single-agent patupilone in patients with advanced solid tumors. J Clin Oncol 2005; 23(36):9120–9129.
29. de Jonge M, Verweij J. The epothilone dilemma. J Clin Oncol 2005; 23(36):9048–9050.
30. Kolman A. Epothilone D (Kosan/Roche). Curr Opin Invest Drugs 2004; 5(6):657–667.
31. Smaletz O, Galsky M, Scher HI, et al. Pilot study of epothilone B analog (BMS-247550) and estramustine phosphate in patients with progressive metastatic prostate cancer following castration. Ann Oncol 2003; 14(10):1518–1524.
32. Galsky MD, Small EJ, Oh WK, et al. Multi-institutional randomized Phase III trial of the epothilone B analog ixabepilone (BMS-247550) with or without estramustine phosphate in patients with progressive castrate metastatic prostate cancer. J Clin Oncol 2005; 23(7):1439–1446.
33. Hussain M, Tangen CM, Lara PN, et al. Ixabepilone (epothilone B analogue BMS-247550) is active in chemotherapy-naive patients with hormone-refractory prostate cancer: a Southwest Oncology Group trial S0111. J Clin Oncol 2005; 23(34):8724–8729.
34. Hussain A, Dipaola RS, Baron AD, et al. A Phase II trial of weekly EPO906 in patients with hormone-refractory prostate cancer (HRPC). Program and Abstracts of the 40th Annual Meeting of the American Society of Clinical Oncology; June 5–8, 2005; New Orleans, Louisiana, Abstract 4563.
35. Christian MC, Spriggs D, Tutsch KD, et al. Phase I trials with Ormaplatin (tetraplatin). In: Howell SD, ed. Platinum and Other Metal Coordination Compounds in Cancer Chemotherapy. New York: Plenum Press, 1991:453–458.
36. Zak F, Turanek J, Kroutil A, et al. Platinum(IV) complex with adamantylamine as noncleaving amine group: synthesis, characterization, and in vitro antitumor activity against a panel of cisplatin-resistant cancer cell lines. J Med Chem 2004; 47(3):761–763.
37. Giandominico CM, Abrams MJ, Murrer BA, et al. Synthesis and reactions of a new class of orally active Pt (IV) antitumor complexes. In: Howell SB, ed. Platinum and Other

Metal Coordination Compounds in Cancer Chemotherapy. New York: Plenum Press, 1991:93–100.

38. Raynaud FI, Mistry P, Donaghue A, et al. Biotransformation of the platinum drug JM216 following oral administration to cancer patients. Cancer Chemother Pharmacol 1996; 38(2):155–162.
39. Carr JL, Tingle MD, McKeage MJ. Rapid biotransformation of satraplatin by human red blood cells in vitro. Cancer Chemother Pharmacol 2002; 50(1):9–15.
40. Reardon JT, Vaisman A, Chaney SG, Sancar A. Efficient nucleotide excision repair of cisplatin, oxaliplatin, and Bis-aceto-ammine-dichloro-cyclohexylamine-platinum (IV) (JM216) platinum intrastrand DNA diadducts. Cancer Res 1999; 59(16):3968–3971.
41. Fink D, Nebel S, Aebi S, et al. The role of DNA mismatch repair in platinum drug resistance. Cancer Res 1996; 56(21):4881–4886.
42. Mellish KJ, Kelland LR. Mechanisms of acquired resistance to the orally active platinum-based anticancer drug bis-acetato-ammine-dichloro-cyclohexylamine platinum (IV) (JM216) in two human ovarian carcinoma cell lines. Cancer Res 1994; 54(23): 6194–6200.
43. Kelland R, Abel G, McKeage M, et al. Preclinical antitumor evaluation of bis-acetato-ammine-dichloro-cyclohexylamine platinum (IV): an orally active platinum drug. Cancer Res 1993; 53(11):2581–2586.
44. Sova P, Mistr A, Kroutil A, et al. Preclinical anti-tumor activity of a new oral platinum (IV) drug. Anti-Cancer Drugs 2005; 16(6):653–657.
45. McKeage MJ, Boxall FE, Jones M, Harrap K. Lack of neurotoxicity of oral bisacetatoamminedichlorocyclohexylamine-platinum (IV) in comparison to cisplatin and tetraplatin in the rat. Cancer Res 1994; 54(3):629–631.
46. Fokkema E, de Vries EGE, Meijer S, Groen HJM. Lack of nephrotoxicity of new oral platinum drug JM216 in lung cancer patients. Cancer Chemother Pharmacol 2000; 45(1):89–92.
47. McKeage MJ, Kelland LR, Boxall FE, et al. Schedule dependency of orally administered bis-acetato-ammine-dichloro-cyclohexylamine-platinum (IV) (JM216) in vivo. Cancer Res 1994; 54(15):4118–4122.
48. Latif T, Wood L, Connell C, et al. Phase II study of oral bis (aceto) ammine dichloro (cyclohexamine) platinum (IV) (JMS-216, BMS-182751) given daily × 5 in hormone refractory prostate cancer (HRPC). Invest New Drugs 2005; 23(1);79–84.
49. Sternberg CN, Whellan P, Hetherington J, et al. Phase III trial of satraplatin, an oral platinum plus prednisone vs. prednisone alone in patients with hormone-refractory prostate cancer. Oncology 2005; 68(1):2–9.
50. Sternberg CN. Satraplatin in the treatment of hormone-refractory prostate cancer. Br J Urol Int 2005; 96(7):990–994.
51. Berthold DR, Sternberg CN, Tannock IF. Management of advanced prostate cancer after first-line chemotherapy. J Clin Oncol 2005; 23(32):8247–8252.
52. Bhandari MS, Petrylak DP, Hussain M. Clinical trials in metastatic prostate cancer-Has there been real progress in the past decade? Eur J Cancer 2005; 41(6):941–953.

19 Molecular Imaging, Clinical Trial Design, and the Development of Emerging Therapies for Metastatic Prostate Cancer

Michael J. Morris and Howard I. Scher
Genitourinary Oncology Service, Department of Medicine, Memorial Sloan-Kettering Cancer Center, New York, New York, U.S.A.

Neeta Pandit-Taksar, Chaitanya Divgi, and Steven Larson
Nuclear Medicine Service, Department of Radiology, Memorial Sloan-Kettering Cancer Center, New York, New York, U.S.A.

INTRODUCTION

Patients with metastatic prostate cancer and their physicians can choose among an unprecedented array of investigational therapeutics whose aim is to alter the basic biology of prostate cancer growth and the metastatic cascade. These drugs can target intracellular signaling, the androgen receptor (AR), apoptosis regulation, angiogenesis, immune surveillance, and other mechanisms of tumor growth and metastatic spread. They can also distinguish prostate cancer cells from normal tissues and can target the bone microenvironment. Many have enhanced antiproliferative or proapoptotic effects on tumor cells relative to normal tissues. Despite these advances in the clinical availability of biologic agents, novel cytotoxics, immunologic manipulations, and targeted therapies, the standard imaging tools to assess both the tumor itself and the effects of drugs on the tumor are relatively primitive.

The usual modalities for imaging solid tumors (tomographic imaging, X-ray, and ultrasound) are not optimal for detecting metastatic lesions, which are most commonly in the skeleton, and poorly delineate treatment effects. Bone scintigraphy shows bone deposition only and not the cancer itself. Bone lesions shown on computerized tomography and plain radiographs generally only appear as sclerotic lesions that may bear little relation to tumor size, nor can they distinguish between the healing effects of successful therapy vs. the osteoblastic response of bone to a tumor that is continuing to progress on therapy.

As a result of all the above limitations, standard imaging hampers drug development for advanced prostate cancer, just as it did when the only treatment options were androgen ablation and chemotherapy. The lack of good imaging methods clouds the identification of active therapies, confuses the decision of when to advance a drug from Phase II to III, and ultimately delays bringing new treatments to patients. Accurate imaging modalities are particularly needed in the age of targeted or biologic therapies, where effective therapies may be cytostatic and may not result in significant prostate-specific antigen (PSA) declines. In such cases, molecular imaging may be the only means by which early biologic activity of a new drug may be detectable in a Phase I or II study. New imaging modalities are under development to allow investigators to identify disease on the basis of aberrant metabolism and the expression of prostate-specific molecules. The prospective testing and validation of these agents is nascent, as is their incorporation into clinical trials. This chapter is a review of these novel imaging modalities that appear to be most relevant for prostate cancer.

PROSTATE CANCER, STANDARD IMAGING, AND CLINICAL TRIAL DESIGN

Distribution of Disease

Prostate cancer is the paradigm of the bone tropic disease. Prostate cancer cells have been shown to produce a host of factors that make it suitable for living in the bone microenvironment, altering osteoblast and osteoclast functionality, and interrupting normal osteoblast and osteoclast communication. These factors include transforming growth factor beta and insulin-like growth factors (1–4), parathyroid hormone-related protein (5–8), osteoprotegrin, and RANK ligand. Prostate cancer cells produce bone matrix proteins such as osteocalcin and osteonectin, alter osteoblast differentiation, bone matrix formation and degradation, and bone remodeling (9–13). As a result, both bone deposition and resorption are altered (14,15), although phenotypically, blastic metastases are the characteristic lesion.

Historically, only 5% to 20% of prostate cancer patients enrolled in trials for castration-resistant disease had tumor masses that were measurable in two dimensions. Even those patients with measurable disease had only a few lesions that generally were small, raising the question of whether they truly represented the primary burden of disease in bone (16–18). However, contemporary Phase III studies have reported an increased number of soft-tissue lesions than have historically been reported. In these studies, as shown in Table 1, as many as half of the patients have been described as having measurable disease, be it in lymph nodes, the viscera, or both. Such a demographic shift would suggest that either the natural history of prostate cancer is perhaps altering, that imaging techniques are improving so that previously undetectable lesions are now measurable, or that investigators have changed their standards of reporting.

Although it is difficult to attribute this shift to any single factor, it does not appear that a change in the true distribution of disease is a major factor. In a retrospective review of 124 patients treated in clinical trials at Memorial Sloan-Kettering

TABLE 1 Distribution of Disease with Contemporary Phase III Studies

	No. of patients	Patients with bone metastases (%)	Patients with nodal disease (%)	Patients with liver or visceral disease (%)
TAX 327 trial (19)	464	90–92	Not stated[a]	22–24
SWOG 99–16 (20)	770	84–88	24–26	18–19
Mitoxantrone/ Prednisone (21)	120	79–86	18	6
MSKCC data set	124	112 (90.3)	48 (38.7)	15 (12.1)

Note: Ranges are given to express the range of percentages across multiple arms of the studies cited.
[a]39–40% had “measurable disease” (including visceral disease).

Cancer Center between 1999 and 2003, 57% were reported as either having soft-tissue disease alone or as having bone and soft-tissue disease. Of these, only 44% had measurable disease by Response Evaluation Criteria in Solid Tumors (RECIST) guidelines using a 2 cm cutoff for defining a target lesion, and 51% had a target lesion >1 cm. Furthermore, a close analysis of these lesions revealed that indeed even in these patients, measurable disease was still not a significant component of patients' overall burden of disease. The median size of all lesions was only 2.5 cm, and was 3 cm if the 2 cm cutoff for defining a target lesion was applied. The median number of such lesions per patient was only 2. Hence, although more than half of the patients were reported as having some form of soft-tissue disease, disease was generally limited to a few small lymph nodes in those who actually had target lesions (22,23).

Prostate cancer is still, therefore, a disease that is characterized by only a minor component of measurable disease, even in the contemporary era. Bone metastases are considered to be nonmeasurable and nontarget by RECIST guidelines (24–28). The primary reservoir of metastatic tumor is, therefore, not measurable using standard techniques.

Bone Scintigraphy Other Standards

Because of the prominent role of new bone formation in metastatic prostate cancer, the archetypal molecular imaging study is the radionuclide bone scan, which targets hydroxyapatite. Bone scintigraphy utilizes technetium-99m (^{99m}Tc) labeled to a polyphosphonate that targets hydroxyapatite, which is the principal component of bone cortex and permits visualization of the entire skeleton. Methylidene diphosphonate is the most commonly used polyphosphonate. Areas of new bone deposition are visualized as foci of increased radioactivity. Bone scanning has excellent sensitivity for bone metastases. However, because only the increased hydroxyapatite turnover is imaged, rather than the cancer itself, the technique lacks true specificity, and other benign lesions including degenerative disease can interfere with the interpretation of these scans. It has greater accuracy at detecting skeletal metastasis in prostate cancer than a clinical evaluation, plain X-ray of the bone, or serum alkaline and acid phosphatase levels (29). Although bone scans are the basis of disease evaluation and management in prostate cancer, it is an imperfect and limited tool for assessing tumor dimensions and treatment response.

Since bone scans detect hydroxyapatite, the turnover of which may also be increased in healing bone, patients who appear to be responding to therapy by virtue of a decline in markers or relief of symptoms can have a paradoxically worsening bone scan. These changes may be the result of an increase in tracer uptake due to treatment-induced changes in blood flow or osteoblast activity rather than an increase in tumor burden. This "flare phenomenon" can be seen in up to 20% of patients (24–26,28,30,31). That does not imply that there is consensus on how to evaluate the remaining 80% patients: some will have stable bone scans, others will have lesions of lesser intensity, and still others will have fewer lesions. There are no definite criteria on what constitutes a "response." Bone scans are therefore limited in indicating treatment effects, though treatment failure can be detected early by demonstrating visualization of new lesions. Progression of disease is therefore easier to detect by bone scintigraphy than is disease regression, and even new lesions may not represent new foci of disease (22).

Detection of bone disease by standard radiographs, especially in the vertebral bodies where many metastases are located due to their rich supply of bone marrow, is insensitive (32,33). Plain radiography and tomography do not contribute significantly to bone scintigraphy in demonstrating metastatic disease. Bone metastases on standard scans are generally represented by areas of sclerosis, the radiographic equivalent of the osteoblastic lesion. However, such sclerosis is not a representation of the tumor itself, but the secondary effects of the cancer on bone. In addition, sclerosis can be seen in noncancer-related processes, and, like bone scintigraphy, can represent bone healing rather than bone injury. For these reasons, standard imaging that is currently available is inadequate and is of limited use to accurately measure tumor volume changes and response to therapy. Other than ruling out vertebral collapse or impending pathologic fracture of long bones, standard imaging contributes little to assessments of tumor involvement in this disease.

Biochemical and Pathology-Based Alternatives to Assessing Measurable Lesions

To compensate for the lack of effective imaging modalities available to indicate whether an agent is effective, investigators have turned to the PSA. Serial PSA levels can be obtained easily and frequently with minimal inconvenience to the patient. Posttreatment declines in PSA have been shown to correlate with survival (34–39). Recently, the prognostic significance of a posttherapy nadir that is undetectable (or <0.2) was reported (29,32,40). Several investigators have proposed that posttherapy PSA changes be used as surrogates for clinical benefits such as time to metastases or prostate cancer-specific mortality in different clinical states (38,41,42). However, the demonstration of an association does not equate with surrogacy, and there remains a large proportion of the association between PSA-based metrics and clinical outcomes that is, as yet, unexplained. Therefore, posttherapy PSA changes have not been adopted by the Food and Drug Administration as an intermediate end point that can be used for an accelerated approval in this patient group.

With the introduction of mechanism-based therapy, the interpretation of a PSA change as a measure of response is made more complex. Some drugs may be effective, yet result in no PSA decline, only a modulation of the PSA rate of rise. Others still may result in PSA stabilization only. For example, zoledronic acid, which alters the bone microenvironment by poisoning osteoclasts, does not alter PSA, yet has been shown to reduce disease-related skeletal events (43). Vaccine therapy that has preliminarily been shown to prolong overall survival (44), does not induce significant PSA declines from baseline and may only alter PSA doubling time (45). Certain biologic therapies, such as calcitriol, may cause cancer cells to release PSA (and thereby elevate levels), yet calcitriol may well have antitumor effects alone, and may even improve overall survival when combined with chemotherapy, even if significant PSA declines are not attained (46).

Even with the availability of the PSA assay, therefore, obtaining an early readout on whether a new drug is effective is still a challenge. At the present time, such indicators of treatment effects are treated independently, with posttreatment alterations in PSA, bone, and soft tissue reported separately. These composite end points have been codified in a series of consensus reports, which are specific to the clinical state for which the drug is being tested. Consensus reports have been issued for patients with castrate metastatic disease and for those who have a rising PSA as their only manifestation of relapse following surgery or radiation (18,47).

Early-phase clinical trials for other solid tumors frequently utilized pathology assays to validate that a targeted or biologic therapy has impacted a given pathway. It is well established, however, that many pathways that may have clinical relevance are variably expressed based on the clinical state of the patient. This is true of HER2, BCL-2, PTEN, the AR, and other therapeutic targets (48–52). Characterizing these pathways for the purposes of drug development is necessary, both to screen appropriate patients for a particular biologic agent and to establish pharmacodynamic effects of therapy. Unfortunately, characterizing these aberrant pathways is difficult, as biopsies from bone marrow in patients with metastatic disease frequently do not yield cancer. For example, in one multicenter, national, cooperative group trial of patients with metastatic androgen-independent prostate cancer, only 25% of patients who underwent a bone marrow biopsy actually yielded a tumor sample, although patients with indices of higher tumor burden were more likely to have a positive biopsy than those who did not (53).

Given that prostate cancer has a paucity of measurable lesions, that PSA is an imperfect tool for assessing treatment effects, and that the acquisition of metastatic tissue is difficult, new methods of assessing the disease are essential to the development of novel therapies. These methods are already under development, and unlike standard imaging modalities, have the potential to directly image the disease, to show the pathways being targeted, and to demonstrate treatment effects.

Molecular Imaging with Radionuclides

Radionuclide imaging can be divided broadly into two categories. The first is single-photon imaging, which is exemplified by bone scanning and refers to imaging based on gamma-emitting isotopes like ^{99m}Tc , indium-111 (^{111}In), and lutetium-177 (^{177}Lu) that may be linked to molecules. The second category is imaging based on positron-emitting isotopes, exemplified by fluorine-18 (^{18}F) or yttrium-86 isotopes, which are imaged by specialized scanners. Positron emission tomographic (PET) imaging has advantage over single-photon imaging as it provides better resolution of images and more accurate dosimetric estimates. The advent of PET and particularly combination PET/CT scanners has significantly enlarged the scope of functional imaging with radiotracers, as exemplified in Figure 1. PET is rapidly emerging as the noninvasive functional imaging modality of choice for assessment of new therapies. PET imaging has the potential to image a variety of metabolic pathways that can be used to assess the presence of a specific target (such as HER2 or the AR) for eligibility or for assessing pharmacodynamic effects.

Using these imaging technologies, nanomolar quantities of radiotracers can be visualized, and can image both bone and soft tissue using a single modality. Another advantage is scanning of the entire body and visualizing both bone and soft tissue in a single scanning procedure. The preferential uptake based on pathophysiology (and hence increased tumor:background ratios) make detection of lesions feasible. By tagging specific molecules, aberrant biological pathways can be also detected. Although nuclear medicine techniques do not have the structural resolution capabilities of MR or CT, the ability to image biologic and physiologic processes make this modality useful in assessment of viable tumor burden and treatment response. A number of molecules can be used for clinical imaging that

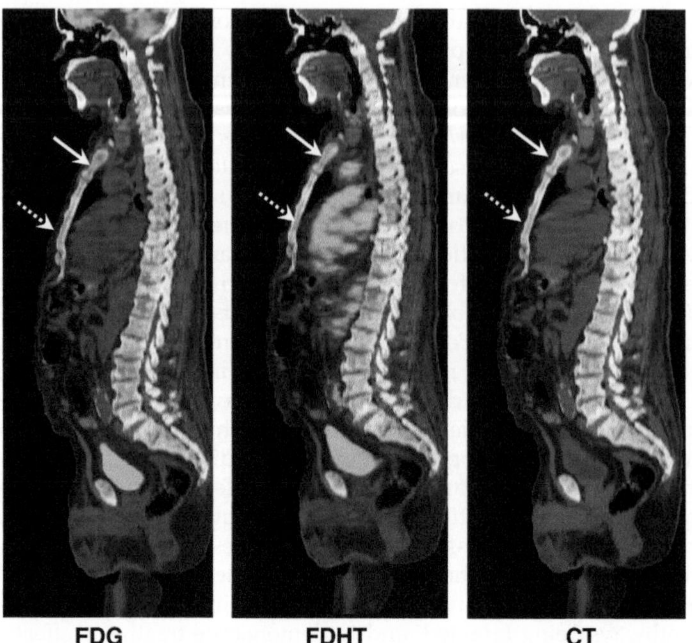

FIGURE 1 (*See color insert*) Shown is a PET CT fusion study of a patient with castrate metastatic prostate cancer. The patient has received [18F] 2-fluoro-d-deoxy-glucose (^{18}FDG) and ^{18}F fluorodihydrotestosterone (FDHT) as tracers. The biological diversity of the tumor is demonstrated. The top arrow shows a sternal lesion that has putatively upregulated glucose transport and androgen receptor overexpression, as it is FDG and FDHT avid. The bottom arrow points to a lesion that does not appear to overexpress the androgen receptor. CT allows for good localization of these lesions seen on positron emission tomographic, but alone illuminates little about the distribution, biology, or activity of the patient's disease. *Abbreviations*: FDG, 2-fluoro-D-deoxy-glucose; FDHT, F fluorodihydrotestosterone; CT, .

can help understand various biologic properties of the cancer. These molecules follow physiologic and metabolic pathways such as glucose metabolism, fatty acid synthesis, cell growth and proliferation, AR expression, and others, as shown in Table 2. For the purposes of discussion, these can be divided into two categories: tracers that demonstrate alterations in growth and metabolism, and those that demonstrate specific targets that are particularly relevant to prostate cancer.

TRACERS THAT DEMONSTRATE METABOLISM AND GROWTH

Glucose Metabolism

PET imaging with [^{18}F] 2-fluoro-d-deoxy-glucose (^{18}FDG) is based upon an increase in glycolytic flux in cancer cells. Uptake in prostate cancer cells may be related to the expression of mRNA and proteins for glucose transporters (54). In prostate cancer, uptake is correlated with PSA levels and PSA velocity, and may be used as a measure of tumor metabolism or aggressiveness (55).

It has been shown to have low sensitivity in the primary staging of prostate cancer, with poor detection of abdominopelvic nodes. Excreted radioactivity

TABLE 2 Selected Tracers Available for Clinical Testing in Prostate Cancer

Tracer	Pathways detected
^{18}FDG	Glucose metabolism
^{11}C-Choline, FEC, FCH	Synthesis of phospholipids, methyl metabolism, lipid cholesterol transport
^{11}C-acetate	Marker of oxygen consumption and lipid synthesis
^{18}F Fluorodihydrotestosterone	Androgen receptor expression
[^{18}F]FLT, FBAU, FMAU	Proliferation
7E11, J591	Prostate-specific membrane antigen
^{99}Tc-annexin, ^{18}F-annexin	Apoptosis
^{18}F-misonidazole, fluorerythronitroimidazole, fluoroetanidazole	Hypoxia
^{11}C-methionine	Amino-acid transport

Abbreviations: ^{18}FDG, [18F] 2-fluoro-D-deoxy-glucose; FEC, fluoro-ethyl-choline; FCH, fluoromethyl-dimethyl-2-hydroxyethylammonium; [^{18}F]FLT, [^{18}F]-fluoro-3-deoxy-3-L-fluorothymidine; FBAU, 2-deoxy-2-fluoro-5-bromo-1-D-arabinofuranosyluracil; FMAU, 2-fluoro-5-methyl-1-D-arabinofuranosyluracil.

in ureters, bladder, and bowel leads to difficulties in interpretation and may be one reason for the low sensitivity (56,57). With the evolution of PET/CT, which allows structural delineation of radioactive distribution, assessment of true disease may be improved. In comparison to bone scans, PET was initially felt to detect fewer lesions and to be less sensitive in patients with prostate cancer (56,58). One explanation for this differential in detecting disease by the two imaging modalities is that FDG-PET imaging may be detecting only active tumor sites or more aggressive cancers.

However, many of the studies examining FDG-PET for prostate cancer have been retrospective studies that have not examined homogeneous groups of patients at the same phase of the disease. For example, there is an often-quoted study by Shreve et al. comparing PET with standard bone scintigraphy in which the sensitivity of PET for detecting metastases was found to be only 65%. Thirty four patients were examined, and were comprised of patients with known metastatic disease who were progressing radiographically or biochemically, patients with equivocal bone scans, and patients with known metastatic disease who were undergoing hormonal therapy (56). Another example is a study by Yeh et al. in which FDG-PET was found to demonstrate only 18% of bony metastases, yet many of these patients were responding to hormonal therapy, which induces apoptosis and cell cycle arrest (59).

Finally, investigators have drawn conclusions about PET on the basis of patients with primary disease rather than metastases. In clinically organ-confined prostate cancer, the uptake of FDG does not correlate with PSA levels, cancer stage, grade, or volume (60), though observations in a preliminary study vary (61). Overall, FDG-PET has proven to be only minimally useful for the evaluation of organ-confined prostate cancer (38,62). Because the biology of bone metastases are significantly different from those of primary prostate cancer, few conclusions can be drawn from the failure of PET as a modality for imaging primary disease in terms of its ability to demonstrate metastases.

By contrast, when FDG-PET is examined in a systematic, prospective manner, for controlling disease state and for disease progression, it appears to be significantly more promising. In a study of patients with progressive metastatic disease, PET was able to distinguish between quiescent and active disease. One hundred thirty four bone lesions were examined. Of those, 71% were detectable by both bone scintigraphy and FDG-PET. At face value, this might appear to confirm that PET does not detect as many bone lesions as bone scans. However, when the bone scans before and after the index scan were examined, PET appeared to be superior to bone scintigraphy in distinguishing active disease. Of the 31 lesions that were not evident on FDG-PET but were evident on bone scintigraphy, 30 proved to be stable on subsequent bone scans. Of the eight lesions that appeared on PET but not on bone scans, all subsequently developed into sites of osseous metastases detectable on bone scintigraphy on subsequent scans. Hence, FDG PET failed to correctly identify only one of the 134 lesions as active disease (63).

Preliminary data have suggested that PET can be used as an effective means of demonstrating treatment effects. Agus and coworkers showed a 38% decrease in FDG uptake by 48 hours that decreased further after 10 days to 32% of baseline in a xenograft model (30). The change in uptake preceded changes in tumor volume or PSA decline. In a clinical study by Oyama et al., FDG-PET performed before and after one to five months of the initiation of therapy showed a decrease in FDG uptake in the prostate gland (12–77%) and in metastatic sites in all patients (64).

FDG-PET has been studied prospectively and compared with posttreatment alterations in PSA and standard imaging, and appeared to capture in a single imaging modality the information usually captured in the composite end point of PSA, bone scintigraphy, and soft-tissue imaging. In a preliminary study, 22 castrate metastatic patients who were registered to clinical trials utilizing antimicrotubule chemotherapy (such as paclitaxel-, docetaxel-, or epothilone-based therapy) were coregistered to an imaging study comparing changes in standardized uptake values (SUV) uptake, PSA, and standard imaging. These patients were followed to progression or death. SUV and PSA were treated identically using a modified form of the PSA Working Group criteria, and the data were dichotomized into categories of either progressing or nonprogressing with treatment. After four weeks of chemotherapy, PET and PSA were in agreement in 86% of cases; in 91% of cases, however, FDG-PET correctly identified whether the patient was progressing. After 12 weeks of therapy, PET, PSA, and standard imaging were compared. In 94% of cases, PET correctly identified the correct clinical status of the patients. These data require validation in a larger data set, but do suggest that FDG-PET, when studied prospectively in a population rigorously controlled for clinical state and disease progression, can effectively be used to demonstrate treatment effects (65).

Cell Membrane Synthesis and Cholesterol Metabolism

Choline is used for a number of physiological processes including synthesis of phospholipids in cell membranes, methyl metabolism and lipid–cholesterol transport, and metabolism. Intracellular choline is metabolized to phosphorylcholine (PC) by the enzyme choline kinase and is trapped within the cell. Prostate cancer is associated with upregulated choline kinase activity, increased choline uptake and elevated levels of PC (66,67). Imaging can be performed as early as three to five minutes after tracer injection, as it is cleared from the blood in approximately seven minutes. The tracer is primarily trapped within cells.

This tracer was first studied labeled with carbon-11 (^{11}C) which has a half-life of 20 minutes. However, the technical challenges presented by a tracer of such a short half-life were formidable, as the radionuclide needed to be produced in a cyclotron on-site, and the chemistry and imaging need to be very well coordinated and performed quickly. ^{18}F-labeled choline compounds have been developed such as [fluoro-ethyl-choline (FEC) and fluoromethyl-dimethyl-2-hydroxyethylammonium (FCH)] with the advantage of a longer half-life (68–71). FCH is taken up and phosphorylated similarly as ^{11}C-choline, but less efficiently than FEC, while the urinary excretion of ^{18}F-FEC and ^{18}F-FCH is comparatively higher than ^{11}C-choline. The concentration of FEC and FCH in the prostate is maximal at 55 and three minutes after injection, respectively. Overall imaging methods are not very different for the various choline agents.

As with other tracers, there has been more attention paid to choline as an imaging agent for localized or nodal disease rather than for bone metastases. Lymph node metastases less than 1 cm in size are poorly visualized, and for nodal staging before prostatectomy a sensitivity of 80% and specificity of 96% has been shown (72). The role of radiolabeled choline as an indicator of biologic aggressiveness or its correlation to tumor grade or Gleason score has not been established. In terms of metastatic disease, preliminary studies suggest that the tracer is indeed able to at least identify sites of disease. Again, from a methodological standpoint these patients were heterogeneous—nine patients were characterized as androgen-independent, and nine as androgen-dependent, although some had metastatic disease, some did not, and some were progressing while others were not. Patients underwent scans with FDG and FCH. FCH was found to have invariably higher uptake than FDG at the primary site, in bone metastases, and in soft tissues. Six patients were found to have lymph nodes imaged; eight patients had bone metastases identified by FCH, seven of whom also had osseous metastases by FDG. These lesions were corroborated either by biopsy or by standard imaging modalities. SUV were over two-fold higher by FCH than by FDG (73). In another study of 23 patients, eight of whom had definitive metastases, all bone and lymph node metastases seen by standard imaging were visualized by ^{11}C-choline PET (74).

^{18}FDG was compared with ^{11}C-choline in 100 subjects with a rising PSA after radical prostatectomy or radiation therapy. Thirty percent of these patients had disease that correlated with either bone scan or CT findings. After prostatectomy or radiation, more lesions were detected with choline than with FDG (47% vs. 27%) and the overall accuracy for detecting local recurrence as well as nodal and distant metastases was greater with choline than with FDG. A negative choline scan was also suggestive of a favorable prognosis (75). Results of studies using ^{18}F-choline to evaluate response to androgen withdrawal therapy in patients with metastatic prostate cancer are encouraging, though more data are needed to confirm this.

Nonspecific uptake of labeled choline compounds have been described in granulocytes, macrophages, reactive lymph nodes, and benign prostatic hyperplasia. Intense bowel activity can interfere in interpretation and fasting may help reduce this (72,76,77).

Indices of Oxygen Consumption and Fatty Acid Synthesis

Acetate accumulates in tumor cells as a result of what appears to be low oxygen consumption and increased lipid synthesis of the cells. Overexpression of fatty acid synthase (FAS) along with increase in fatty acid synthesis and accumulation occurs in prostate cancer (78). This can occur early in cancer development and is more pronounced in hormone-responsive tumors with advanced stage and progression. FAS-mediated lipid synthesis mainly affects lipids in membrane rafts that are associated with signal transduction processes and are relevant for tumor growth and metastasis (79,80). Certain prostate tumors prefer acetate to glucose as a substrate for cellular metabolism. In prostate cancer, a high concentration of ^{11}C-acetate in primary and metastatic lesions has been seen (81,82). It has been shown that ^{11}C-acetate accumulates not only in prostate tumors but also in normal prostate glands of patients under 50 years of age, and in benign prostatic hyperplasia, with essentially no difference in uptake between hyperplasia (mean SUV of 2.1) and cancer (mean SUV of 1.9). Longer acquisition times are needed to study the tracer kinetics of ^{11}C-acetate in normal as well as in pathologic prostate tissue, as cancer has a higher early-to-late activity ratio of SUVs than normal or hyperplastic tissue (83).

One advantage of ^{11}C-acetate is that it is metabolized and incorporated into the cellular lipid pool, mainly phosphatidylcholine and neutral lipids which correlate with cellular growth activity as measured by ^{3}H-thymidine incorporation. The remaining fraction of ^{14}C-acetate is converted into CO_2 and amino acids (84,85). It is not excreted by the kidneys, which is of particular advantage for imaging at least primary or nodal disease. The relationship between intensity of acetate uptake in prostate cancer is currently unclear. Acetate is currently labeled with ^{11}C and thus imaging needs to be performed early: dynamic and/or static images up to 20 minutes are usually obtained. Due to its short half-life, imaging with other tracers such as FDG can be easily combined.

In a study by Oyama et al., dual tracer imaging was undertaken in 46 patients with a rising PSA after prostatectomy or radiation. Thirty percent of the ^{11}C-acetate studies had findings highly suspicious for tumor, as compared to only 9% of the FDG-PET studies. Unfortunately, only four total patients had findings suspicious for bone metastases by ^{11}C-acetate PET, and bone scintigraphy was not performed in all cases to confirm. Hence, this study does not inform the investigator interested in using this modality for metastatic disease as to whether this is an avenue worth pursuing (86). Fricke et al. studied ^{11}C-acetate and FDG-PET in 25 patients who represented primary disease, patients with biochemical relapse, or metastatic disease. Eight of these patients had distant metastases, and it appeared that 75% of these patients had positive FDG-PET scans, and 50% had positive ^{11}C-acetate scans (87). Significantly, more work will need to be performed in a prospective manner focusing on metastatic disease before ^{11}C-acetate could be characterized as an accurate indicator of activity of metastatic lesions.

Amino-Acid Transport and Protein Synthesis

Uptake of ^{11}C-labeled methionine appears related to amount of viable tumor and active tumor proliferation as it is based on amino-acid transport and protein synthesis (88,89). Methionine is rapidly cleared from the blood pool, metabolized in the liver and pancreas, with no significant renal excretion. This makes it more suitable than FDG in imaging pelvic disease. Encouraging results from the first observations of its use in prostate cancer by Nilsson et al. led to further exploration of its potential use in prostate cancer (90). In a study of 12 patients with progressive castrate metastatic prostate cancer, 348 metastatic lesions seen by standard imaging were tracked. Using standard imaging modalities as a "gold standard," the sensitivity of FDG-PET was 48% and of ^{11}C-methionine was 72%. The ^{11}C-methionine was able to visualize significantly more lesions that the FDG-PET. Specifically, ^{11}C-methionine identified 227 of 325 bone metastases. Although the total number of patients was low, the fact that ^{11}C-methionine was well able to visualize metastatic disease by virtue of amino-acid transport is promising, and efforts to prospectively assess this tracer for demonstrating antitumor effects are underway.

Proliferation

Imaging and measuring proliferation in vivo is a relatively new field in molecular imaging, offers a novel insight into tumor physiology, and can also be a means of assessing antitumor effects of new agents. Although little has been published regarding the use of PET tracers in evaluating tumor proliferation in prostate cancer in humans, these agents are of increasing interest and will likely be extensively investigated in the near future.

Initially, thymidine was investigated as a PET tracer, and was labeled with ^{11}C. Increasingly, though, proliferation has been assessed using the novel tracer [^{18}F]-fluoro-3-deoxy-3-l-fluorothymidine ([^{18}F]FLT). [^{18}F]FLT is a thymidine analogue that is taken up by the cell via both passive diffusion and facilitated transport by Na^+-dependent carriers. Thymidine kinase-1 (TK_1) is a principal enzyme in the salvage pathway of DNA synthesis and its activity is maximum in the late G_1 and S phases of the cell cycle of proliferating cells (91). TK_1 phosphorylates [^{18}F]FLT into [^{18}F]FLT-monophosphate, which then becomes trapped in the cell. [^{18}F]FLT can be used as a PET tracer to distinguish cancer cells from normal cells, because neoplastic tissues have three to four times higher TK_1 activity and have deregulated TK_1 activity due to impaired degradation caused by mutation of TK_1. A strong association has been shown between [^{3}H]-thymidine uptake and [^{3}H]-FLT uptake suggesting that [^{3}H]-FLT uptake represents the salvage pathway even though it is not incorporated into the DNA (92). Its role in determining proliferation has been shown in other cancers and the uptake was found to correlate with Ki-67 immunohistochemistry (93).

Several studies have examined [^{18}F]FLT-PET in prostate cancer animal models. In one, investigators utilized the androgen-dependent CWR22 mouse model. Imaging with [^{18}F]FLT-PET showed good uptake in the tumor, and subsequent androgen ablation using diethylstilbesterol, resulted in a significant decline in tumor implant uptake. The tracer was rapidly cleared from the blood; highest uptake and longer retention of tracer was seen in the tumor in comparison to all organs. Uptake into the tumor had the highest activity of all organs, and was retained longer ($0.69 \pm 0.14\%$ ID/g at 2 hours postinjection) than in normal organs (94). FLT does detect the proliferative activity of bone marrow, and therefore has a significant amount of uptake in bone in humans. For example, the SUV of the bone marrow of the vertebral column can be 5.5 (95). This may be a limiting factor in imaging bone metastases in humans, but it has not been sufficiently studied to be able to define how limiting this problem may be.

Newer nucleoside tracers like 2-deoxy-2-fluoro-5-bromo-1-d-arabinofuranosyluracil and 2-fluoro-5-methyl-1-d-arabinofuranosyluracil (FMAU) are also pyrimidine analogues that are incorporated in DNA and may reflect DNA synthesis directly. FMAU is less excreted in bladder enabling better evaluation of pelvis though normal liver uptake may lower sensitivity for detecting liver lesions.

IMAGING INDIVIDUAL PROTEINS RELEVANT TO PROSTATE CANCER

^{18}F Fluorodihydrotestosterone

All of the above strategies focus on assessing prostate cancer on the basis of general metabolic properties, be they glucose metabolism, amino-acid transport, or fatty acid synthesis. Although these tracers may well be useful for screening drugs for antitumor effects in early-phase studies, they are not prostate-specific. The AR, by contrast, is still highly functional and signaling even in the castrate state, and is still a major source of tumor growth despite the absence of its ligand dihydrotestosterone. It can be mutated, overexpressed, and activated by nonligand means (96). A number of novel therapies are designed to target the AR. For example, the ansamycins inhibit heat-shock protein 90 (hsp90) and therefore disrupt normal AR folding (97). Histone deacetylase inhibitors also have anti-AR effects, and are under clinical testing (98,99). Imaging the AR has the potential to identify patients who might benefit from such therapies, and could demonstrate pharcodynamic effects in early-phase studies.

16β-^{18}F-Fluoro-5α-dihydrotestosterone (FDHT) is a radiolabeled analog of dihydrotestosterone, the predominant AR ligand. An initial study of FDHT and FDG in seven patients with progressive castrate metastatic prostate cancer examined 59 lesions seen on standard imaging studies. Ninety-seven percent of these lesions were seen on FDG; 78% were seen on FDHT-PET scans (100). Similar results were seen in a more recent study where FDHT-PET had sensitivity of 63% and a lesion detection rate of 86%. Positive FDHT-PET studies were associated with higher PSA levels and thus, presumably, with greater tumor burden. Importantly, a decrease in tumor FDHT uptake was seen 24 hours after flutamide with a drop in SUV from 7.0 ± 4.7 to 3.0 ± 1.5 (101). FDHT is now being investigated prospectively in patients with castrate metastatic disease receiving antimicrotubule chemotherapy.

Prostate-Specific Membrane Antigen

Antibodies that are directed to prostate-specific targets have applications as imaging and therapeutic agents. As the purpose of this chapter is to review novel imaging modalities only, the therapeutic applications of such antibodies will not be discussed, except to say that such approaches using naked antibodies, radioconjugates, and chemoconjugates have been shown to be safe and to induce PSA declines (102–105).

As imaging agents, antibodies have a number of roles. First, as discussed earlier, prostate cancer is a disease with a paucity of means of directly imaging the tumor. Most standard modalities detect changes caused by the tumor rather than the tumor itself, for example, the tumor's impact on bone to detect disease and drug effects. However, antibodies can localize to the cancer itself, and thereby distinguish noncancer-related bone abnormalities (such as arthritis, trauma, infection, or Paget's disease) from those that are tumor related. Therefore, one can define the presence of the target as a means of eligibility, as well as posttreatment alterations in target expression. One can also correlate antitumor effects with pre- and posttreatment target expression levels.

PSMA is one such target. It is a 100 kDa type 2 transmembrane glycoprotein on prostate epithelial cells (106), with a large external domain ($PSMA_X$) comprised of over 700 amino acids responsible for its enzymatic action as a hydrolase (107). PSMA is expressed in almost all prostate cancer cells, from primary to metastatic disease, and appears to be maximally expressed following androgen withdrawal. The antigen is found in low levels in some nonprostate tissues, notably liver and Schwann cells (108–111). Antibodies against PSMA thus may hold promise, if labeled with radionuclides, as diagnostic agents. It is, in many ways, an ideal therapeutic target.

PSMA has been utilized for a number of treatment strategies, including those involving radioisotope and chemo-conjugated antibodies. However, a number of other strategies are being developed as well. For example, DNA vaccines that encode either the entire open reading frame or portions of PSMA are in Phase I and II studies. The scientific basis of such studies is to increase antigen presentation and thereby induction of anti-PSMA humeral and cell-mediated immune activity (112,113). RNA anti-PSMA vaccines have also been explored, as have vaccines using PSMA protein (114). The capacity to image the target could validate its presence before therapy, and could be used to correlate treatment effects with target expression.

ProstaScint® (capromab pendetide) consists of an intact murine monoclonal antibody, 7E11-C5.3 to which a linker chelator (GYK-DTPA-HCL) is bound; the chelator permits labeling with ^{111}In. A new antibody using 1,4,7,10-tetraazacyclododecane-*N*, *N′*, *N″*, *N‴*-tetraacetic acid (DOTA) as a linker is now available for study as well, allowing for conjugation with such radiometals as ^{177}Lu.

The antibody, 7E11, targets the intracellular epitope of PSMA, a transmembrane molecule. This has been hypothesized to limit its detection to membrane-permeable cells or necrotic tissue (115). Scintigraphic (gamma camera and SPECT) imaging with ^{111}In-capromab pendetide has been used to detect tumor of prostatic origin. Although the antibody does not bind viable LNCaP cells in vitro, several studies have demonstrated specific accumulation of antibody in vivo to histologically demonstrated viable tumor foci.

The overall sensitivity and specificity of detecting disease using ProstaScint has been widely variable in reported studies (116–120). These studies demonstrated average sensitivities of 60%, specificities of 70%, positive predictive values of 60%, and negative predictive values of 70%. In a meta-analysis, ^{111}In-labeled capromab pendetide studies in 2154 patients from 15 institutions were analyzed. Overall sensitivity for detection of tumor in biopsy-proven primary carcinoma was 80.1%. The sensitivities were variable, ranging between 75.2% and 99% due to significant inter-reader variability. Kahn et al. studied 183 patients with biochemical recurrence following radical prostatectomy. ^{111}In-labeled capromab pendetide imaging was positive in 29/59 patients with a positive fossa biopsy. The sensitivity of the technique was 49% and the positive predictive value for fossa recurrence was 50% (121). As a result of these mixed results, ProstaScint is not routinely used as an imaging agent for prostate cancer staging, nor is it incorporated into standard pretreatment predictive models of outcome, whether in the setting of initial treatment or salvage therapy (122–125).

In addition to the drawbacks described above, this modality also suffers from the shortcomings common to other indium-labeled antibodies including nonspecific accumulation of radioactivity in the normal blood pool, bowel, and bone marrow. In addition, there is uptake of the antibody or radiolabel in the liver, and slow clearance results in background activity that makes lesion detection difficult. The inherent low resolution of gamma camera/SPECT imaging further limits utility. Finally, there is limited anatomic information in the images and location of the abnormal foci can only be approximated. Sometimes "pooling" of radiolabeled antibodies in a tumor with high blood content can give positive scan.

As discussed above, the initial exploration of 7E11 to stage patients before radiation or surgery has had only checkered results. Almost no attention has been paid to it as a means of either imaging patients with advanced disease or as a means of developing drugs. ProstaScint has not undergone rigorous prospective testing in patients with known progressive metastatic disease. In one study of patients with metastatic disease, some treated and others not, patients received escalating doses of ^{111}In-CYT-356 (0.1, 0.2, 0.5, 1, and 5 mg doses per cohort, using 5 mCi of ^{111}In). Thirty-eight patients had known bone metastases. Of these patients, 55% demonstrated uptake at metastatic sites. However, it was noted that the sensitivity of antibody imaging was lowest (25%) for the patients who received the lowest dose of antibody, highest for patients who received 0.2 mg (90%), and intermediate for doses at 0.5 mg and higher (46%). No biopsies were performed or subsequent bone scans analyzed to confirm that the patients who had a negative ProstaScint and positive bone scan indeed had active cancer at those sites. In two patients, the ProstaScint-imaged disease that was not evident on bone scans, but was evident on other imaging modalities (126). The relationship between disease detection, dose, and treatment using this antibody remains unclear. In another trial, this one with therapeutic intent using yttrium-90 (^{90}Y)-labeled CYT-356, 12 patients with hormone-refractory metastatic disease were treated with escalating doses of ^{90}Y. The antibody mass was fixed at 0.5 mg, and ^{111}In was used as an imaging agent, as ^{90}Y cannot be imaged due to lack of significant gamma emissions. Although bone metastases were imaged in seven of 12 patients, only a minority of total individual lesions were detected (127).

A possible explanation for these findings is that the internal domain of PSMA is not accessible to the antibody; studies to determine whether chemotherapy can enhance access of the antibody by altering the localization of PSMA in the cell and by disrupting the cell membrane are being planned. In addition, the use of blood pool subtraction with ^{111}In-capromab pendetide imaging may help in delineating vascular radioactivity from true uptake in lesions. SPECT/CT combination scanners may offer a more practical and efficient imaging and help improve diagnostic accuracy.

Hamilton et al. (128) initially used a semiautomated technique of coregistering separate ProstaScint images with CT scans; Ellis et al. (129), using a similar technique, found ^{111}In-labeled capromab pendetide imaging to have a sensitivity of 79%, a specificity of 80%, and an overall accuracy of 80%. Recently, a hybrid SPECT–CT scanner was used for ^{111}In-labeled capromab pendetide imaging in 35 patients. The availability of CT images helped by reducing imaging time, provided more accurate anatomic correlation and better differentiation of activity in prostate gland versus neighboring organs and blood pool, and helped in differentiating postoperative and other post-therapy changes (130). These technologies, along with imaging in the context of therapies likely to disrupt the prostate cell membrane in controlled patient populations, will allow for more systematic and accurate study of 7E11 for imaging distant metastases in this disease.

In addition, antibodies are available that target the external domain of PSMA. J591 (MLN591; Millennium Pharmaceuticals, Cambridge, MA, U.S.A.) is one such antibody, and is a monoclonal IgG_1 molecule that targets $PSMA_X$ (131). The constant regions of the murine antibody were replaced by human IgG_1 sequences, and the antibody "deimmunized" by replacing amino-acid sequences in the antibody variable domains, without loss of specificity or affinity. J591 has been covalently coupled with DOTA, with targeting of ^{111}In-labeled antibody to metastatic prostate cancer in several studies aimed at radioimmunotherapy. These studies have demonstrated antibody localization to known disease (103,104). A clinical trial of ^{90}Y-DOTA-J591 demonstrated that 89% of patients with bone metastases by standard imaging also had uptake using the antibody; a study of ^{177}Lu-DOTA J591 demonstrated targeting of metastatic disease in all patients with distant lesions, and in some cases the antibody localization appeared to image a greater number of bone lesions than did standard imaging; a study of ^{111}In-DOTA-J591, all patients had good localization of the antibody to distant sites. In all of these studies, detailed lesional analyses have not yet been published (102–104).

New targets for antibody-based imaging are under development. Radiolabeled anti-HER2 antibodies can be used to detect posttreatment effects of therapies that induce HER2 degradation by targeting hsp90 (132). Antibodies targeting prostate stem cell antigen (133,134) have been developed for clinical testing, and may have a role in disease detection in the future. Whether these antibodies will be primarily used for therapy or for drug development remains to be seen.

SUMMARY AND FUTURE DIRECTIONS

Prostate cancer is a singularly ripe field for developing improved imaging modalities, as standard imaging cannot directly visualize the tumor and is inadequate in assessing tumor size and burden. There are no standard means of directly visualizing the cancer in order to assess its true dimensions, PSA is not an ideal index of antitumor effects, and tissue cannot be acquired with ease. Presently, imaging the tumor on the basis of a number of biological properties is feasible. These include glucose metabolism, fatty acid metabolism, proliferation, AR expression, cell membrane synthesis, and others. Specific targets can be imaged using radiolabeled antibodies. Hence, while there is an abundance of new biologic agents to test in clinical trials, there is also a host of imaging modalities that can be used in clinical trials to test these agents.

A major challenge for the field is prioritizing which of these agents should be pursued, and which abandoned. Such selection will likely rest on several criteria. The physical properties of the radioisotope is an important criterion. For example, ^{11}C has a relatively short half-life of approximately 20 minutes. To study ^{11}C-based tracers usually requires in-house cyclotron facilities or their equivalent, given that the time from tracer synthesis to injection and imaging is necessarily short. This limitation, which impacts feasibility and commercial viability, must be considered in deciding whether to advance tracers such as ^{11}C-methionine, ^{11}C-acetate, or ^{11}C-choline. By comparison, ^{18}F-based tracers have already been shown to be practical and commercially viable. A related concern is the feasibility and stability of the ligand, as opposed to the isotope. For example, FDHT can be challenging to synthesize, and the precursor can be unstable. Such concerns may present economic and logistical challenges that limit the widespread implementation of a tracer for routine clinical use.

Biodistribution is another factor that must be considered in prioritization. Tracers such as FDG that are renally excreted may be unacceptable for staging patients with primary disease, because they obscure the pelvic lymph nodes.

However, a renally-excreted tracer may be appropriate for evaluating patients with metastatic disease, given that bone metastases are the primary reservoir of the disease, and usually any pelvic adenopathy at that point is clinically a secondary issue. By the same token, FLT, which can have significant uptake in the bone marrow due to its high proliferative index, may have at least hypothetical limits for evaluating patients with bone metastases.

Yet another factor in tracer selection will be the target tissue. Given the biologic variability of prostate cancer, a tracer for the patient with androgen-dependent local disease may be of little use for patients with castration-resistant disease that has metastasized to bone. Although it may seem self-evident that tracers should be tested on patients who are at the same point in the natural history of the disease, such a methodology has traditionally not been implemented in studies of new tracers. Many of these agents are being tested by scanning patients who, although they may all have prostate cancer, represent a heterogeneous group.

By contrast, testing of new therapies is, by consensus, performed on patients who represent one of several discreet clinical states: localized disease, a rising PSA after surgery or radiation therapy, or metastatic disease. The latter two states are frequently subcategorized as either progressing before or despite androgen deprivation. Patients can only enter clinical trials if they meet specific criteria for progression, including that of progressing through antiandrogen withdrawal (18,47,135). These standards were developed in recognition that the biology of prostate cancer is highly variable, not only within states, but between them. Imaging studies of novel agents have, in large part, not adhered to these standards.

Future investigations of these agents must focus on prospective studies that strictly control for progression and for clinical state. In addition, the patient population must match the question being asked. For example, studies that focus on the rising PSA population should not be the basis for drawing conclusions regarding disease detection; by definition, these patients do not have detectable disease. By the same token, studies of patients with localized disease are not the population by which to define the ability of a modality to detect distant disease. Only when the sophistication of the trial designs match those of the imaging studies themselves will the full potential of these valuable tools be met. While such imaging modalities offer a great promise in terms of either detecting disease, identifying patients with specific pathways, assessing drug effects, or prognostication, such promise cannot be fulfilled unless the testing of these agents matures.

REFERENCES

1. Ignotz RA, Endo T, Massague J. Regulation of fibronectin and type I collagen mRNA levels by transforming growth factor-beta. J Biol Chem 1987; 262:6443–6446.
2. Sporn MB, Roberts AB, Wakefield LM, de Crombrugghe B. Some recent advances in the chemistry and biology of transforming growth factor-beta. J Cell Biol 1987; 105:1039–1045.
3. Steiner MS, Zhou ZZ, Tonb DC, Barrack ER. Expression of transforming growth factor-beta 1 in prostate cancer. Endocrinology 1994; 135:2240–2247.
4. Guise TA, Mundy GR. Cancer and bone. Endocr Rev 1998; 19:18–54.
5. Wu G, Iwamura M, di Sant'Agnese PA, Deftos LJ, Cockett AT, Gershagen S. Characterization of the cell-specific expression of parathyroid hormone-related protein in normal and neoplastic prostate tissue. Urology 1998; 51:110–120.
6. Iwamura M, di Sant'Agnese PA, Wu G, et al. Immunohistochemical localization of parathyroid hormone-related protein in human prostate cancer. Cancer Res 1993; 53:1724–1726.

7. Asadi F, Farraj M, Sharifi R, Malakouti S, Antar S, Kukreja S. Enhanced expression of parathyroid hormone-related protein in prostate cancer as compared with benign prostatic hyperplasia. Hum Pathol 1996; 27:1319–1323.
8. Abou-Samra AB, Juppner H, Force T, et al. Expression cloning of a common receptor for parathyroid hormone and parathyroid hormone-related peptide from rat osteoblast-like cells: a single receptor stimulates intracellular accumulation of both cAMP and inositol trisphosphates and increases intracellular free calcium. Proc Natl Acad Sci USA 1992; 89:2732–2736.
9. Koeneman KS, Yeung F, Chung LW. Osteomimetic properties of prostate cancer cells: a hypothesis supporting the predilection of prostate cancer metastasis and growth in the bone environment. Prostate 1999; 39:246–261.
10. Li J, Sarosi I, Yan XQ, et al. RANK is the intrinsic hematopoietic cell surface receptor that controls osteoclastogenesis and regulation of bone mass and calcium metabolism. Proc Natl Acad Sci USA 2000; 97:1566–1571.
11. Hsu H, Lacey DL, Dunstan CR, et al. Tumor necrosis factor receptor family member RANK mediates osteoclast differentiation and activation induced by osteoprotegerin ligand. Proc Natl Acad Sci USA 1999; 96:3540–3545.
12. Nakagawa N, Kinosaki M, Yamaguchi K, et al. RANK is the essential signaling receptor for osteoclast differentiation factor in osteoclastogenesis. Biochem Biophys Res Commun 1998; 253:395–400.
13. Romas E, Sims NA, Hards DK, et al. Osteoprotegerin reduces osteoclast numbers and prevents bone erosion in collagen-induced arthritis. Am J Pathol 2002; 161:1419–1427.
14. Noguchi M, Yahara J, Noda S. Serum levels of bone turnover markers parallel the results of bone scintigraphy in monitoring bone activity of prostate cancer. Urology 2003; 61:993–998.
15. Brown JE, Cook RJ, Major P, et al. Bone turnover markers as predictors of skeletal complications in prostate cancer, lung cancer, and other solid tumors. J Natl Cancer Inst 2005; 97:59–69.
16. Scher HI, Yagoda A. Clinical trials in prostatic cancer: Methodology and controversies. In: Bruce AW, Trachtenberg J, eds. Adenocarcinoma of the Prostate. New York: Springer-Verlag, 1987:197–220.
17. Figg WD, Ammerman K, Patronas N, et al. Lack of correlation between prostate-specific antigen and the presence of measurable soft tissue metastases in hormone-refractory prostate cancer. Cancer Invest 1996; 14:513–517.
18. Bubley GJ, Carducci M, Dahut W, et al. Eligibility and response guidelines for phase II clinical trials in androgen-independent prostate cancer: recommendations from the PSA Working Group. J Clin Oncol 1999; 17:1–7.
19. Tannock IF, de Wit R, Berry WR, et al. Docetaxel plus prednisone or mitoxantrone plus prednisone for advanced prostate cancer. N Engl J Med 2004; 351:1502–1512.
20. Petrylak DP, Tangen CM, Hussain MH, et al. Docetaxel and estramustine compared with mitoxantrone and prednisone for advanced refractory prostate cancer. N Engl J Med 2004; 351:1513–1520.
21. Berry W, Dakhil S, Modiano M, Gregurich M, Asmar L. Phase III study of mitoxantrone plus low dose prednisone versus low dose prednisone alone in patients with asymptomatic hormone refractory prostate cancer. J Urol 2002; 168:2439–2443.
22. Pollen JJ, Shlaer WJ. Osteoblastic response to successful treatment of metastatic cancer of the prostate. Am J Roentgenol 1979; 132:927–931.
23. Scher HI, Morris MJ, Kelly WK, Schwartz LH, Heller G. Prostate cancer clinical trial end points: "RECIST"ing a step backwards. Clin Cancer Res 2005; 11:5223–5232.
24. Pollen JJ, Witztum KF, Ashburn WL. The flare phenomenon on radionuclide bone scan in metastatic prostate cancer. Am J Roentgenol 1984; 142:773–776.
25. Citrin DL, Cohen AI, Harberg J, Schlise S, Hougen C, Benson R. Systemic treatment of advanced prostatic cancer: development of a new system for defining response. J Urol 1981; 125:224–227.
26. Langhammer H, Sintermann R, Hor G, Pabst HW. Serial bone scintigraphy for assessing the effectiveness of treatment of osseous metastases from prostatic cancer. Nuklearmedizin 1978; 17:87–91.

27. Therasse P, Arbuck SG, Eisenhauer EA, et al. New guidelines to evaluate the response to treatment in solid tumors. European Organization for Research and Treatment of Cancer, National Cancer Institute of the United States, National Cancer Institute of Canada. J Natl Cancer Inst 2000; 92:205–216.
28. Fossa SD, Heilo A, Lindegaard M, Skinningrud A, Ous S. Clinical significance of routine follow-up examinations in patients with metastatic cancer of the prostate under hormone treatment. Eur Urol 1983; 9:262–266.
29. Gerber G, Chodak GW. Assessment of value of routine bone scans in patients with newly diagnosed prostate cancer. Urology 1991; 37:418–422.
30. Levenson RM, Sauerbrunn BJ, Bates HR, Newman RD, Eddy JL, Ihde DC. Comparative value of bone scintigraphy and radiography in monitoring tumor response in systemically treated prostatic carcinoma. Radiology 1983; 146:513–518.
31. Johns WD, Garnick MB, Kaplan WD. Leuprolide therapy for prostate cancer. An association with scintigraphic "flare" on bone scan. Clin Nucl Med 1990; 15:485–487.
32. Beekman K, Morris M, Slovin S, et al. Androgen deprivation for minimal metastatic disease: threshold for achieving undetectable prostate-specific antigen. Urology 2005; 65:947–952.
33. Jacobs SC. Spread of prostatic cancer to bone. Urology 1983; 21:337–344.
34. Kelly WK, Steineck G, Mazumdar M, Vlamis V, Dnistrian A, Scher H. Post-therapy changes in biochemical markers in patients with androgen independent prostate cancer. Proc Am Soc Clin Oncol 1995; 14.
35. Scher HI, Kelly WK, Zhang Z-F, et al. Post-therapy serum prostate specific antigen level and survival in patients with androgen-independent prostate cancer. J Natl Cancer Inst 1999; 91:244–251.
36. Vollmer RT, Kantoff PW, Dawson NA, Vogelzang NJ. A prognostic score for hormone-refractory prostate cancer: analysis of two Cancer and Leukemia Group B studies. Clin Cancer Res 1999; 5:831–837.
37. Vollmer RT, Montana GS. Predicting tumor failure in prostate carcinoma after definitive radiation therapy: limitations of models based on prostate-specific antigen, clinical stage, and gleason score. Clin Cancer Res 1999; 5:2476–2484.
38. D'Amico AV, Moul JW, Carroll PR, Sun L, Lubeck D, Chen MH. Surrogate end point for prostate cancer-specific mortality after radical prostatectomy or radiation therapy. J Natl Cancer Inst 2003; 95:1376–1383.
39. D'Amico AV, Cote K, Loffredo M, Renshaw AA, Schultz D. Determinants of prostate cancer-specific survival after radiation therapy for patients with clinically localized prostate cancer. J Clin Oncol 2002; 20:4567–4573.
40. Stewart A, Scher H, Chen M, et al. The clinical significance of a PSA Nadir >0.2 to patients with a rising post-operative state or post-radiation PSA treated with androgen deprivation. Proc Am Soc Clin Oncol 2005; 23:389s.
41. Kelloff GJ, Coffey DS, Chabner BA, et al. Prostate-specific antigen doubling time as a surrogate marker for evaluation of oncologic drugs to treat prostate cancer. Clin Cancer Res 2004; 10:3927–3933.
42. D'Amico AV, Moul J, Carroll PR, Sun L, Lubeck D, Chen MH. Prostate specific antigen doubling time as a surrogate end point for prostate cancer specific mortality following radical prostatectomy or radiation therapy. J Urol 2004; 172:S42–S46; discussion S46–S47.
43. Saad F, Gleason DM, Murray R, et al. A randomized, placebo-controlled trial of zoledronic acid in patients with hormone-refractory metastatic prostate carcinoma. J Natl Cancer Inst 2002; 94:1458–1468.
44. Small EJ, Schellhammer PF, Higano C, Neumanaitis J, Valone F, Herschberg RM. Immunotherapy (APC8015) for androgen independent prostate cancer (AIPC): final survival data from a phase 3 randomized placebo-controlled trial. Proceedings of the Multidisciplinary Prostate Cancer Symposium, abstract 264, 2005.
45. Beinart G, Rini BI, Weinberg V, Small EJ. Antigen-presenting cells 8015 (Provenge) in patients with androgen-dependent, biochemically relapsed prostate cancer. Clin Prostate Cancer 2005; 4:55–60.

46. Strother JM, Lopez CD, Beer TM, Blanke CD. A phase II trial of weekly high-dose calcitriol and docetaxel in patients with locally advanced or metastatic pancreatic adenocarcinoma. Proc Am Soc Clin Oncol, abstract 94, 2005.
47. Scher HI, Eisenberger M, D'Amico AV, et al. Eligibility and outcomes reporting guidelines for clinical trials for patients in the state of a rising prostate-specific antigen: recommendations from the Prostate-Specific Antigen Working Group. J Clin Oncol 2004; 22:537–556.
48. Nelson WG, De Marzo AM, Isaacs WB. Prostate cancer. N Engl J Med 2003; 349: 366–381.
49. Signoretti S, Montironi R, Manola J, et al. Her-2-neu expression and progression toward androgen independence in human prostate cancer. J Natl Cancer Inst 2000; 92:1918–1925.
50. Whang Y, Wu X, Suzuki H, et al. Inactivation of the tumor suppressor PTEN/MMAC1 in advanced human prostate cancer through loss of expression. Proc Natl Acad Sci USA 1998; 95:5246–5250.
51. McDonnell TJ, Troncoso P, Brisbay SM, et al. Expression of the protooncogene bcl-2 in the prostate and its association with emergence of androgen-independent prostate cancer. Cancer Res 1992; 52:6940–6944.
52. Colombel MC, Symmans F, Chopin D, Benson M, Olsson C, Buttyan R. The apoptosis-suppressing oncoprotein, bcl-2 is expressed in germinal layers of human prostate gland in various stages of prostatic oncogenesis. 1992 International Symposium on Biology of Prostate Growth, 101, 1992.
53. Ross RW, Halabi S, Ou SS, et al. Predictors of prostate cancer tissue acquisition by an undirected core bone marrow biopsy in metastatic castration-resistant prostate cancer—a Cancer and Leukemia Group B study. Clin Cancer Res 2005; 11:8109–8113.
54. Chandler JD, Williams ED, Slavin JL, Best JD, Rogers S. Expression and localization of GLUT1 and GLUT12 in prostate carcinoma. Cancer 2003; 97:2035–2042.
55. Seltzer MA, Barbaric Z, Belldegrun A, et al. Comparison of helical computerized tomography, positron emission tomography and monoclonal antibody scans for evaluation of lymph node metastases in patients with prostate specific antigen relapse after treatment for localized prostate cancer. J Urol 1999; 162:1322–1328.
56. Shreve PD, Grossman HB, Gross MD, Wahl RL. Metastatic prostate cancer: initial findings of PET with 2-deoxy-2[F-18]fluoro-D-glucose. Radiology 1996; 199:751–756.
57. Sanz G, Robles JE, Gimenez M, et al. Positron emission tomography with ^{18}fluorine-labelled deoxyglucose: utility in localized and advanced prostate cancer. BJU Int 1999; 84:1028–1031.
58. Yeh S, Imbriaco M, Larson S, et al. Detection of bony metastases of androgen independent prostate cancer by PET-FDG. Nucl Med Biol 1996; 23:693–697.
59. Agus DB, Cordon-Cardo C, Fox W, et al. Alterations of cell cycle regulators in prostate cancer: response to androgen withdrawal and development of androgen independence. J Natl Cancer Inst 1999; 91:1869–1876.
60. Liu IJ, Zafar MB, Lai YH, Segall GM, Terris MK. Fluorodeoxyglucose positron emission tomography studies in diagnosis and staging of clinically organ-confined prostate cancer. Urology 2001; 57:108–111.
61. Hermann K, Schoeder H, Eberhard S. FDG PET for the detection of recurrent/metastatic prostate carcinoma in patients with rising PSA after radical prostatectomy. J Nucl Med 2004; 45:359.
62. Hoh CK, Seltzer MA, Franklin J, deKernion JB, Phelps ME, Belldegrun A. Positron emission tomography in urological oncology. Urology 1998; 159:347–356.
63. Morris MJ, Akhurst T, Osman I, et al. Fluorinated deoxyglucose positron emission tomography imaging in progressive metastatic prostate cancer. Urology 2002; 59:913–918.
64. Oyama N, Akino H, Suzuki Y, et al. FDG PET for evaluating the change of glucose metabolism in prostate cancer after androgen ablation. Nucl Med Commun 2001; 22:963–969.

65. Morris MJ, Akhurst T, Larson SM, et al. Fluorodeoxyglucose positron emission tomography as an outcome measure for castrate metastatic prostate cancer treated with antimicrotubule chemotherapy. Clin Cancer Res 2005; 11:3210–3216.
66. Hara T, Kosaka N, Shinoura N, Kondo T. PET imaging of brain tumor with [methyl-11C]choline. J Nucl Med 1997; 38:842–847.
67. Hara T, Kosaka N, Kishi H. PET imaging of prostate cancer using carbon-11-choline. J Nucl Med 1998; 39:990–995.
68. Hara T, Kosaka N, Kishi H. Development of (18)F-fluoroethylcholine for cancer imaging with PET: synthesis, biochemistry, and prostate cancer imaging. J Nucl Med 2002; 43:187–199.
69. DeGrado TR, Coleman RE, Wang S, et al. Synthesis and evaluation of 18F-labeled choline as an oncologic tracer for positron emission tomography: initial findings in prostate cancer. Cancer Res 2001; 61:110–117.
70. DeGrado TR, Baldwin SW, Wang S, et al. Synthesis and evaluation of (18)F-labeled choline analogs as oncologic PET tracers. J Nucl Med 2001; 42:1805–1814.
71. DeGrado TR, Reiman R, Price DT. Pharmacokinetics and radiation dosimetry of 18F-fluorocholine. J Nucl Med 2002; 43:92–96.
72. de Jong IJ, Pruim J, Elsinga PH, Vaalburg W, Mensink HJ. Preoperative staging of pelvic lymph nodes in prostate cancer by 11C-choline PET. J Nucl Med 2003; 44:331–335.
73. Price DT, Coleman RE, Liao RP, Robertson CN, Polascik TJ, DeGrado TR. Comparison of [18 F]fluorocholine and [18 F]fluorodeoxyglucose for positron emission tomography of androgen dependent and androgen independent prostate cancer. J Urol 2002; 168:273–280.
74. Kotzerke J, Prang J, Neumaier B, et al. Experience with carbon-11 choline positron emission tomography in prostate carcinoma. Eur J Nucl Med 2000; 27:1415–1419.
75. Picchio M, Messa C, Landoni C, et al. Value of [11C]choline-positron emission tomography for re-staging prostate cancer: a comparison with [18F]fluorodeoxyglucose-positron emission tomography. J Urol 2003; 169:1337–1340.
76. Wyss MT, Weber B, Honer M, et al. 18F-choline in experimental soft tissue infection assessed with autoradiography and high-resolution PET. Eur J Nucl Med Mol Imaging 2004; 31:312–316.
77. Sutinen E, Nurmi M, Roivainen A, et al. Kinetics of [(11)C]choline uptake in prostate cancer: a PET study. Eur J Nucl Med Mol Imaging 2004; 31:317–324.
78. Armbrecht JJ, Buxton DB, Schelbert HR. Validation of [1-11C]acetate as a tracer for noninvasive assessment of oxidative metabolism with positron emission tomography in normal, ischemic, postischemic, and hyperemic canine myocardium. Circulation 1990; 81:1594–1605.
79. Heemers H, Vanderhoydonc F, Roskams T, et al. Androgens stimulate coordinated lipogenic gene expression in normal target tissues in vivo. Mol Cell Endocrinol 2003; 205:21–31.
80. Swinnen JV, Roskams T, Joniau S, et al. Overexpression of fatty acid synthase is an early and common event in the development of prostate cancer. Int J Cancer 2002; 98:19–22.
81. Shreve P. Carbon-11 acetate PET imaging of prostate cancer [abstr]. J Nucl Med 1999; 40 (suppl).
82. Oyama N, Akino H, Kanamaru H, et al. 11C-acetate PET imaging of prostate cancer. J Nucl Med 2002; 43:181–186.
83. Kato T, Tsukamoto E, Kuge Y, et al. Accumulation of [11C]acetate in normal prostate and benign prostatic hyperplasia: comparison with prostate cancer. Eur J Nucl Med Mol Imaging 2002; 29:1492–1495.
84. Yoshimoto M, Waki A, Yonekura Y, et al. Characterization of acetate metabolism in tumor cells in relation to cell proliferation: acetate metabolism in tumor cells. Nucl Med Biol 2001; 28:117–122.
85. Swinnen JV, Van Veldhoven PP, Timmermans L, et al. Fatty acid synthase drives the synthesis of phospholipids partitioning into detergent-resistant membrane microdomains. Biochem Biophys Res Commun 2003; 302:898–903.

86. Oyama N, Miller TR, Dehdashti F, et al. 11C-acetate PET imaging of prostate cancer: detection of recurrent disease at PSA relapse. J Nucl Med 2003; 44:549–555.
87. Fricke E, Machtens S, Hofmann M, et al. Positron emission tomography with 11C-acetate and 18F-FDG in prostate cancer patients. Eur J Nucl Med Mol Imaging 2003; 30:607–611.
88. Schober O, Duden C, Meyer GJ, Muller JA, Hundeshagen H. Non selective transport of [11C-methyl]-L-and D-methionine into a malignant glioma. Eur J Nucl Med 1987; 13:103–105.
89. Hatazawa J, Ishiwata K, Itoh M, et al. Quantitative evaluation of L-[methyl-C-11] methionine uptake in tumor using positron emission tomography. J Nucl Med 1989; 30:1809–1813.
90. Nilsson S, Kalkner K-M, Ginman C, et al. C-11 methionine positron emission tomography in the management of prostatic carcinoma. Antibody, Immunoconjugates Radiopharmaceut 1995; 8:23.
91. Munch-Petersen B, Cloos L, Jensen HK, Tyrsted G. Human thymidine kinase 1 regulation in normal and malignant cells. Adv Enzyme Regul 1995; 35:69–89.
92. Rasey JS, Grierson JR, Wiens LW, Kolb PD, Schwartz JL. Validation of FLT uptake as a measure of thymidine kinase-1 activity in A549 carcinoma cells. J Nucl Med 2002; 43:1210–1217.
93. Buck AK, Halter G, Schirrmeister H, et al. Imaging proliferation in lung tumors with PET: 18F-FLT versus 18F-FDG. J Nucl Med 2003; 44:1426–1431.
94. Oyama N, Ponde DE, Dence C, Kim J, Tai YC, Welch MJ. Monitoring of therapy in androgen-dependent prostate tumor model by measuring tumor proliferation. J Nucl Med 2004; 45:519–525.
95. Shields AF. PET imaging with 18F-FLT and thymidine analogs: promise and pitfalls. J Nucl Med 2003; 44:1432–1434.
96. Scher HI, Sawyers CL. Biology of progressive, castration-resistant prostate cancer: directed therapies targeting the androgen-receptor signaling axis. J Clin Oncol 2005; 23:8253–8261.
97. Solit DB, Zheng FF, Drobnjak M, et al. 17-Allylamino-17-demethoxygeldanamycin induces the degradation of androgen receptor and HER-2/neu and inhibits the growth of prostate cancer xenografts. Clin Cancer Res 2002; 8:986–993.
98. Chen L, Meng S, Wang H, et al. Chemical ablation of androgen receptor in prostate cancer cells by the histone deacetylase inhibitor LAQ824. Mol Cancer Ther 2005; 4:1311–1319.
99. Butler LM, Agus DB, Scher HI, et al. Suberoylanilide hydroxamic acid, an inhibitor of histone deacetylase, suppresses the growth of prostate cancer cells in vitro and in vivo. Cancer Res 2000; 60:5165–5170.
100. Larson SM, Morris M, Gunther I, et al. Tumor localization of 16beta-18F-fluoro-5alpha-dihydrotestosterone versus 18F-FDG in patients with progressive, metastatic prostate cancer. J Nucl Med 2004; 45:366–373.
101. Dehdashti F, Picus J, Michalski JM, et al. Positron tomographic assessment of androgen receptors in prostatic carcinoma. Eur J Nucl Med Mol Imaging 2005; 32:344–350.
102. Morris MJ, Divgi CR, Pandit-Taskar N, et al. Pilot trial of unlabeled and indium-111-labeled anti-prostate-specific membrane antigen antibody J591 for castrate metastatic prostate cancer. Clin Cancer Res 2005; 11:7454–7461.
103. Milowsky MI, Nanus DM, Kostakoglu L, Vallabhajosula S, Goldsmith SJ, Bander NH. Phase I trial of yttrium-90-labeled anti-prostate-specific membrane antigen monoclonal antibody J591 for androgen-independent prostate cancer. J Clin Oncol 2004; 22: 2522–2531.
104. Bander NH, Milowsky MI, Nanus DM, Kostakoglu L, Vallabhajosula S, Goldsmith SJ. Phase I trial of 177lutetium-labeled j591, a monoclonal antibody to prostate-specific membrane antigen, in patients with androgen-independent prostate cancer. J Clin Oncol 2005.
105. Galsky MD, Eisenberger M, Moore-Cooper S, et al. Phase I trial of MLN2704 in patients with castrate-metastatic prostate cancer (CMPC). Proc Am Soc Clin Oncol 23:403, abstract 4592, 2004.

106. Israeli RS, Powell CT, Fair WR, Heston WD. Molecular cloning of a complementary DNA encoding a prostate-specific membrane antigen. Cancer Res 1993; 53:227–230.
107. Ghosh A, Heston WD. Tumor target prostate specific membrane antigen (PSMA) and its regulation in prostate cancer. J Cell Biochem 2004; 91:528–539.
108. Sweat SD, Pacelli A, Murphy GP, Bostwick DG. Prostate-specific membrane antigen expression is greatest in prostate adenocarcinoma and lymph node metastases. Urology 1998; 52:637–640.
109. Silver DA, Pellicer I, Fair WR, Heston WD, Cordon-Cardo C. Prostate-specific membrane antigen expression in normal and malignant human tissues. Clin Cancer Res 1997; 3:81–85.
110. Wright GL Jr., Grob BM, Haley C, et al. Upregulation of prostate-specific membrane antigen after androgen-deprivation therapy. Urology 1996; 48:326–334.
111. Chang SS, Reuter VE, Heston WD, Bander NH, Grauer LS, Gaudin PB. Five different anti-prostate-specific membrane antigen (PSMA) antibodies confirm PSMA expression in tumor-associated neovasculature. Cancer Res 1999; 59:3192–3198.
112. Mincheff M, Tchakarov S, Zoubak S, et al. Naked DNA and adenoviral immunizations for immunotherapy of prostate cancer: a phase I/II clinical trial. Eur Urol 2000; 38: 208–217.
113. Gregor PD, Wolchok JD, Turaga V, et al. Induction of autoantibodies to syngeneic prostate-specific membrane antigen by xenogeneic vaccination. Int J Cancer 2005; 116: 415–421.
114. Slovin SF. Prostate-specific membrane antigen vaccines: naked DNA and protein approaches. Clin Prostate Cancer 2005; 4:118–123.
115. Smith-Jones PM, Vallabahajosula S, Goldsmith SJ, et al. In vitro characterization of radiolabeled monoclonal antibodies specific for the extracellular domain of prostate-specific membrane antigen. Cancer Res 2000; 60:5237–5243.
116. Hinkle GH, Burgers JK, Neal CE, et al. Multicenter radioimmunoscintigraphic evaluation of patients with prostate carcinoma using indium-111 capromab pendetide. Cancer 1998; 83:739–747.
117. Haseman MK, Reed NL, Rosenthal SA. Monoclonal antibody imaging of occult prostate cancer in patients with elevated prostate-specific antigen: positron emission tomography and biopsy correlation. Clin Nucl Med 1996; 21:704–713.
118. Texter JH Jr., Neal CE. The role of monoclonal antibody in the management of prostate adenocarcinoma. J Urol 1998; 160:2393–2395.
119. Babaian RJ, Sayer J, Podoloff DA, Steelhammer LC, Bhadkamkar VA, Gulfo JV. Radioimmunoscintigraphy of pelvic lymph nodes with 111-indium-labeled monoclonal antibody CYT-356. J Urol 1994; 152:1952–1955.
120. Polascik T, Manyak M, Haseman M, et al. Comparison of clinical staging algorithms and 111indium-capromab pendetide immunoscintigrapy in the prediction of lymph node involvement in high risk prostate carcinoma patients. Cancer 1999; 85:1586–1592.
121. Kahn D, Williams RD, Manyak MJ, et al. 111Indium-capromab pendetide in the evaluation of patients with residual or recurrent prostate cancer after radical prostatectomy. The ProstaScint Study Group. J Urol 1998; 159:2041–2046; discussion 2046–2047.
122. Kattan M, Stapleton A, Wheeler T, Scardino P. Evaluation of a nomogram used to predict the pathologic stage of clinically localized prostate carcinoma. Cancer 1997; 79:528–537.
123. Kattan MW, Eastham JA, Stapleton AMF, Wheeler TM, Scardino PT. A preoperative nomogram for disease recurrence following radical prostatectomy for prostate cancer. J Natl Cancer Inst 1998; 90:766–771.
124. Kattan MW, Zelefsky MJ, Kupelian PA, Scardino PT, Fuks Z, Leibel SA. Pretreatment nomogram for predicting the outcome of three-dimensional conformal radiotherapy in prostate cancer. J Clin Oncol 2000; 18:3352–3359.
125. Stephenson AJ, Shariat SF, Zelefsky MJ, et al. Salvage radiotherapy for recurrent prostate cancer after radical prostatectomy. JAMA 2004; 291:1325–1332.
126. Wynant GE, Murphy GP, Horoszewicz JS, et al. Immunoscintigraphy of prostatic cancer: preliminary results with 111In-labeled monoclonal antibody 7E11-C53 (CYT-356). Prostate 1991; 18:229–242.

127. Deb N, Goris M, Trisler K, et al. Treatment of hormone-refractory prostate cancer with 90Y-CYT-356 monoclonal antibody. Clin Cancer Res 1996; 2:1289–1297.
128. Hamilton RJ, Blend MJ, Pelizzari CA, Milliken BD, Vijayakumar S. Using vascular structure for CT-SPECT registration in the pelvis. J Nucl Med 1999; 40:347–351.
129. Ellis RJ, Kim EY, Conant R, et al. Radioimmunoguided imaging of prostate cancer foci with histopathological correlation. Int J Radiat Oncol Biol Phys 2001; 49:1281–1286.
130. Wong TZ, Turkington TG, Polascik TJ, Coleman RE. ProstaScint (capromab pendetide) imaging using hybrid gamma camera-CT technology. Am J Roentgenol 2005; 184: 676–680.
131. Liu H, Moy P, Kim S, et al. Monoclonal antibodies to the extracellular domain of prostate-specific membrane antigen also react with tumor vascular endothelium. Cancer Res 1997; 57:3629–3634.
132. Smith-Jones PM, Solit DB, Akhurst T, Afroze F, Rosen N, Larson SM. Imaging the pharmacodynamics of HER2 degradation in response to Hsp90 inhibitors. Nat Biotechnol 2004; 22:701–706.
133. Reiter RE, Gu Z, Watabe T, et al. Prostate stem cell antigen: a cell surface marker overexpressed in prostate cancer. Proc Natl Acad Sci USA 1998; 95:1735–1740.
134. Gu Z, Thomas G, Yamashiro J, et al. Prostate stem cell antigen (PSCA) expression increases with high gleason score, advanced stage and bone metastasis in prostate cancer. Oncogene 2000; 19:1288–1296.
135. Scher HI, Heller G. Clinical states in prostate cancer: towards a dynamic model of disease progression. Urology 2000; 55:323–327.

Index

T - #0110 - 111024 - C352 - 229/152/16 - PB - 9780367390181 - Gloss Lamination